# Breast Imaging Techniques for Radiographers

Cristina Poggi

# Breast Imaging Techniques for Radiographers

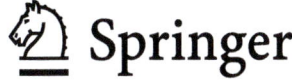 Springer

Cristina Poggi
Oncological Prevention Center E. Martini
Prato, Italy

ISBN 978-3-031-63313-3    ISBN 978-3-031-63314-0  (eBook)
https://doi.org/10.1007/978-3-031-63314-0

This Springer imprint is published by the registered company Springer Nature Switzerland AG
The registered company address is: Gewerbestrasse 11, 6330 Cham, Switzerland

If disposing of this product, please recycle the paper.

*To Bianca and Duccio*

# Foreword

I met Cristina a long time ago, as part of a training programme, and it was immediately obvious how important the quality of the work and the level of performance was for her, how much she did to acquire specific skills in the field, and how she wanted to share them, with great generosity and passion.

In the following years, we often collaborated in the training of breast radiographers around Italy, and I have been working in the field for 38 years! Since 2018, Cristina has become the reference member for the Azienda USL Toscana Centro, in the Breast Radiographers Working Group of the Regional Screening Centre.

She is a person who has always believed in her profession, with a tactful and competent approach to the patient, along the process of breast cancer diagnosis: this book, which is the fruit of many years of hard work and study, is a tangible evidence of this.

I believe that this Handbook contains a real "treasure" for breast radiographers: it deals with the "core" issues of breast radiology in an exhaustive manner, offering itself as a basis for supporting colleagues who are about to work in the field, but also for those who want to improve their performance with awareness. In other words, the book makes it possible to work with knowledge of the facts: in the pages you are about to read, Cristina provides answers to many questions; in addition, the iconography she made available shows the relationship between images and anatomical reality, outlining the fundamental role played by the radiographer in the process leading to diagnosis.

This text demonstrates that Radiographers' profession, in general, but here it is the Senology branch that is taken into consideration, is a highly complex science, and not an art.

It is a book written by a Radiographer for Radiographers, which we really needed!

Institute for the Study, Prevention,                                     Eva Carnesciali
and the Oncological Network
Florence, Italy

# Preface

This text has been designed for radiographers who intend to devote themselves, or who already do, to Senology.

The idea that prompted me to write it was to collect precise, but at the same time non-dispersive information, on most of the competences required for those working in this field. The problem, which is personally perceived as its greatest appeal, is that Senology includes various imaging examinations, as well as a much important relationship with the patient, than in other branches of diagnostic imaging.

Therefore, many texts must be read to learn what is needed, which makes it perfectly clear why it is so difficult to profile this specialised professional figure.

The goal of this manual, very high and perhaps unattainable, is to provide the breast radiographer with the basis of knowledge and the know-how, in a single book. We are talking about advanced competences, needed to make her/him participate with full awareness in the path of diagnosis and surveillance of breast cancer.

In particular, mammography and breast MRI examinations are treated extensively, drawn from my long working experience and from the studies carried out.

A new method of patient management in mammography, from positioning to image evaluation, is also offered: it involves categorising patients according to three parameters, with the intention of predicting, and thus minimising, the most common positioning errors.

The other aim of this text is to provide a thorough understanding of the correlations between anatomy and radiographic anatomy. Indeed, it revolves around a pivotal topic: the quality of image, especially the one correlated to the mammographer's performance, also called *clinical quality*. It is described by only two factors: the positioning technique and the compression process. Mammography examination continues to be the gold standard for early diagnosis of breast cancer, and this makes the training of the Radiographer working in the Senology department crucial. Performance must therefore be subject to constant and careful monitoring.

Prato, Italy                                                                                         Cristina Poggi

# Acknowledgements

During the drafting of this text, I drew on the valuable professional support of colleagues (and friends):

- **Tommaso Prioreschi**, Radiographer, musculoskeletal imaging expert, Pescia Hospital, Tuscany Centre Area
- **Lucia Arezzini**, Head of Laboratory Technicians, Pathologic Anatomy, Tuscany South East Area
- **Stamatia Papathanasiou,** Lecturer in Radiography, Radiation Protection Supervisor, School of health and Psychological Sciences, City, University of London
- **Vincenzo Mazzalupo**, Breast Radiographer, IT System Administrator, Head of Technical-health Coordination centre, ISPRO, Florence
- **Andrea Fattori**, Radiographer, Specialist in MRI, Tuscany Centre Area
- **Rosa Anna Amoruso**, Breast Radiographer, Tuscany Centre Area
- **Paola Bagnoli**, Physiotherapist CPSS, Referee Upper limb-hand surgical Rehabilitation, Tuscany Centre Area

Also:

- **Silvana "Silvia" Salimbeni**, former Breast radiographers' Manager, Bellaria Hospital, Bologna
- **Silvia Sozzi,** Radiographer, P.O. Responsible for technical processes and procedures in MRI, University of Florence professor, PO SOS Diagnostic Imaging Activities Florence, Tuscany Centre Area
- **Eva Carnesciali**, Breast Radiographer, I.F. Head of Technical Sanitary Area, ISPRO
- **Stefania Bracciali**, Radiographer, Specialist in MRI, Breast Radiographer, Director of Professional Diagnostic Imaging Department, Chief Quality and Accreditation, Department PTSRP, Tuscany South East Area
- **Christina Malamateniou**, Radiographer, Associate Professor, City, University of London

*…to whom I owe my heartfelt thanks.*
C.P.

# About This Book

This textbook is intended to give most of the information a Mammographer should have to understand and successfully perform breast imaging techniques.

It is structured in seven parts, dealing with: (I) Basic theory on anatomy, breast cancer, treatment and organisational features of breast screening programme; (II) Technical quality, on the mammographic unit and image; (III) Clinical quality, mammography positioning and quality assessment; (IV) On the report, digital breast tomosynthesis (DBT), stereotaxis, artefacts, surgical specimen management, contrast-enhanced spectral mammography (CESM), molecular breast imaging (MBI), radio protection in the Senology department and breast magnetic resonance imaging (BMRI); (V) Ergonomics in the Senology department, radiographer academic training and communication skills; (VI) Advanced information in evaluating and producing high-quality mammograms and about the Poggi method; (VII) Two annexes on clinical and technical quality in mammography and one about collecting historical data in breast MRI.

Each part is divided into chapters, made up of short paragraphs with very specific titles, to give the reader the opportunity to find the answer to her/his question easily. Furthermore, in every chapter references to other chapters, dealing with the same topic but from a different point of view, are provided, so that a more complete picture could be obtained.

Much importance is given to the image produced, which should be characterised by a very high level of diagnostic information, to allow the reader to find the lesion, if it is there, as early as possible. The book it dealt with the topic of how to produce the image and also to assess thoroughly and appropriately the quality of it. Giving this in-depth knowledge was the aim of this work.

The book covers up-to-date information about breast imaging and the surveillance pathway of the patient with breast cancer; it is therefore of significant interest to Radiographers, Technologists, Radiologists and Breast nurses. Also to radiographers students, both undergraduate and postgraduate.

# Contents

**Part IV   On the Report, Other Breast Imaging Modalities; Radiation Protection in Senology**

## Part VI The Poggi Method

# About the Author

**Cristina Poggi** has had a permanent position as Radiographer since 1994, after getting the Bachelor's degree in Radiologic and Imaging Science at the University of Florence in 1993 (ratified by DM 19/2/2009). In the last 20 years, she devoted herself to the work of Breast Radiographer. She took a master course (first level) in Magnetic Resonance Imaging in 2013. She has pursued the career of educator and trainer in Senology since 2010, building her expertise taking advanced courses, held both in Italy and in Europe, including some by professor Tabar L., MD (FACR). She also keeps up to date consulting the latest news in this field, from European Commission on Breast Cancer (ECBC) and American College of Radiology (ACR). She gave many lectures on quality in mammography and breast MRI in Italy.

During the pandemic outbreak, she started giving lectures online, in Italian and in English, through a YouTube dedicated channel. She collaborated with Mammography Educators by Louise Miller R.T. (R) (M) (ARRT). She worked in Federazione delle Associazioni Scientifiche dei Tecnici di radiologia (FASTER), Scientific Associations of Radiographers Federation, from 2018 to March 2023, as member of the Scientific Committee for Senology. During that period, she participated in some of the European Federation of Radiographer Societies (EFRS) projects. She is currently teaching Senology at the University of Florence, also as a thesis advisor. She was part of the team in the project "Mammographer in A… ×3, in South East Tuscany area, leader Stefania Bracciali, Dr. Radiographer, winner of the first prize Lean Healthcare Award, November 2022.

# List of Figures

and back of the hand resting on the table with fingers
flexed into a fist, open the fingers one at a time and then
close them one at a time, returning to the starting position.
(**n**) Stretching: extend the arm with the palm outwards and
the fingers towards the floor, grasp all four fingers with the
other hand. Pull the fingers towards you without forcing
them. Remain in this position for 20 s, and repeat two
times on each side. (**o**) Open and stretch your fingers on
the table and gently pull your first finger in the opposite
direction to your index finger. Remain 15 s and repeat three
times per hand. (**p**) Activation: from a sitting position,
hands on knees, inhale by bringing the pelvis forward,
arching the back, then exhale by performing the opposite
movement (pelvis back, arching the back). Perform the
sequence slowly and repeat five times. (**q**) Relaxation:
standing upright, keeping your feet firmly on the floor and
with your hands on your hips, bring your pelvis forward.
Hold the position for a few seconds, then return to the

# List of Tables

# Part I

# Basic Theory

# Epidemiology

## 1.1 Principles of Basic Epidemiology

Modern epidemiology is a complex science, strongly related to statistics. It is a healthcare branch of focal importance, as it studies the onset of diseases in human beings, looking for cause-effect links with what causes them. It is not an easy task, given the presence of multiple confounding factors. It describes the frequency of *events*, which are the diseases under study, and how these are distributed in the sample population. Very simply, we can say that there are two aims in an epidemiological study. The estimation of the frequency of events, which is the object of **descriptive epidemiology**, and the identification of the determinants of disease, the aim of **analytic epidemiology**. Epidemiological studies assess what impact the adoption of **preventive measures, early diagnosis** and specific therapies has on the population. Measures that are implemented by public healthcare in Europe. Epidemiology has therefore an increasing importance for what concerns the planning of the healthcare services provided, especially for screening programmes.

**Frequency** and **effect** are epidemiological measures. *Incidence* and *prevalence* are part of frequency. **Incidence** measures the frequency with which a certain disease, e.g. breast cancer, is diagnosed. This is done in a given population in a specific time interval. We are talking about new events, which obviously change in number depending on the period of time chosen for the measurement. It is therefore a dynamic measure. It assesses the direct risk (probability) of contracting that disease and also the impact of new risk factors. On the other hand, **prevalence** measures the number of events presents in the sample population at the time of measurement. It provides the number of people who have been diagnosed with breast cancer, out of the total population, in the distant and recent past. It is a static measure, a kind of snapshot of the situation for that disease. *Prevalence is a key indicator for public health planning. This is because it measures the penetration (breakthrough) of the studied disease in the territory. It thus quantifies the demand for healthcare services.* Considering a single individual instead of the entire population, there is another epidemiological measure to mention: the **risk**. For breast cancer in particular, it is important to know what is the probability of developing this disease over the life time. This is conventionally calculated between 0 and 84 years and is called **cumulative or lifetime risk**. Risk is a measure of *effect*, and it is used to compare incidence in *different* groups, that is to say, exposed to different risk factors. **Survival** is another important epidemiological indicator. It describes the probability of surviving the disease, after a certain amount of time from diagnosis. It thus represents **prognosis,** defined as the prediction of the development

C. Poggi, *Breast Imaging Techniques for Radiographers*, https://doi.org/10.1007/978-3-031-63314-0_1

and of the expected outcomes of the disease. *The survival rate is the main indicator of the severity of the disease itself,* as is easily understood. *It is also an important index of how effective is the health intervention implemented.*

Epidemiological data are not absolute values. They are related to a sample population, usually of a size of 100,000 individuals, and they must always be assessed with appropriateness. This is why we speak of a *gold standard (the tested method deemed most reliable)* for epidemiological studies. Appropriateness is not only linked to sample size but also to the length of the observation period [1–3].

## 1.2 Epidemiological Data on Breast Cancer BC: Italian, European and International Sources

Most of the organisations analysing breast cancer data are listed in Table 1.1.

**Table 1.1** Epidemiological data sources

| Name | Source origin | Description |
| --- | --- | --- |
| AIRTUM reports | Italy | They are the CANCER REGISTERS, which are not nationwide |
| CCM | Italy | Centre for Disease Prevention and Control, Ministry of Health |
| AIOM | Italy | Italian Medical Oncology Association: publishes every year "The number of cancer in Italy," free to download from the website |
| WHO | International | World Health Organization (OMS in Italian) |
| IARC | International | International Agency for Research on Cancer (AIRC in Italian) |
| ECO-EUCAN | Europa | European Cancer Observatory: national data |
| ISTAT | Italy | Italian National Institute of Statistics |
| SDO | Italy | Hospital discharge cards |
| ENCR | Europe | European Network of Cancer Registry |
| ECIS | Europe | European Cancer Information System |
| GLOBOCAN | International | Global Cancer Observatory: interactive platform for cancer statistical information, monitoring and research |
| ECIBC | Europe | European Commission Initiative on Breast Cancer: it develops guidelines based on EBP (Chap. 24) for breast screening programme and diagnosis GDC Guidelines Development Group (Chap. 6) |
| GICR | Europe | Global Initiative for Cancer Registry Development: to address and resolve inequalities between countries, through education strategies (Train the Trainer) and capacity building |

## 1.3 Epidemiological Data on BC in Italy and Comparison with Other Countries; Cure, Survival and Prevalence

Breast cancer is the most commonly diagnosed cancer in women, in Italy. It accounts for 30.3% of all cancers in women. This is applied to all age groups: 41% from 0 to 49 years, 35% from 50 to 69 and 22% from 70 years onwards. Breast cancer is also the first cause of oncological death in women in Italy, both by summing up all ages and by breaking them down into groups. It accounts for the 17% of the total of the female oncological deaths [4]. It is 28% in the age group of 0–49 years, 20% for the 50–69 years group and 14% from 70 years onwards. *The cumulative risk in Italy is high, about 1 woman out of 8 are at risk of developing breast cancer. This is more than 12%* [5].

The incidence of **male breast cancer MBC** is very high in Italy too, considering that we are talking about a rare disease. The cumulative risk is 1 in 599. It is especially high when compared to other European and non-European countries. According to *Breast Cancer Research Foundation (BCRF)*, in a recent update of January 2022 [6], MBC stands at 1 in 833 in America, and on average worldwide is about 1 in 1000 [7]. Interestingly, although outdated, an article by Ly et al. [8], in which Italy ranked third in the world of incidence of this cancer in men (1988–2002 data). See Chap. 14.

Getting back to women, risk is strongly dependent on age. It is more likely in the 50–69 years bracket, 1 in 20, than in the 0–49 years bracket, 1 in 40, and in the over 70, 1 in 25 [4]. There are still differences between one region and the other, in Italy, in terms of both incidence and mortality. However, many aspects must be considered. First of all, access to an organised breast screening programme (Chap. 6). In regions where the adherence is low, incidence appears falsely lower and mortality higher. In regions where the programme works well, *overdiagnosis* needs to be taken into account: a percentage that is difficult to calculate. Breast screening detractors define it as very high (Chap. 6). Survival is higher in Tuscany than in North Europe (Scandinavian Countries), which is

considered to have a very high quality of care [4]. Overall, however, it must be said that some of the Italian programmes show difficulties in guaranteeing high quality over time [9, 10].

One can speak of **cure** from a neoplastic disease, and this occurs a certain number of years after diagnosis, which depends on the type of neoplasia. When this specific number of years has passed, the patient's probability of dying is practically superimposed on that of the general population. It is said that **zero excess mortality** related to that disease has been reached.

One can also speak of **complete prevalence** to indicate the proportion of people who have been diagnosed with (breast) cancer during their lifetime and are still alive at the study reference date. Particular indicators are used to measure complete prevalence. They are based on statistical models; hence, they express a probability. These models are the **cure fraction** and the **time to cure**. The former indicates the proportion of patients who received the diagnosis of breast cancer, and the estimates say they will be cured, out of all the diseased patients. The latter is the number of years that need to elapse since diagnosis, in order to be considered cured. The proportion of survivors, or complete prevalence, is high for breast cancer. *It can definitely be said that breast cancer has a long-term survival rate.* The cure fraction is strongly influenced by age, it is better for women between 45 and 49 years, in comparison with the younger group, and maybe more surprisingly, also in comparison with the older group. The time to cure is very long: a significative excess of mortality persists, up to 17 years after diagnosis. The time to cure for colon cancer, for example, is 9 years (for female patients) [11].

## 1.4 Notes on Epidemiological Data on BC in Europe and Worldwide

Breast cancer is the most frequently diagnosed cancer among women in Europe as well, and the leading cause of cancer death in women, as it is in Italy [12–17] (Fig. 1.1). The **5-year net survival rate** has increased everywhere, thanks to

**Fig. 1.1** Overall breast cancer incidence and mortality rates in Europe, for selected countries. Incidence in light green and mortality in dark green, age standardized, per 100,000 population sample (Adapted from ECIS 2020 [22])

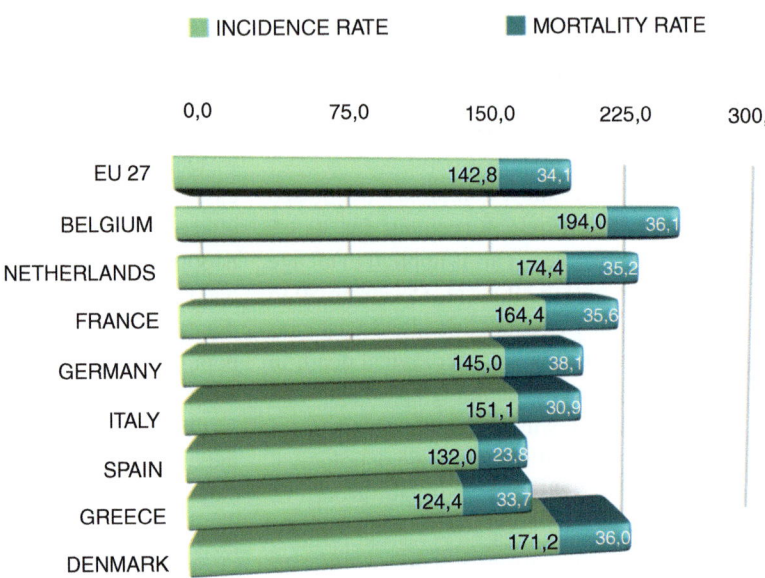

screening programmes, but above all, according to the opinion of many scientists, thanks to timely access to treatment. Treatments have indeed made extraordinary progresses [18]. Incidence is increasing not only in high-income but also in low-middle-income countries. Mortality rate is decreasing in the former, rising in the latter [19]. Worth mentioning is the importance of **breast cancer awareness** and the high rate of survival, if diagnosed early. Despite the ongoing debate about breast screening, mammography is still the best method to achieve a significant reduction in mortality. Studies about it are based on a large amount of data.

Likewise, in the United States, breast cancer is the most commonly diagnosed, being 30% of all cancers [20]. It is 31% according to the 2023 figs [21]. However, it is not the leading cause of oncological death, standing at 15%, while death from lung cancer is about 22% in both men and women (2023 estimates reduce the figure to 21%).

# References

1. Pandolfi P. Appunti di epidemiologia. Servizio Sanitario Regionale Emilia-Romagna. https://www.studocu.com/it/document/universita-degli-studi-del-piemonte-orientale-amedeo-avogadro/epidemiologia/appunti-epidemiologia/13423120.

2. Beaglehole R, et al. Epidemiologia di base, Italian edition cured by Aggazzotti G, Editoriale Ferdinando Folini. isbn:88-7266-031-9 published by WHO 1993 with the title Basic Epidemiology.

3. Principles of Epidemiology in Public Health Practice, CDC, 3rd ed., self-study course SS1000. https://stacks.cdc.gov/view/cdc/6914/cdc_6914_DS1.pdf.

4. I numeri del cancro in Italia 2019 AIOM Working Group, PASSI.

5. I numeri del cancro in Italia 2020, AIOM AIRTUM, SIAPEC-IAP, Intermedia editore.

6. What to know about male breast cancer. https://www.bcrf.org/blog/male-breast-cancer-statistics-research/.

7. Gao Y, et al. Breast cancer screening in men. J Breast Imaging. 2023;5:104–11, SBI. https://doi.org/10.1093/jbi/wbac095.

8. Ly D, et al. An international comparison of male and female breast cancer incidence rates. Int J Cancer. 2013;132(8):1918–26. https://doi.org/10.1002/ijc.27841.

9. Rapporto sul 2019 ONS. https://www.osservatorion-azionalescreening.it/content/rapporto.

10. Battisti F, et al. Key performance indicators of breast cancer screening programmes in Italy, 2011-2019. Ann Its Super Sanità. 2022;58(4):244–53. https://doi.org/10.4415/ANN_22_04_04.

11. I numeri del cancro in Italia 2022 AIOM, AIRT, ONS, Intermedia editore.

12. Sung H, et al. Global Cancer Statistics 2020: GLOBOCAN estimates of incidence and mortality worldwide for 36 cancers in 185 countries. CA Cancer J Clin. 2021;71:209–49. ACS. https://doi.org/10.3322/caac.2160.

13. Smolarz B, et al. Breast cancer-epidemiology, classification, pathogenesis and treatment (review of literature). Cancers. 2022;14:2569. https://doi.org/10.3390/cancers14102569.

14. Ferlay J, et al. Cancer incidence and mortality patterns in Europe: estimates for 40 countries and 25 major cancers in 2018. EJC. 2018;103:356–87. https://doi.org/10.1016/j.ejca.2018.07.005.

15. Altobelli E, et al. Breast cancer in European union: an update of screening programmes as of March 2014 (review). Int J Oncol. 2014;45:1785–92. https://doi.org/10.3892/IJO.2014.2632.

16. Breast cancer statistics 2020, WCRF. https://www.wcrf.org/cancer-trends/breast-cancer-statistics/.

17. The Global Cancer Burden in 2018 -framing global cancer control, PPT, IARC, World Cancer Congress Kuala Lumpur, Malaysia 1–4 Oct 2018 UICC.

18. Narod SA, et al. Why have breast cancer mortality rates declined? J Cancer Policy. 2018;5:8–17. https://doi.org/10.1016/j.jcpo.2015.03.002.

19. Francies FZ, et al. Breast cancer in low-middle income countries: abnormality in splicing and lack of targeted treatment options. Am J Cancer Res. 2020;10(5):1568–91. www.ajcr.us/ISSN:2156-6976/ajcr0113159

20. Cancer Facts&Figures 2021 ACS. https://www.cancer.org/research/cancer-facts-statistics/all-cancer-facts-figures/cancer-facts-figures-2021.html.

21. Siegel RL, et al. Cancer statistics, 2023. CA Cancer J Clin. 2023;73:17–48. https://doi.org/10.3322/CAAC.21763.

22. Cancer burden statistics and trend across Europe/ECIS. https://ecis.jrc.ec.europa.eu.

# Breast Cancer Risk Factors

**2**

## 2.1 Introduction

Breast cancer is an extremely complex disease. Therefore, finding definite links between disease and risk factors is not an easy task. *Risk factors could be defined as particular conditions that may promote the initiation and progression of a neoplastic disease.* Each case is discussed by a team which includes many different professional figures, in the Multi-Disciplinary (Team) Meeting (MDM). It is called *GOM* in Italy, see Chap. 6.

## 2.2 BC Risk Factors [1–5]

Epidemiological data have shown undoubtedly that the main risk is gender. That is, women are far more likely of getting breast cancer than men. It is also known that advancing age entails an increased risk of developing cancers. This is because some compensatory and regulatory mechanisms start to fail [6, 7].

It is a risk factor to have been diagnosed with certain benign proliferative lesions, such as *Atypical Ductal Hyperplasia (ADH). ADH* is associated with an approximately fourfold higher risk compared to those who have not had this lesion. Another risk is having a personal history of breast cancer. We are not talking about a recurrence, but for developing a new one, in the same breast or in the contralateral. This is calculated to be 3–4 times higher than in the general population.

Having a high **mammographic density** is a well-defined risk. It is considered one of the highest, so much that a women with extremely dense breasts is 4–6 times more likely to develop breast cancer than one with very low density. *The term mammographic density refers to the proportion of breast made up of fibro-glandular tissue (FGT) in relation to the total area, in a mammographic image*. Dense tissue contains higher concentrations of certain growth factors and hormones which are hypothesised to abnormally stimulate the FGT. It could explain, at least in part, the density-related increased risk of cancerous transformation [8, 9].

An International Consortium on Mammographic Density has been set up [10] to study *variations in mammographic density, and how these correlate to variation of breast cancer incidence rates, cit*. This is done at an international level, and more than 20 countries have been included in the project [11].

It appears that not only a larger amount of gland but also a slower involution rate is related to an increased risk of developing breast cancer. This was highlighted in a recent study published by Jiang et al., in April 2023 [12]. It would suggest the need for monitoring, with a re-assessment of the risk for the individual patient at each examination.

C. Poggi, *Breast Imaging Techniques for Radiographers*,
https://doi.org/10.1007/978-3-031-63314-0_2

It would seem to increase the risk of breast cancer taking **hormone replacement therapy (HRT)**, especially if it is combined and continuous, i.e. when both oestrogen and progesterone are administered without interruption. The data came from a major epidemiological study, carried out in America by the *Women Health Initiative (WHI)* association. It was supposed to last for 9 years, but was stopped after 5, as the results led to the decision that it would be unethical to pose healthy people at risk. According to this study, HRT would increase also the risk of developing cardiovascular diseases and pulmonary embolism. The excellent breast cancer survival rate and cure results in America have also been ascribed to the cessation of HRT prescription thereafter (since the publication of the data in 2002) [13]. More recent studies [14] seem to confirm the increased risk for breast cancer, precisely for combined treatments and for longer duration of HRT use.

The so-called **reproductive factors**, i.e. how long one has been exposed to endogenous oestrogens and progestogens, are also crucial. Early menarche, late menopause and not having full-term pregnancies are therefore risk factors. Conversely, late menarche, early menopause and having had more full-term pregnancies are **protective factors**. Some studies have found a positive association between late pregnancy (after the age of 30) and breast cancer, if the pregnancy is the first. Breastfeeding is confirmed to be a protective factor, but only if it is prolonged and before the age of 30.

A high **Body Mass Index (BMI)**, the parameter that correlates height and body fat, in menopause, is considered to be a risk factor. This is because body fat produces oestrogens during menopause, and this would expose one to an increased risk [15]. Furthermore, increased fat may emphasise an inflammatory state, which in turn affects the level of circulating hormones. This is thought to facilitate pro-carcinogenic events (see Chap. 4) [5].

The *Continuous Update Project* (CUP) is an international project, whose aim is to analyse how physical activity, nutrition, diet and obesity affect all types of cancer [16]. Also in Italy, a similar surveillance system has been set up, called *PASSI Progressi per le Aziende Sanitarie per la Salute in Italia* [17].

Having been treated with chest radiotherapy at a young age (below the age of 30), such as *mantle irradiation for Hodgkin lymphoma*, significantly increase the lifetime risk of developing breast cancer. In fact, these women are included in the high-risk group. For them is recommended annual screening with MRI exams (Chap. 22).

Also important are those **genetic alterations (mutations)** associated with an increased risk of having breast and ovarian cancer. They were discovered in 1994, on specific chromosomes (see Chaps. 4 and 5). These mutations are hereditable and expose carriers to a very high risk [18]. These people are in fact screened every year with MRI examination. These patients appear to be particularly sensitive to ionising radiation and should be directed to imaging modalities that do not use X-rays. See Chap. 21 on radiation protection. *The percentage of hereditary breast cancer of all breast cancers is low. It could however exceed 10%, according to recent studies* [19].

## 2.3 What Do Incidence and Survival Depend On?

Incidence depends on genetic predisposition, risk and protective factors and on the screening programme.

Regarding the survival rate, we could surely say that screening allows early diagnosis, and this in turn allows many patients to be cured. An early diagnosis means also a timely access to the most effective surgical and therapeutic protocols that have been standardised worldwide.

The main risk factors are summarised in Table 2.1.

**Table 2.1** Main breast cancer risk factors

| Sorted by quote |
| --- |
| 1 Belonging to the female birth-gender |
| 2 Advancing age |
| 3 Having been diagnosed with proliferative benign but predisposing lesions for the development of breast cancer, such as ADH |
| 4 Having had breast cancer and/or relatives that have had it |
| 5 Having a high mammographic density (perhaps even a slow involution rate of it) |
| 6 Having taken combined HRT, for a long time |
| 7 Early menarche |
| 8 Late menopause |
| 9 Not having had full-term pregnancies |
| 10 High BMI |
| 11 Having being treated with chest radiotherapy, at a young age (as in the case of Hdgk. lymphoma) |
| 12 Having predisposing genetic alterations and/or family members who have them |
| 13 Having had ovarian cancer, and/or family members that have had it |

# References

1. https://www.cancer.org/cancer/types/breast-cancer/risk-and-prevention.html.
2. Linee guida Neoplasie della Mammella, edizione 2021. AIOM. https://www.aiom.it/wp-content/uploads/2021/11/2021_LG_AIOM_Neoplasie_Mammella_11112021.pdf.pdf
3. Weir R, et al. Risk factors for breast cancer in women: a systematic review of the literature. NZHTA Report. 2007;10(2). isbn:978-1-877455-12-4.
4. Jemal A, et al. The cancer atlas, 3rd ed. ACS; 2019. isbn:978-1-60443-265-7.
5. Łukasiewicz S, et al. Breast cancer-epidemiology, risk factors, classification, prognostic markers, and current treatment strategies—an updated review. Cancers (Basel). 2021;13:4287. https://doi.org/10.3390/cancers13174287.
6. Dong Q, et al. Aging is associated with an expansion of CD49f^hi mammary stem cells that show a decline in function and increased transformation potential. Aging (Albany NY). 2016;8:2754–76.
7. Dall GV, Britt KL. Estrogen effect on the mammary gland in early and late life and breast cancer risk. Front Oncol. 2017;7:110. https://doi.org/10.3389/fonc.2017.00110.
8. Mirette H, et al. Is mammographic density a biomarker to study the molecular causes of breast cancer? In: Uchiyama N, editor. Mammography, recent advances. isbn:978-953-51-0285-4 tech 2012. https://www.intechopen.com/chapters/31636.
9. Bodewes FTH, et al. Mammographic breast density and the risk of breast cancer: a systematic review and meta-analysis. Breast. 2022;66:62–8. https://doi.org/10.1016/j.breast.2022.09.007.
10. McCormack V, et al. International consortium on mammographic density: methodology and population diversity captured across 22 countries. Cancer Epidemiol. 2016;40:141–51. https://doi.org/10.1016/j.canep.2015.11.015.
11. https://mdpool.iarc.who.int/.
12. Jiang S, et al. Longitudinal analysis of change in mammographic density in each breast and its association with breast cancer risks. JAMA Oncol. 2023;9(6):808–14. https://doi.org/10.1001/jamaoncol.2023.0434.
13. Largest women's health prevention study ever. Women's Health Initiative. https://www.womenshealth.gov/30-achievements/25.
14. Vinogradova Y, et al. Use of hormone replacement therapy and risk of breast cancer: nested case-control studies using research and CPRD database. BMJ. 2020;371:m3873. https://doi.org/10.1136/bmj.m3873.
15. Breast cancer screening/IARC Working Group on the evaluation of cancer-preventive interventions, 2014, 2nd ed. (IARC handbooks of cancer prevention, vol 15); 2016. isbn:978-92-832-3017-5.
16. World Cancer Research Fund International/American Institute for Cancer Research. Continuous update project report: diet, nutrition, physical activity and breast cancer, 2017. WCRF. wcrf.org/breast-cancer-2017.
17. Sovrappeso e obesità in Italia: dati Passi (2010–2013) e Passi d'Argento. 2012. EPICENTRO. www.epicentro.iss.it/passi, www.epicentro.iss.it/passi-argento.
18. Breast Cancer Association Consortium. Breast cancer risk genes—association analysis in more than 113,000 women. N Engl J Med. 2021;384:428–39. https://doi.org/10.1056/NEJMoa1913948.
19. Inherited risk factors and hereditary breast cancer: ongoing areas of focus for BCRF. Breast Cancer Research Foundation. https://www.bcrf.org/blog/hereditary-breast-cancer-how-bcrf-researchers-are-uncovering-inherited-risk-factors/.

## 3.1    Anatomy of the Breast [1–3]

The breast is an even, symmetrical organ with a hemispherical shape, located on the thorax. It extends from the third to the sixth or seventh rib vertically and from the sternum to the anterior/median axillary line, horizontally.

The base of the breast lies on the upper anterior wall of the thorax: 2/3 on the pectoralis major muscle and the remaining third (approximately) on the serratus anterior. This is a muscle that covers a large part of the upper lateral wall of the thorax. Below the *pectoralis major muscle*, also known as the *grand pectoral muscle*, is the *pectoralis minor muscle*. It is not visible on the mammogram, however, because it is too deep.

The **pectoralis major muscle** consists of three bundles, arranged from top to bottom. The middle one is important in mammography, because it can act as a guide for choosing the right obliquity of mammographic unit C-arm, performing the mediolateral oblique (MLO) projection. It is an object that can be seen and is palpable when the patient lifts her arm. The bundle is the one indicated by the red-dotted line in Fig. 3.1a.

The **latissimus dorsi** (or *grand dorsal*) is also an important muscle in mammography. It is a large lamina that covers much of the lateral and inferior wall of the thorax, posteriorly. Its central and lower portions should not be included in the image. On the other hand, its presence in the upper inner corner of the image as a triangle is desirable. It appears with greater radio-opacity than the pectoralis major. It indicates that deep superior lateral tissue of the axillary cavity has been included, given that the latissimus forms part of the posterior axillary wall. This muscle represents an overall important anatomical landmark for central and inferior tissues too. Indeed, the radiographer should include in the image all the tissues anterior to it, up to, and not beyond, the **mid-axillary line**, which is located just in front of the latissimus (Fig. 3.1b, red-dotted line). See also Chap. 9.

The breast has a well-defined lower limit, below the lower margin of the pectoralis major muscle, called the **inframammary fold, IMF** or

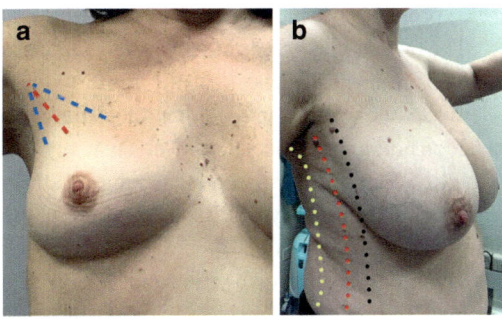

**Fig. 3.1** Anatomy: (**a**) frontal view of the torso: the three bundles of the pectoralis muscle, in red the intermediate bundle, which is helpful to choose the right obliquity of the mammographic unit arch; (**b**) sagittal oblique view of the torso: the anterior (in black) and middle (in red) axillary lines, in front of the latissimus dorsi; in yellow the posterior one

**Fig. 3.2** Erect, flat, retracted or inverted nipple, axial and coronal view

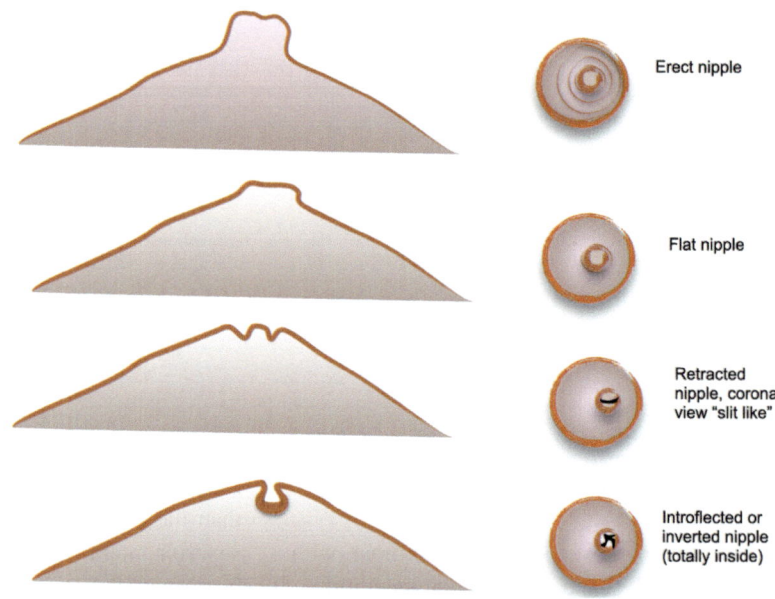

Erect nipple

Flat nipple

Retracted nipple, coronal view "slit like"

Introflected or inverted nipple (totally inside)

**IMA** (InfraMammary Angle). The upper one is shaded. The documentation of a fold-free IMF is one of the most difficult to meet quality criteria for the MLO projection. This is according to a high percentage of breast radiographers internationally. Medially, there is the *intermammary cleft or sulcus* (or *cleavage*). The documentation of this portion, or rather of the deep medial portion of the breast looking towards it, is the most important quality criterion of the cranio-caudal (CC) projection (Chaps. 11, 25, 27 and Annex 1).

The breasts can be asymmetrical in shape, size and position on the chest, in the same woman. Between one woman and another, the differences are considerable, especially in consistency and mobility. Both these parameters have a strong impact on the quality of the mammogram that can be produced (Chap. 26).

The breast is covered by thin skin. It has a pigmented areola in the centre, at the apex of which is the nipple. Both vary enormously in shape, size and colour between one woman and another. The areola has a rough surface due to the presence of small protrusions called *Morgagni's tubercles*. Modified *sebaceous glands* called *Montgomery's* glands open in the tubercles. The Montgomery's glands task is to provide elasticity for sucking. The nipple is the site of the outlet of a variable number of galactophore ducts, through which milk reaches the outside. The areola and nipple form the **nipple-areolar complex (NAC)**.

The **nipple is** said to be **retracted** when only part of it folds inwards. The **nipple is** said to be **inverted** when is completely retracted, Fig. 3.2. Retractions of varying degrees can occur. That is to say that the nipple, when stimulated, may return more or less partially to the outside, or remain inside. This characteristic may be congenital or come about gradually over time, sometimes first one nipple and then the other. However, it is a sign that, especially when it happens within a short period of time, must be reported to readers. This is as it may indicate the presence of a breast lesion (see also Chap. 16). It is a responsibility of the breast radiographer, who in a screening programme may be the only health worker the patient meets.

## 3.2  Subdivision into Quadrants

The breast is divided into *quadrants*, looking at it frontally: **Outer Quadrants OQ**, laterally to the line passing vertically from the nipple and **Inner Quadrants IQ**, medially to the same line (Fig. 3.3).

**Fig. 3.3** Breast subdivision into quadrants: UOQ, UIQ, LOQ, LIQ. Axillary lobe or axillary tail, or Tail of Spence, right breast

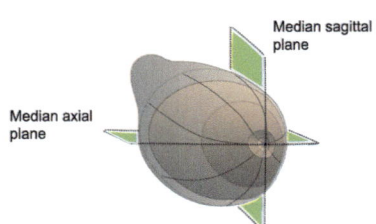

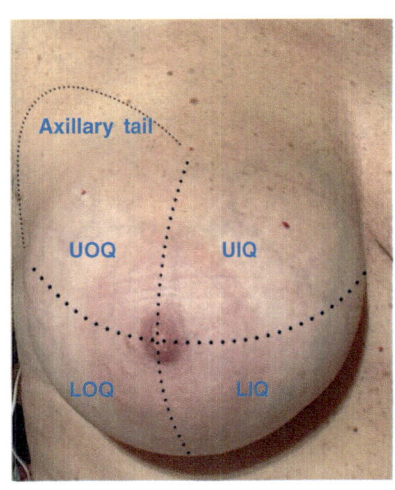

A distinction is therefore made between the **UQ Upper Quadrants**, which are above the line passing horizontally from the nipple, and the **LQ Lower Quadrants**, below. Four quadrants are therefore outlined: *UOQ Upper-Outer quadrant; UIQ Upper-Inner quadrant; LOQ Lower-Outer* and *LIQ Lower-Inner quadrants.* In addition, there is an approximately triangular formation pushing towards the axillary fossa, called **axillary extension** or **tail**, or **lobe,** or *Tail of Spence*. Additional information is given in Chap. 25. The breast can also be subdivided according to the mid-axial plane passing by the nipple, into **superior and inferior parts.** Considering the mid-sagittal plane, also passing through the nipple, into **medial and lateral parts,** the medial and superior parts are fixed to the bony and muscular components with denser connective fibres, and the skin is also thicker, compared to the inferior and lateral parts. This has an important effect on the positioning technique (Chap. 9), and above all, on the results achievable for each individual patient (Chap. 26).

## 3.3   Internal Anatomy [4–6]

The deepest part of the skin is the *hypodermis* or *subcutaneous fat.* Skin and hypodermis make up the **skin envelope.** This is the anatomical part that encases the breast externally and anchors it to the thorax. For the impact of the *skin envelope*

on image quality, see Chap. 26. Beneath the hypodermis is a connective layer that wraps around the whole breast. It consists actually of two layers, one superficial and one deep, and it is called *fascia.* The only part not covered by it is the nipple. Connective ligaments, known as **Cooper's ligaments**, branch off from the subcutaneous tissue with an anteroposterior course. They attach to the subcutaneous fat anteriorly and reach the pectoralis major muscle posteriorly. They have a supportive function, but are not rigid: This allows the natural movement of the breast and the radiographer to document the majority of the breast tissue in the mammographic examination.

With age, the ligaments become looser, particularly those in the upper quadrants, and this contributes to *breast ptosis.* Cooper's ligaments are seen in a physiological setting as thin, curved, radio-opaque lines. However, they can be affected by a lesion, which distorts and stiffens them (see *desmoplastic effects,* Chap. 4). Sometimes the distortion is such to induce *local skin retraction.* This sign must absolutely be described to the professional reading the images and is called *dimpling.* Observed in Fig. 3.4: from the bottom (posterior) to the top (anterior): (1) the radio-opaque lunette-shaped object is the **pectoralis major muscle**; (2) the radio-lucent zone in front of it and behind the glandular body is the **retromammary space,** which is filled with fat; (3) the gland or glandular body, of varying density,

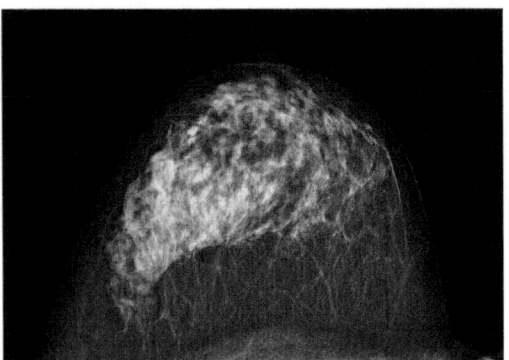

**Fig. 3.4** Mammography in CC projection, left breast

quantity and distribution; (4) the **subcutaneous fat** or **hypodermis,** which may or may not be thick, also radio-lucent; (5) the **skin edge** and the **nipple-areolar complex.**

The most easily visualised Cooper's ligaments are those of the anterior portion, running from the hypodermis to the gland. They are also called **ridges or crests of Duret** (see Chap. 25).

They are observed in Fig. 3.5, in the posterior-anterior direction:

1. The latissimus dorsi muscle, which appears as a very radio-opaque triangle in the top right angle of the image;
2. axillary lymph nodes;
3. the pectoralis major muscle, which is radio-opaque but less so than the latissimus; the retromammary space;
4. the gland.

One can study the glandular tissue below and above the pectoralis major muscle (optimal contrast); in the bottom right corner of the image, the IMF is shown, well stretched.

See also Chap. 25 and Annex 1.

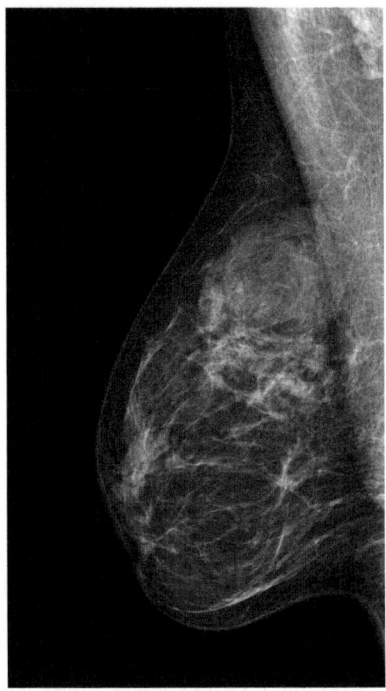

**Fig. 3.5** Right MLO projection

There may be glandular tissue in the retromammary space, which follows Cooper's ligaments, as shown in Fig. 3.5. Consequently, it is essential that the contrast of the image is such that this tissue can be seen through the pectoralis muscle. This is actually the densest and therefore most radio-opaque structure normally present in the mammogram, not counting the latissimus dorsi, which cannot always be documented. This is an absolutely indispensable parameter of technical quality (see Chaps. 7 and 8).

The retromammary space contributes to the mobility of the breast in relation to the chest wall and is used by breast radiographers as a pivot during positioning (Fig. 3.6).

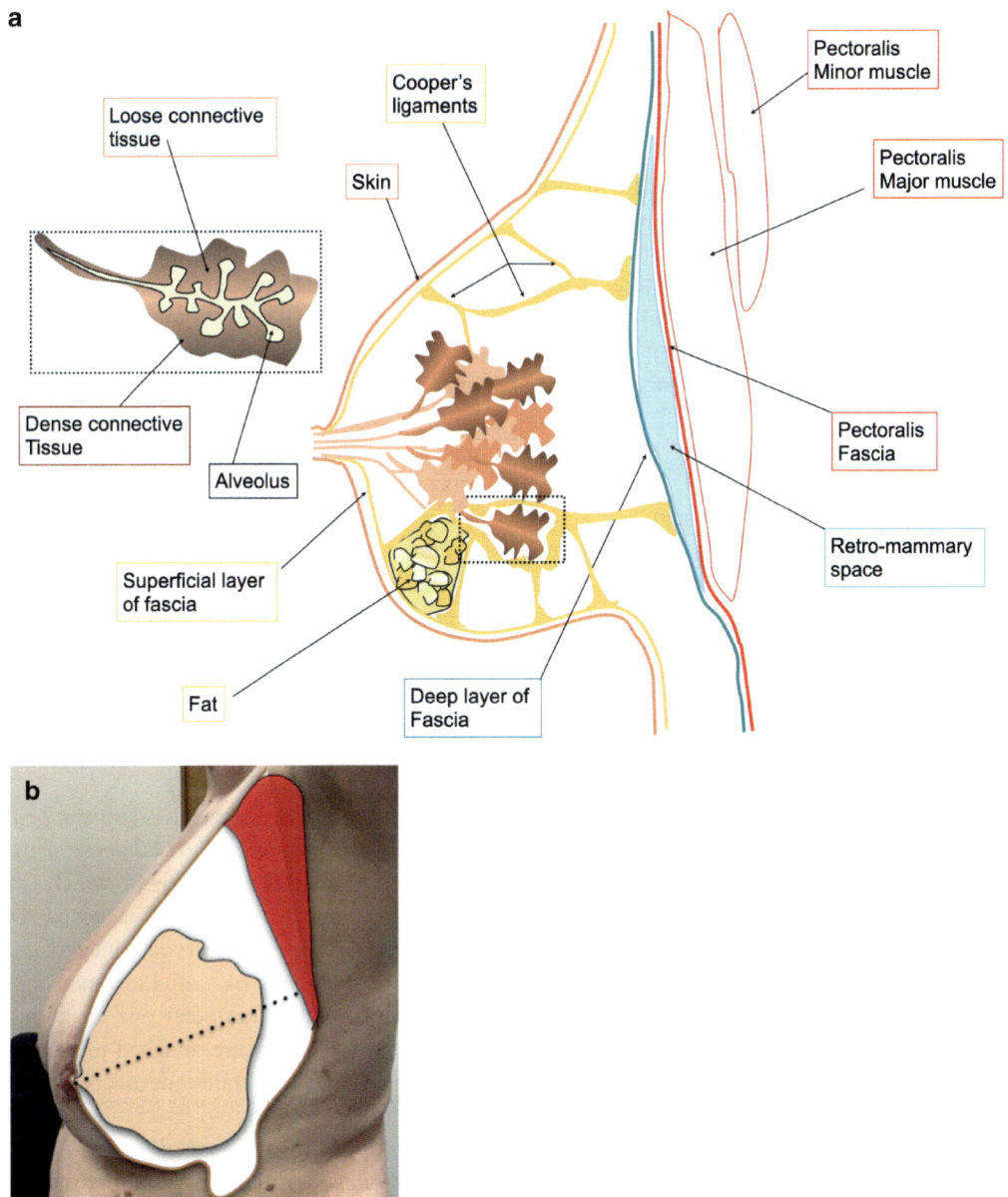

**Fig. 3.6** (**a**) Simplified graphic representation for teaching purposes of the microscopic anatomy of the breast, median sagittal plane (**b**)

## 3.4    Breast Vascularisation

The breast is a highly vascularised organ. The arterial supply is mainly provided by the *internal thoracic artery*, once called the internal mammary artery. It derives from the *subclavian*. The arteries branch out to form a rather florid plexus around the areola. Venous drainage is mainly provided by the *axillary vein* and the *internal thoracic vein*, whose course follows that of the arteries. There are direct connections with the vertebral venous system, which accounts for the fact that metastases from breast cancer commonly form in the vertebrae and pelvis.

## 3.5    Lymphatic Drainage

Drainage begins at the glandular level, reaches the areolar site, and from there, it departs distally. It consists of two intercommunicating planes. There is a predominance of lymphatic drainage towards the axilla. This is why the area is tested as the first site in metastases research.

**Lymph nodes** are filtering structures and are subdivided into groups. The surgical subdivision into levels is often used, first, second and third, depending on their position in relation to the pectoralis minor muscle.

There are also inframammary lymph nodes. They are usually found in the OQ. They are easily recognisable on mammography and have an oval shape and a radio-lucent hilum (fat). However, the hilum needs to be taken in axial view in order to be seen.

## 3.6    Histological Anatomy

The two main tissues are **glandular**, mixed with connective, fibrous tissue and **fat**. The connective or stromal tissue is formed by the progressive subdivision of Cooper's ligaments. They depart in a perpendicular direction from the main ones and continue to subdivide successively, enveloping the glandular tissue externally and internally, in a dense multi-directional intertwining. Fat is present everywhere, especially in the posterior area, the retromammary space. It decreases as it proceeds anteriorly and disappears completely behind the nipple. In this way, the gland has a direct outlet to the skin. It is the amount of fat that determines the overall volume of the breast.

*The mammary gland therefore has two components, a functional and a supporting one, stemmed by Cooper's ligaments. They are so intertwined that they form a single whole, the* *fibro-glandular tissue FGT.* The human mammary gland is exocrine, apocrine, with a compound branched tubulo-alveolar structure. It consists of a *secreting part* from which the secretory ducts, called the *draining part*, branch off. The set of secretory ducts constitutes the **ductal tree.** The gland is organised in **lobes.** They are not arranged radially in an orderly fashion as was once thought, and their number varies, about 20, as indicated by Sir Astley Paston Cooper, the pioneer of breast studies, in the mid-nineteenth century [7, 8]. The number of main ducts is less than the number of lobes, and those that flow into the nipple seem to number about ten. Each lobe consists of a group of **lobules**; each lobule is formed by a group of **acini or alveoli** (Figs. 3.6 and 3.7).

*The mammary gland is a very dynamic organ. It is active only during pregnancy and lactation.* For the rest of the time, the gland is inactive (after puberty). In fact, one should only speak of acini when the gland is active, since it is the location where milk is produced and stored. The acinus represents the evolution of the most distal part of the ductal tree.

The *acinus*—when present—the *intralobular duct* and the *extralobular duct* compose the **terminal Duct Lobular Unit** *TDLU*, which is the histological unit of the breast. The walls of the ducts are lined with two rows of epithelial cells: (1) an inner one that looks into the lumen, called *luminal cells,* and (2) an outer one, made up of *basal cells*, since they are attached to the *basal membrane*, which separates the ducts from the stroma.

*It is thought that almost all breast tumours start from these epithelial cells.* Furthermore, the invasion of tumour cells through the basal membrane distinguishes the so-called in situ *tumour* from the *invasive or infiltrating tumour*. This distinction significantly impacts the likelihood of survival (Fig. 3.7 and Chap. 5).

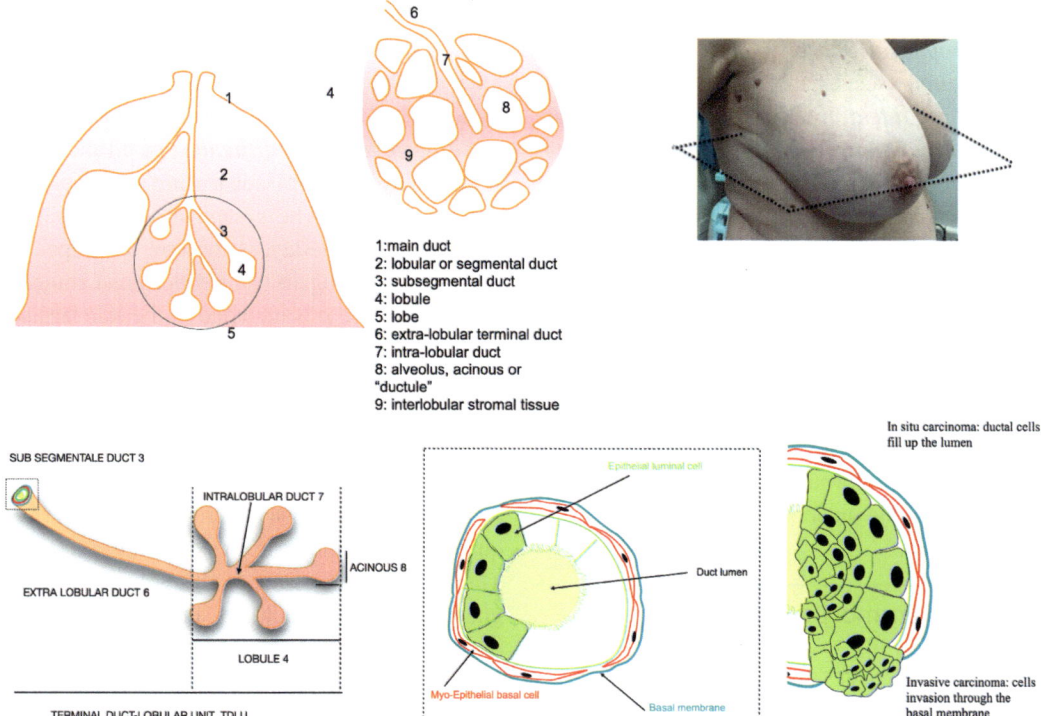

1:main duct
2: lobular or segmental duct
3: subsegmental duct
4: lobule
5: lobe
6: extra-lobular terminal duct
7: intra-lobular duct
8: alveolus, acinous or "ductule"
9: interlobular stromal tissue

**Fig. 3.7** Ductal tree and detail on lobule, median axial plane; TDLU and epithelial cells lining ducts; tumour in situ and infiltrating

## 3.7   Development and Physiology of the Breast

Development begins during embryonic life. Two *ridges* known as *milk lines* form, starting at the armpits and running down to the groin. They recede completely apart from the areas where the breasts will appear. Along these ridges, it is possible to see **accessory nipples**: They are usually located in the inframammary fold, sometimes associated with glandular tissue. In this case, we speak of **accessory breasts,** more usually located in the axilla. The latter is a genetic condition more likely in women of Asian origin than in European of Caucasian origin.

The breast is immature until puberty, when it begins to grow under the influence of hormones, oestrogen, growth hormone and then progesterone. The breast continues to change with each menstrual cycle until the age of 30–35 years of age, when the first involutional phenomena begin.

The most important changes are obviously those associated with pregnancy and breastfeeding.

With regard to hormonal influence during the fertile phase, it is noted that the *follicular phase* (the first 2 weeks after the first day of menstruation) corresponds to the proliferative phase for the uterus. Instead, it is quiescent for breast tissue. Therefore, it is probably the best phase to do a mammography, also for radiation protection reasons. The *luteal phase* (after ovulation) is the proliferative phase for the breast and corresponds to a sharp increase in progesterone. The breast can become very sore, so mammography is not recommended for those with high breast sensitivity, although it is not specifically contraindicated. On the other hand, the MRI of the breast is extremely sensitive to progesterone-induced changes. Foci can be formed from contrast medium uptake that can pose differential diagnostic doubts to the reporter (see Chap. 22).

*The breast undergoes changes also during the menopausal phase.* In fact, unless *HRT* is administered (see Chap. 2), which delays this process, *the ductal tree is subjected to progressive involution and replaced by fat* [9–11]. Fat is no longer considered an inert tissue, as was once thought: It has endocrine capabilities and it can produce hormones and other substances. During menopause, it promotes oestrogen biosynthesis, converting androgens into oestrogens, via an enzyme called aromatase. The amount of fibroglandular tissue FGT therefore varies with age. It is mainly in the retro-areolar area and in the UOQ. The involution process starts from the depth, heading towards the nipple, generally starting from the inner quadrant.

## 3.8   Mammographic Density

The amount of FGT in relation to the total area of the breast represents the *mammographic density* (it is a ratio). We have already mentioned it as an important risk factor (Chap. 2). It is also one of the few that can be modified: There are therapies that can decrease it, although the associated side effects should not be underestimated. It is also perhaps the most important deterrent factor for mammography sensitivity. *It is responsible for the summation or masking artefact, caused by* *the fact that mammography is a two-dimensional investigation of a three-dimensional organ. This is to say, tissues overlap along the beam direction, and in the case of dense breast, reading it becomes more difficult.* For all these reasons, many ways of measuring it have been devised [12–14]. The system most widely used worldwide, still today, is the one developed by American radiologists (*ACR American College of Radiology*), and it is included in the standardised breast imaging report *BI-RADS®* [15]. It provides also four density classes, associated with a short description (an example in Fig. 3.8). This is a purely qualitative system, the subdivision is done simply by looking at the mammographic image and is in fact not easily reproducible. Currently, quantitative volumetric systems are preferred: They provide estimates of the volume of fibroglandular tissue, which are, among other things, implemented automatically [16].

*Density measurement is important for risk stratification.* So much so that in America (in 38 states), there is legislation on the subject. It deals with the doctor's obligation to inform patients with dense breasts that they are at higher risk, and possibly recommend other imaging modalities besides mammography. Recently (March 2023), the *Food and Drug Administration (FDA)* strengthened the recommendation of density notification [17]. In addition, this measure, if

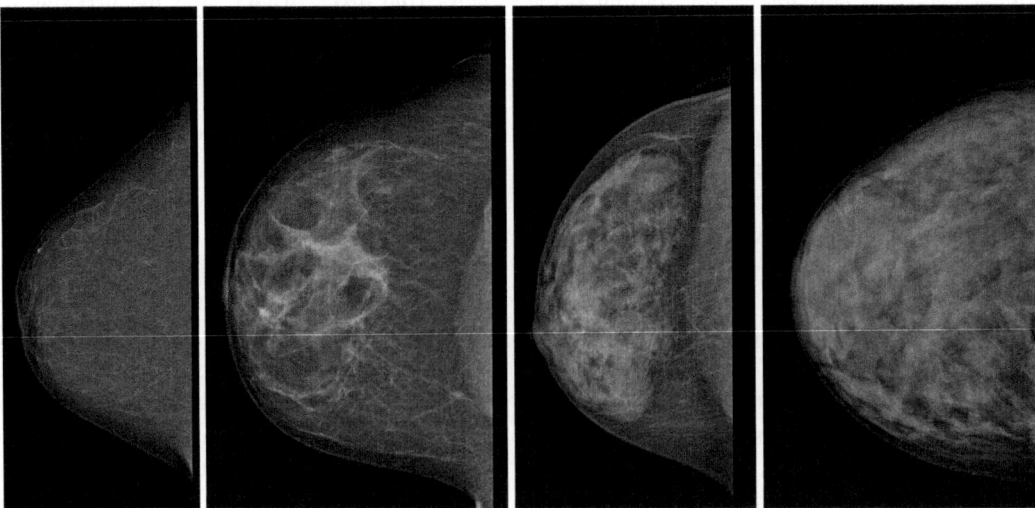

**Fig. 3.8** Increasing mammographic density, from left to right

monitored over time, could provide data for a better risk assessment in the individual patient [18]. See also Chap. 1.

*In measuring density, the following are crucial: (1) positioning, for the inclusion of the maximum part of the breast tissue; (2) compression: if adequate allows a more exact evaluation, for the consequent improvement of spatial resolution. In other words, the quality of the breast radiographer's work is very important.*

# References

1. Macea JR, Tavares Guerreiro Fregnani JH. Anatomy of the thoracic wall, axilla and breast. Int J Morphol. 2006;24(4):691–704.
2. Hamdi M, et al. Anatomy of the breast: a clinical application; 2005. http://eknygos.Ismuni.It/springer/477/1-8.pdf.
3. Jesinger R. Breast anatomy for the interventionalist. Techn Vasc Interv Radiol. 2014;17(1):3–9, open access by US Department of Defense at DigitalCommon@university of Nebraska-Lincoln.
4. Haakensen VD. Biology of the normal breast: relation to mammographic density and risk of breast cancer. 2011. Thesis, Oslo Universitessykehus. isbn:978-82-8264-155-5.
5. Hassiotou F, et al. Anatomy of the human mammary gland: current status of knowledge. Clin Anat. 2013;26:29–48. https://doi.org/10.1002/ca22165.
6. Geddes DT. The anatomy of the lactating breast: latest research and clinical application. Infant. 2007;3(2):59–63. https://www.infantjournal.co.uk/pdf/inf_014_lbt.pdf.
7. Cooper APB. Structure of the breast in human female. On the anatomy of the breast, 1840, Paper 6. https://jdc.jefferson.edu/cooper/6.
8. Cooper APB. Of the structures of the constituent parts of the breast. On the anatomy of the breast, 1840, Paper 7. https://jdc.jefferson.edu/cooper/7.
9. Watson CJ. Key stages in mammary gland development involution: apopthosis and tissue remodeling that convert mammary gland from milk factory to a quiescent organ. Breast Cancer Res. 2006;8:203. https://doi.org/10.1186/bcr1401.
10. Martinez MJ, et al. Adipose tissue and desmoplastic response in breast cancer, chart 21, from: Breast cancer: carcinogenesis, cell growth and signalling pathways. IntechOpen; 2011. pp. 447–454.
11. Britt K, et al. The pathobiology of mammographic density. J Cancer Biol Res. 2014;2(1):1021.
12. Astley SM, et al. A comparison of five methods of measuring mammographic density: a case-control study. Breast Cancer Res. 2018;20:10. https://doi.org/10.1186/s13058-018-0932-z.
13. Gastounioti A, et al. Beyond breast density: a review on the advancing role of parenchimal texture analysis in breast cancer risk assessment. Breast Cancer Res. 2016;18:91. https://doi.org/10.1186/s13058-016-0755-8.
14. Chiarelli AM, et al. Influence of patterns of hormone replacement therapy use and mammographic density on breast cancer detection. Cancer Epidemiol Biomarkers Prev. 2006;15(10):1856–62. https://doi.org/10.1158/1055-9965.EPI-06-0290.
15. ACR BI-RADS® II. Reporting system. https://www.acr.org/-/media/ACR/Files/RADS/BI-RADS/Mammography-Reporting.pdf.
16. Fieselmann A, et al. Volumetric breast density measurement for personalized screening: accuracy, reproducibility, consistency, and agreement with visual assessment. J Med Imaging. 2019;6(3):031406. https://doi.org/10.1117/1.JMI-6.3.031406.
17. Updates mammography regulation to require reporting of breast density information and enhance facility oversight; FDA. 2023. https://www.fda.gov/news-events/press-announcements/fda-updates-mammography-regulations-require-reporting-breast-density-information-and-enhance.
18. Jiang S, et al. Longitudinal analysis of change in mammographic density in each breast and its association with breast cancer risks. JAMA Oncol. 2023;9(6):808–14. https://doi.org/10.1001/jamaoncol.2023.0434.

# Carcinogenesis

**4**

## 4.1 Introduction

*Carcinogenesis is the process by which a tumour forms and evolves.* It generally takes a very long time for cells to become increasingly differentiated from those from which they originate, multiplying uncontrollably through mutations in their DNA. There are compensatory and regulatory mechanisms that most of the time are able to block this process.

The word cancer comes from the Latin *cancer*, meaning crab, referring to the ramifications of this lesion. The term *neoplasia* comes from the Greek *neos*, new, and *plasis*, formation. It was originally coined in 1846 by pathologists who wanted to indicate in this way the new abilities developed by the tumour in comparison with healthy tissue. Tumour comes from the Latin *tumor-tumoris*, and from *tumere*, which means to be swollen [1].

## 4.2 Cancer as a Genetic Disease

Breast cancer is one of the most complex cancers, whose mechanisms are not yet fully understood. It is known that all cancers, including breast cancer, are genetic diseases, meaning that they are caused by alterations in genes. These may affect (1) somatic cells, and in this case are not heritable by offspring; (2) germ cells, and in this case are heritable. Somatic mutations are the vast majority and can be induced by environmental factors, lifestyles, or occur spontaneously. However, breast cancer is a genetically heterogeneous disease, as it requires mutations in different genes. There are diseases that are mono-genetic. Moreover, many mutations are required to accumulate for the process of tumour development to begin.

## 4.3 Genome and DNA

The *genome* is the haploid, i.e., a single-copy or single set of chromosomes, of DNA that is contained in a cell. It consists of *genes*, which are portions of the genome, or segments of DNA. The genome contains information to produce proteins, each gene a specific protein, through which many important cellular functions are controlled, as proliferation and DNA damage repair.

The study of genetics has changed medicine profoundly. For example, *human molecular genetics* is a branch of medicine that has undergone considerable development in recent years. It specifically focuses on the transfer of genetic information from DNA and RNA, and how the alteration of this process correlates with the development of diseases. It allows the identification of individuals at increased risk of developing cancer and is the basis of *predictive medicine*. In particular, the aim is to understand why two people who have the same disease and are treated

C. Poggi, *Breast Imaging Techniques for Radiographers*,
https://doi.org/10.1007/978-3-031-63314-0_4

surgically and therapeutically in the same way, can have very different outcomes. Knowledge of the precise genotypic identity of the tumour is fundamental to successfully curing it. Some scholars think that this information should also be complemented by knowledge of the patient's personality. This defines *personalised medicine (tailor-made)*, on which a special commission has been set up in the European Parliament, and which has been much debated in recent years.

Great progress has been made since the complete mapping of human DNA, mentioned in a world-famous article (Nature 2003), actually completed afterwards (Science, March 2022). *Mapping* means getting knowledge of the position of genes, and in which chromosome they are located. Genetic alterations in cancer cells are also studied using state-of-the-art methods. For example, there is a catalogue of somatic mutations in cancer called *COSMIC (Cancer Gene Census)*. It is made available to the international scientific community [2].

## 4.4  Tumour Evolution and Breast Carcinogenesis Theories

Very summarily, we can say that cancer evolves through a cascade of events, which we divide for simplicity into time stages, *initiation, formation* and *progression.* They are extremely variable from one tumour to another. This evolution is particularly well observed in colorectal cancer that of breast cancer is more complex. Evolution is driven by various factors, including an accumulation of certain sequential genetic alterations that are called *drivers.* These allow the cancer to acquire a number of characteristics that enable it to survive, expand and eventually colonise distant locations [3, 4].

Many theories on breast carcinogenesis have been proposed. The best known is based on a stochastic model. In this, cancer is assumed to develop from a healthy cell through successive alterations, with a selection of the most successful cell clone. This is the one that will eventually lead to the tumour. There is another theory, equally well known, involving the development of cancer from modified stem cells. These would give rise to various cell populations, not all cancerous. Such cells, called *Breast Cancer Stem Cells (BCSCs),* have indeed been identified, and they are said to be responsible for recurrences. This is because they are able to enter a quiescent phase for many years, and eventually come back and reproduce. Some scientists promote a hypothesis that contains features of both theories [5–8].

Another theory on carcinogenesis that is important to know about is that suggested by Harold Dvorak (M.D.). In it, the tumour is seen as *a wound that does not heal* [9]. The aetiology of breast cancer is not based on inflammatory mechanisms, but recent studies suggest that most, but perhaps all, solid tumours induce an inflammatory response. This is in order to create a proto-tumorigenic environment. The inflammatory response is part of the host's physiological defence; however, it appears that prolonged exposure to certain substances in the inflammatory process may promote carcinogenic transformation [6, 10].

A fundamental characteristic of cancer is its cellular heterogeneity, and thus its overall complexity [3]. It can be explained as the lesion's search for effective solutions to overcome host resistance. *Genetic instability* is very important too, the neoplastic lesion increases the frequency of mutations and becomes more sensitive to them, so as to obtain favourable ones for its growth. It is a kind of Darwinian evolutionary process. Another of the salient features of cancer is *chronic proliferation.* Normal tissue controls cell division very carefully, so as to maintain normal tissue architecture and function. It is a process called *homeostasis.* That is, almost all our cells respond to a network of inhibiting and stimulating signals. Cancer deregulates this mechanism following a totally autonomous evolutionary path. *Oncogenes* are genes that regulate growth function under physiological conditions, stimulating cell reproduction. Mutations in them are always activating, and the result is hyperstimulation. *Oncosuppressor* are genes whose function is to block cell reproduction. A mutation in them is always inactivating, i.e., the reproduction can progress unbridled.

*Mutations do not actually affect genes directly, but rather their function, the production of proteins, also known as gene expression.* Another important aspect of mutations is that they are irreversible and can be inherited by daughter cells. Mention was made earlier of the control mechanisms that are most often capable of blocking tumour evolution. These are mechanisms that can prevent the cell from progressing from one phase to the next, in the presence of DNA damage, until it is repaired. There are proteins, the *cyclins*, whose absence at a specific stage of the reproduction cycle induces a forced DNA replication, even in the presence of damage [11]. After mitosis, in the absence of stimulating signals, the cell enters a quiescent phase, called *G0*. The majority of cells in an adult organism are in this phase. Cells have a short life span, undergoing a few mitotic cycles and then go into senescence where they can no longer reproduce. Finally into *apoptosis*, which is the process of programmed cell death. It has been found that in many organs, there are *stem cells* not only in organ undergoing a high cell turnover, as was once thought. They never leave the reproduction cycle and have the task of compensating for physiological or pathological losses in a tissue. They can therefore accumulate more oncogenic alterations. From these, cancer stem cell BCSCs can evolve.

A further tumour characteristic to mention is the acquisition of the ability to evade cell death, i.e. the assumption of immortality. It is a battle with the host organism which most often wins, causing tumour evolution to abort. On the other hand, if the lesion manages to survive and proliferate, the process of *neoangiogenesis* develops. A vascular network is created around the lesion to meet its own nutritional needs, which are disproportionate to those of healthy tissue. The actuating drive of exams like breast MRI and CESM is indeed based on *neoangiogenesis.* See Chaps. 22 and 20, respectively. Not all breast lesions are highly vascularised though, and that makes their diagnosis more difficult. The operating mechanism of PET is instead based on the metabolism of the tumour cell that takes place via *aerobic glycolysis* (*Warburg effect*, see Chap. 20). In fact, radioactive glucose is administered [12]. The

involvement of the environment outside the lesion, the so-called *stromal microenvironment*, is also crucial for tumour growth. Studies have shown that it undergoes pathological changes at the same time as the tumour epithelial cells. The change in composition and function of the microenvironment results in *fibrosis* through *desmoplastic effects.* They are responsible for the hard and dense consistency of the tumour mass. The reaction of the stroma manifests itself in more or less visible signs on the mammogram, firstly with *architectural distortions* (Chap. 13). Subsequent tumour growth eventually leads to local compression and/or dislocation of adjacent tissues (*mass effect*) [13]. The compression and dislocation process can eventually lead to dimpling (Chap. 3). It should also be recalled that the tissue ecosystem that hosts the tumour is not a closed environment. The external environment in which the human being lives, her/his lifestyle, and possible exposure to carcinogens are also important.

## 4.5   Hereditary Mutations

There are mutations that are heritable by offspring. Thus, there are people who from birth are carriers of specific mutations associated with an increased risk of developing breast (and ovarian) cancer. The most likely are **BRCA 1 and 2 (BReast CAncer genes 1, 2)**. They are 50% heritable from offspring, both male and female, and can also be inherited from the father. Those who have this mutation do not necessarily develop the disease, but the probability can be very high. The BRCA *mutation* is in fact a *high-penetrance mutation,* that is to say, it is associated with a high probability of disease manifestation [14–17].

Breast cancers can therefore be divided into three major groups: (1) **sporadic cancers**, where there are no cases of breast or ovarian cancer in the family; (2) **familial cancers**, in which there are cases, but no associated mutations have been proven; however, the risk in this group is higher than in the general population; (3) **hereditary cancers**, in which the mutation has been proven by testing. Quantifying the risk of a carrier of a specific chromosome abnormality for breast and ovarian cancer is very difficult, as many factors are involved. These people follow a different diagnostic-therapeutic pathway from that of the general population. It begins with a *genetic counselling*, in which a family history is taken by means of a *family tree*. In it, the number of relatives with breast and ovarian cancers and the age of onset are transcribed. Hereditary cancers show typically an early onset. For the **degree of familiarity**, see Fig. 4.1.

*Multi-genomic tests* have been developed to estimate the likelihood of carrying these mutations [16–19]. They may become decisive in the choice of treatment, defining themselves as *prognostic and predictive tools*. For example, they help in choosing or not chemotherapy, and assessing whether and how much is the risk of recurrence. People who are to be referred to genetic testing may not receive a conclusive answer, i.e., either positive or negative. This is especially true when the search concerns an unknown mutation. They may receive the Variant of Uncertain Significance (VUS) response. It indicates the presence of a variant whose health-associated risk is unclear, or uncertain. It is easier if the mutation is known, i.e., if a family member has already been tested with a positive result. *In the case of an established (and specific) predisposing syndrome, prophylactic surgery may be proposed.*

It is still very difficult to choose the right combination of genes to test in the case of suspected genetic predisposition. There is an international debate aiming to reach a consensus [16]. In Italy, a Decree was signed in July 2021 to allocate a specific fund for **genomic testing** free of charge for breast cancer. Their use is currently very uneven between regions. There is an increase in the testing fund in the *National Oncology Plan 2023–2027*, adopted on the 26th of January, 2023.

**First degree**: All family members sharing 50% of the genes with the person tested, i.e. par-

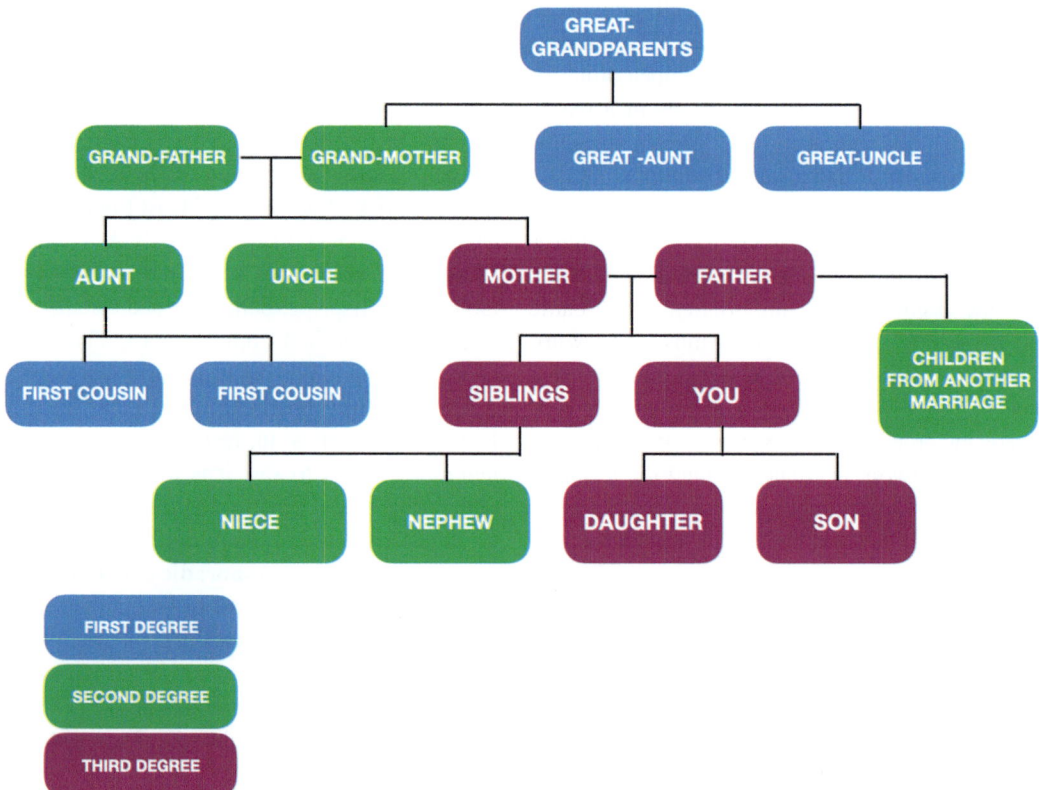

**Fig. 4.1** Degrees of relative risk in breast cancer: family history

ents, children, sisters (brothers). **Second degree**: all family members sharing 1/4 (25%) of the genes: maternal or paternal uncles or aunts, grandparents, children of another marriage, nieces and nephews, and grandchildren. **Third degree**: all relatives who share 1/8 (12.5%) of the genes: first cousin, great-aunts/uncles, and great-grandparents and great-grandchildren.

See also Chap. 16.

## References

1. Lukong KE. Understanding breast cancer—The long and winding road. BBA Clin. 2017;7:64–77. https://doi.org/10.1016/j.bbacli.2017.0.001.
2. Sondka Z, et al. The COSMIC cancer gene census: describing genetic dysfunctions across all human cancers. Nat Rev Cancer. 2018;18(11):696–705. https://doi.org/10.1038/s41568-018-0060-1.
3. Hanahan D, Weinberg AR. Hallmarks of cancer: the next generation. Cell. 2011;144:646. https://doi.org/10.1016/j.cell.2011.02.013.
4. Jinyao A. Carcinogenesis as a defect in the cell interactions. J Clin Exp Pathol. 2021;11:6. https://www.omicsonline.org/open-access/carcinogenesis-as-a-defect-in-the-cell-interactions.pdf.
5. Greaves M, Maley CC. Clonal evolution in cancer. Nature. 2012;481(7381):306–13. https://doi.org/10.1038/nature10762.
6. Colotta F, et al. Cancer-related inflammation, the seven hallmarks of cancer: links to genetic instability. Carcinogenesis. 2009;30(7):1073. https://doi.org/10.1093/carcin/bgp127.
7. Wang K, et al. Cancer stem cell theory: therapeutic implications for nanomedicine. Int J Nanomedicine. 2013;8:899–908. https://doi.org/10.2147/IJN.S38641.
8. Lopez-Lazaro M. Stem cell division theory of cancer. Cell Cycle. 2015;14(16):2547–8. https://doi.org/10.1080/15384101.2015.1062330. issn:1551-4005 (Online).
9. Byun JS, Gardner K. Wounds that will not heal pervasive cellular reprogramming in cancer. Am J Pathol. 2013;182:1055–64. https://doi.org/10.1016/j.ajpath.2013.01.009.
10. Grivennikov SI, et al. Immunity, inflammation, and cancer. Cell. 2010;140(6):833–99. https://doi.org/10.1016/j.cell.2010.01.025. https://pubmed.ncbi.nlm.nih.gov/20303878/.
11. Ozhand A, et al. Variation in inflammatory cytokine/growth-factor genes and mammographic density in premenopausal women aged 50–55. PLoS One. 2013;8(6):e65313. https://doi.org/10.1371/journal.pone.0065313.
12. Østergaard L, et al. The relationship between tumor blood flow, angiogenesis, tumor hypoxia, and aerobic glycolysis. Cancer Res. 2013;73(18):5618–24. AACR.
13. Martinez J, Ciguentes M. Adipose tissue and desmoplastic response in breast cancer, breast cancer—Carcinogenesis, cell growth and signaling pathways. In: Gunduz M, editor. InTech. isbn:978-953-307-714-7.
14. National Cancer Institute Cancer Genetics Overview PDQ®-health professional version, NIH. Updated March 16, 2023. https://www.cancer.gov/about-cancer/causes-prevention/genetics/overview-pdq.
15. Shiovitz S, Korde LA. Genetics of breast cancer: a topic in evolution. Ann Oncol. 2015;26(7):1291–9. https://doi.org/10.1093/annonc/mdv022.
16. Angeli D, et al. Genetic predisposition to breast and ovarian cancers: how many and which genes to test? Int J Mol Sci. 2020;21:1128. https://doi.org/10.3390/ijms21031128.
17. Duffy SW, et al. Mammographic density and breast cancer risk in breast screening assessment cases and women with a family history of breast cancer. EJC. 2018;88:48–56. https://doi.org/10.1016/j.ejca.2017.10.022.
18. Tung N, et al. Frequency of mutations in individuals with breast cancer referred for BRCA1 and BRCA2 testing using next-generation sequencing with a 25-gene panel. Cancer. 2015;121:25–33. https://doi.org/10.1002/cm.
19. Gustavsson E, et al. Genetic testing for breast cancer risk, from BRCA1/2 to a seven gene panel: an ethical analysis. BMC Med Ethics. 2020;21:102. https://doi.org/10.1186/s12910-020-00545-8.

# Classification of Neoplastic Breast Diseases: Notes on Surgical and Therapeutic Treatments

**5**

## 5.1 Introduction

Breast cancer is complex and heterogeneous. We speak of distinct entities; i.e., there are **different types of breast cancer**. All of them have different biological features and different clinical behaviour. This means that the response patterns to treatment are different, despite the fact that almost all of them start from the TDLU, the *terminal duct-lobular unit*. See Chap. 3, Sect. 3.6 and Figs. 3.6 and 3.7.

## 5.2 Histopathological Classification

The histopathological classification based on tumour morphology has seen an important evolution in recent years. Although still relevant, it requires the evaluation of other factors for a meaningful stratification of treatment and outcome (see below). The WHO classification, fourth edition, 2019 [1], includes also the so-called *tumours* in situ. These are referred to as pre-cancerous lesions, but they confer an increased risk of developing a neoplasm and may coexist with infiltrating or invasive lesions. Among the invasive, the most frequent is what was once called *invasive ductal carcinoma (IDC)*, currently referred to as no special type

NST. Second in frequency is the *lobular* (part of the special types) [2]. The other types are rarer.

There are then metastatic tumours and inflammatory tumours.

## 5.3 Histological Grade and Staging

The histological grade analyses the differentiation of the tumour, i.e. how much the tumour cell (1) has diversified from the starting healthy cell, in a morphological sense; and (2) how fast it proliferates. There are three grades: *G1*, *G2* and *G3* (Table 5.1). The grade of the in situ tumour that may be present with the invasive pathology must also be considered.

The spread extent of the disease is then assessed. The system used internationally is still the *TNM*, where T stands for tumour, N for lymph node and M for metastasis. It has recently been updated with

**Table 5.1** Histological grades

| | |
|---|---|
| G1 | The cells resemble the starting cells, the *mitotic count* (= proliferation rate, now expressed in mm$^2$) is low: it is the least dangerous degree |
| G2 | Intermediate grade |
| G3 | The cells have differentiated so much from the starting cell that they are sometimes not recognisable; the mitotic count is high |

data relating to biological factors. The number next to the T indicates the growing tumour size.

The number next to the N indicates the number of lymph nodes involved in the disease increasing. M0 indicates that no metastases were found, and M1 indicates that they were found. All the information gathered is put together to form the *stages*. There are 5, ranging from 0 to 4: at stage 0, there are tumours in situ; and at stage 4, tumours are metastatic [2–4].

## 5.4  Hormone Receptors (Biomarkers) and Clinical Classification

To predict what the clinical response of the lesion will be, i.e. whether and how it will respond to treatment, a number of markers are measured. Oncologists are thus able to make the right choices. Specifically, *hormone receptors* are tested. A hormone receptor is defined as a protein that is present inside the cell, binding hormones as they diffuse within, and this is the physiological situation. Some breast tumours are dependent on these hormones, which are mainly oestrogen and progesterone, and in these lesions, the hormone receptors are amplified, i.e., in greater numbers than normal. This makes it possible to divide tumours into three groups, this time according to a *clinical classification,* which assesses their response to treatments. The first group is the oestrogen- and progesterone-positive **HR+** group, where the specific receptors are amplified. There are also **HR negatives.** The second is HER2 positive (**HER2+**): it is a growth factor. There are also **HER2 negative**, with generally better biological features than the positive. The third is negative for all three of these markers and is called triple negative (TN) [5–8] (Table 5.2).

An Italian research project on a protein, *p140Cap*, was recently published in the journal

**Table 5.2** Clinical classification of breast tumours with biomarkers

| Type | Characteristics |
| --- | --- |
| HR+/− | Hormone receptor positive: these make up the vast majority: they respond well to endocrine therapies and can be treated well, and the prognosis is favourable |
| HER2+/− | They do not respond to endocrine therapies; however, there are specific treatments; in general, they are less treatable than HR+, but the prognosis is steadily improving; HER2− shows better features than HER2+ |
| TN | They do not respond to the treatments used in the first and second groups, tend to be more aggressive, and are often associated with young, BRCA-mutated women. The prognosis tends to be poorer than in the other two groups |

*Nature*. Its presence is correlated with a more favourable outcome in the HER2 group [9]. A *genomic prognostic-predictive test* for this type of breast cancer became available very recently (see Chap. 4).

## 5.5  Molecular Classification and Subdivision into Subtypes

Lately, another type of classification of invasive cancers called *molecular classification* has gained ground. It is based on mRNA gene expression levels, and it would seem to shed more light on the clinical behaviour of the disease than the histopathological one. *The Cancer Genome Atlas (TCGA)* has identified many breast cancer types, profiled for their DNA, RNA and protein levels [10, 11]. The use of gene profiling tests with the identification of the subtypes shown in Table 5.3 has not yet come into practice, for various reasons. Tumours should anyway be grouped into subtype surrogates by routine histological study and IHC (immunohistochemical) data.

**Table 5.3** Table of breast cancer subtypes according to mRNA molecular classification and correlation with clinical classification

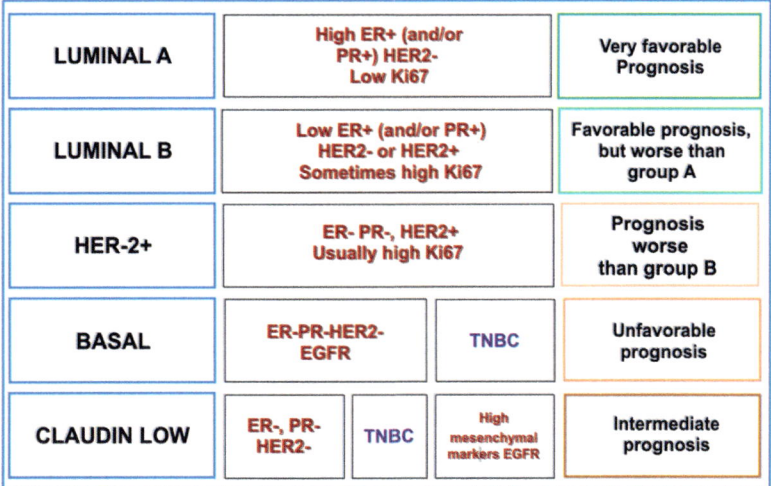

| LUMINAL A | High ER+ (and/or PR+) HER2- Low Ki67 | | | Very favorable Prognosis |
| LUMINAL B | Low ER+ (and/or PR+) HER2- or HER2+ Sometimes high Ki67 | | | Favorable prognosis, but worse than group A |
| HER-2+ | ER- PR-, HER2+ Usually high Ki67 | | | Prognosis worse than group B |
| BASAL | ER-PR-HER2- EGFR | TNBC | | Unfavorable prognosis |
| CLAUDIN LOW | ER-, PR- HER2- | TNBC | High mesenchymal markers EGFR | Intermediate prognosis |

*Ki-67* nuclear protein found during certain phases of the cell cycle, which indicates cell proliferation, *EGFR* epidermal growth factor receptor, *TNBC* triple-negative breast cancer

## 5.6   The Surgical Procedure [12, 13]

As soon as the multidisciplinary team has evaluated all the information at its disposal, the surgical-therapeutic course of action is determined. In most cases, *conservative surgery* is chosen: currently, it involves the exeresis of the lesion and a small amount of healthy tissue around it. It may or may not be combined with *lymphadenectomy* or *axillary lymph node dissection (ALND)*. ALND is generally preceded by *the sentinel lymph node biopsy (SLNB),* usually carried out by injecting a radioactive tracer in the periareolar or peritumoral site. The lymph nodes that have become infiltrated are identified with a special probe, taken and biopsied (see Chap. 20). Dissection is only carried out if they are positive.

Many factors count when choosing between *conservative surgery BCS, quadrantectomy* or *lumpectomy,* and radical surgery, or *mastectomy.* Among these factors: (a): the type of disease; (b): the patient's age; (c): the extent of the lesion in relation to the total breast volume. For example, a *multifocal cancer,* where there are several foci in the same quadrant, allows a conservative choice. A *multicentric cancer,* where the foci are in different quadrants, could lead to radical surgery.

As is well known, **conservative surgery combined with radiotherapy** dates back to 1973, when it was proposed by Professor Umberto Veronesi, medical oncologist doctor and scientific director emeritus of the European Institute of Oncology (IEO), Milan. To date, around 70% of women diagnosed with breast cancer benefit from this method. It has evolved over time, in terms of both incisions and the possibility of avoiding removal of the skin overlying the lesion. Due to the attention that is now also paid to the aesthetics of the result, we speak of *oncoplastic surgery.* This aspect is also taken into account when the patient has to proceed with an extension of the exeresis: this happens for instance when the surgical specimen has *positive margins,* i.e., when tumour cells are found at its edges. See Chap. 19. A mastectomy may be followed by *reconstructive surgery.* It may involve, as a first step, the placement of an *expander,* filled with saline solution to the desired size. The point at which the expander is filled is often magnetic, which prevents these patients from undergoing an MRI examination (Chap. 22). In any case, the surgeon gives the patient a guide with all the data concerning her safety, including MRI compatibility. In recent times, other types of reconstruction are becoming more common, with *muscle-cutaneous flaps,* sometimes with *lipofill-*

*ing. **Scars can be redundant and are very easily shown up on mammography. Especially disturbing is the retraction effect. This is why radiographers must describe them accurately by position and extent.** See Chap. 16.*

## 5.7    The Therapeutic Treatment

There are many types of surgical-therapeutic treatments. It can be said that generally conservative surgery is almost always followed by *RT radiotherapy* (as indicated by Prof. Veronesi). If the tumour is hormone-sensitive, **endocrine therapy** is also prescribed. It may be combined with so-called **analogue** drugs, which inhibit oestrogen production by the ovaries and consequently block the menstrual cycle. **Chemotherapy** is associated with more aggressive cancers and is usually administered post-operatively. When it is administered before, it is called **neoadjuvant chemo** and has a cytoreductive purpose. That is to say, it could allow conservative surgery even in cases of large tumours. **Biological** or **target therapy** is usually associated with the treatment of patients with HER2+ cancers and can be administered before or after surgery [14].

## 5.8    Radiotherapy RT Treatments: Overview

RT radiation therapy aims to reduce the incidence of recurrence in the surgically treated breast. In recent years, studies have reportedly revealed the effectiveness of the conservative approach *partial breast irradiation (PBI),* in which the treatment field is reduced to the tumour bed only. This has been made possible by CT-3D planning. It is regarded as a valid alternative to *whole breast irradiation (WBI).* The toxicity of RT should always be carefully balanced in terms of the cost-benefit ratio, i.e., in the case of patients at low risk of recurrence, omitted. In case of mastectomy, RT (to the chest wall) is only offered in selected cases. Post-surgical radiation treatment should begin within 12–20 weeks, and 4 weeks after chemotherapy, if performed [15, 16]. Many different data

have to be taken into account in the treatment setup phase. As far as anatomical data are concerned, they are acquired by means of CT scans. This imaging methodology allows accurate delineation of volumes of interest and critical organs in the area. The radiographer-radiotherapist is therefore an important professional figure, even though there is no dedicated educational pathway in Italy. The role of the radiographer-radiotherapist is undergoing an important evolution, given the implementation of *artificial intellingence (AI)* (Chap. 24) in RT planning.

## 5.9    Side Effects of RT

RT for breast cancer has various side effects, both acute and long term, that can more or less impact the mammographic image. *Telangiectasia,* a dilatation of small vessels visible on the skin, is very common. RT erythema, which is a kind of burn, is also possible. *Lymphoedema* is often a consequence of irradiation of the axillary lymph nodes: it is a swelling and functional impairment of the arm on the same side as the surgery. These side effects are usually minor and seen much more rarely than they used to be, due to the current prevalence of the systemic approach and improved radiotherapy techniques. Telangiectasia and erythema are part of *radiodermatitis,* which is the result of the radiotherapy-induced toxic effect on the skin.

On the mammogram performed on a patient after radiotherapy, a more or less pronounced *fibrosis* can be observed. Moreover, an oedema of the tissues and thickening of the skin can also be observed. It may be necessary then to switch to the manual technique, increasing both kV and mAs. Otherwise, the image may result in underexposed (see Chap. 7). These effects are present although attenuated on average for 3–4 years after irradiation. The subjective differences are considerable (Fig. 5.1).

Most side effects last a few days or weeks. On the other hand, tiredness may last for months after the end of the treatment. There are also very severe late sequelae, which can appear even after many years. Cardiovascular complications are

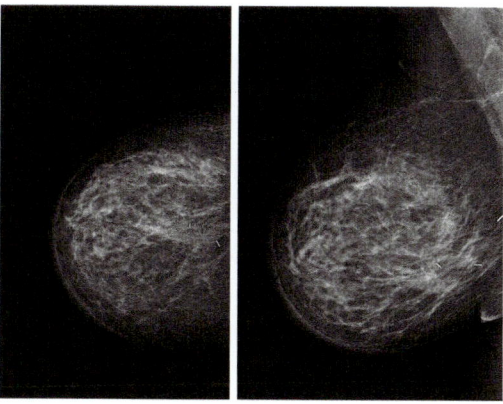

**Fig. 5.1** Post-acute mammography after RT treatment. Fibrosis and thickening of the skin. Presence of metal clips in the surgical site

especially important. The risk of secondary cancer induced by different RT techniques is also widely discussed [17].

Two aspects arising from breast cancer irradiation need to deepen understanding: (1) the risk of hypothyroidism, which has only been hypothesised for the time being; and (2) the impact on *fertility* and equal access to its preservation for all young cancer patients. *Fertility preservation* was discussed in the European Parliament in February 2023 and is the subject of encouraging studies [18]. It is also one of the requirements listed in the Manual of Breast Cancer Service (ECIBC) (see Chap. 6).

# References

1. Tan HP, et al. The 2019 World Health Organization classification of tumors of the breast. Histopathology. 2020;77:181–5. https://doi.org/10.1111/his.14091.
2. Łukasiewicz S, et al. Breast cancer-epidemiology, risk factors, classification, prognostic markers, and current treatment strategies—An updated review. Cancers (Basel). 2021;13:4287. https://doi.org/10.3390/cancers13174287.
3. Rakha E, et al. Breast cancer prognostic classification in the molecular era: the role of Histhological grade. Breast Cancer Res. 2010;12(4):207. https://doi.org/10.1186/bcr2607. Epub 2010 Jul 30. https://pubmed.ncbi.nlm.nih.gov/20804570/.
4. Weigelt B, et al. Histological types of breast cancer: how special are they? Mol Oncol. 2010;4:192–208. https://doi.org/10.1016/j.molonc.2010.04.004.
5. Li J, et al. Clinicopathological classification and traditional prognostic indicators of breast cancer. Int J Clin Exp Pathol. 2015;8(7):8500–5. https://pubmed.ncbi.nlm.nih.gov/26339424/.
6. Williams C, Lin CY. Oestrogen receptors in breast cancer: basic mechanisms and clinical implication. Ecancermedicalscience. 2013;7:370. https://doi.org/10.3332/ecancer/2012.370.
7. Duffy MJ, et al. Clinical use of biomarkers in breast cancer: updated guidelines from the European Group on Tumor Markers (EGTM). Eur J Cancer. 2017;75:284–98. https://doi.org/10.1016/j.ejca.2017.01.017.
8. Teng CT, et al. Chapter 14. Estrogen-related receptors and breast cancer: a mini review, breast cancer. Carcinogenesis, cell growth and signaling pathway. IntechOpen; 2011. pp. 313–322.
9. Salemme V, et al. p140Cap inhibits beta-catenin in the breast cancer stem cell compartment instructing a protective anti-tumore immune response. Nat Commun. 2023;14:2350. https://www.nature.com/articles/s41467-023-37824-y.
10. Kalecky K, et al. Integrative analysis of breast cancer profiles in TCGA by TNBC subgrouping reveals novel microRNA-specific clusters, including miR-17-92a, distinguishing basal-like 1 and basal-like 2 TNBC subtypes. BMC Cancer. 2020;20:141. https://doi.org/10.1186/s12885-020-6600-6.
11. Thennavan A, et al. Molecular analysis of TCGA breast cancer histologic types. Cell Genom. 2021;1:100067. https://doi.org/10.1016/j.xgen.2021.100067.
12. Breast Cancer Surgery Patient Handbook Comprehensive Cancer Center Medicine, University of Michigan Health System (UMHS), last revised 2016.
13. Riis M. Modern surgical treatment of breast cancer. Ann Med Surg. 2020;56:95–107. https://doi.org/10.1016/j.amsu.2020.06.016.
14. ESMO interactive guidelines 2019. https://interactiveguidelines.esmo.org/esmo-web-app/gl_toc/index.php?GL_id=73.
15. Shah C, et al. Advance in breast cancer radiotherapy: implication for current and future practice. JCO Oncol Pract. 2021;17(12):697–706, ascopubs.org/journal/op. https://doi.org/10.1200/OP.21.00635.
16. Polgar C, et al. Radiotherapy of breast cancer-professional guideline 1st Central-Eastern European Professional Consensus Statement on Breast Cancer. Pathol Oncol Res. 2022;28:1610378. https://doi.org/10.3389/pore.2022.1610378.
17. Zhang Q, et al. Secondary cancer risk after radiation therapy for breast cancer with different radiotherapy techniques. Sci Rep. 2020;10:1220. https://doi.org/10.1038/s41598-020-58134-z.
18. Giordano SH. Positive results for breast cancer survivors who desire pregnancy. N Engl J Med. 2023;388:1709–10. https://doi.org/10.1056/NEJMe2301139.

# Theoretical Basis of Mammography Screening Programmes and Clinical Mammography: The Breast Screening Centres

## 6.1 Introduction

*The concept of a screening programme refers to a method of early diagnosis applied to an asymptomatic population. The aim is precisely to detect a disease in its early stages, so that its evolution can be modified, thereby reducing mortality.* Action is thus taken in the area of *secondary prevention*. The population targeted by the programme is theoretically chosen on the basis of its risk and benefit, where the *prevalence* of the disease in question is high (see also Chap. 1).

The term *primary prevention* refers to that set of measures aimed at preventing a disease from occurring. S*econdary prevention* refers to that set of diagnostic and therapeutic instruments aimed at preventing the disease from progressing. *Tertiary prevention* refers to the sum of all those therapeutic steps aimed at preventing the disease from recurring, once the subject has been cured, or at helping the patient to cope with chronic illness.

Breast cancer is a disease in which early diagnosis significantly improves the prognosis.

## 6.2 Sojourn Time, Lead Time and the Breast Screening Programme Target

Breast cancer is a progressive disease. The time interval in which the neoplastic breast lesion can be detected by screening, before it becomes symptomatic, is called **sojourn time**. The **lead time** is the time interval between when the lesion is diagnosed through screening and when it would have become symptomatic (Fig. 6.1). Screening aims to increase the lead time (retrograde the diagnosis, making it earlier and earlier) and thus halt the stage of disease progression [1].

Even today, there is still a heated debate about the clinical results of screening, i.e., on its real effectiveness.

In particular, *overdiagnosis* is indicated as the most important side effect of breast screening (Fig. 6.2). **Overdiagnosis** *refers to the early diagnosis of a cancerous lesion that would never have displayed clinical signs of itself throughout the subject's lifetime, had it not been screened* [2]. The almost inevitable consequence is **overtreatment** [3].

The *Scientific Institute for Prevention and the Oncological Network* [4] represents Italy for screening programmes in the European project EU4Health 2023-JA-06 [5]. In one of its projects, called "IMPATTO", it is hypothesised that four types of breast cancerous lesions could be considered, characterised by different growth rates: fast, slow, very slow and non-progressive. The former are those that quickly progress to the clinical (symptomatic) phase and produce metastases. Breast screening can detect them, but it is not easy, and they often appear as **interval cancers** (**IC**) between screening sessions. The systematic offering of the test is more accurately called

C. Poggi, *Breast Imaging Techniques for Radiographers*,
https://doi.org/10.1007/978-3-031-63314-0_6

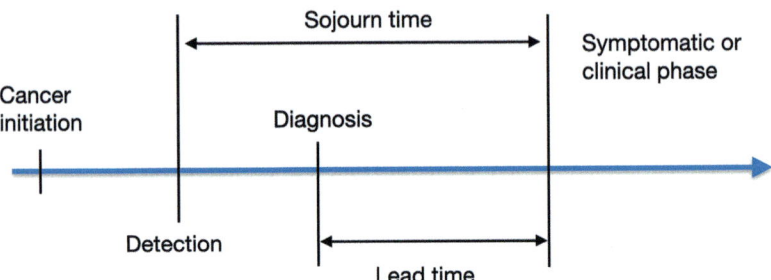

**Fig. 6.1** Sojourn time and lead time

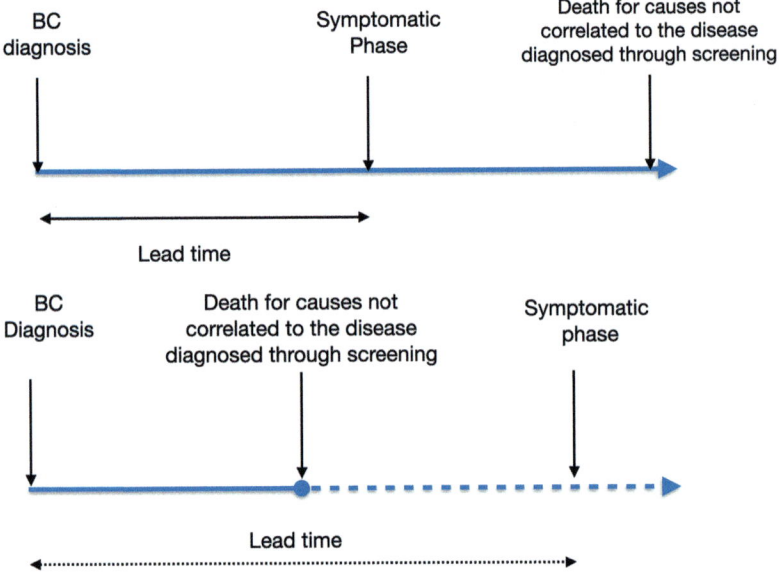

**Fig. 6.2** Overdiagnosis

**round** or **pass**. Slow-growing tumours are the real target of screening: the validity of the programme is indeed high when the tumour has a long growing phase. Very slow and non-progressive tumours are the ones that can lead to overdiagnosis.

### 6.3 Organisational Features of Breast Screening Centres, Frequency of Testing in the Organised Programme, by Age Group

*The only imaging procedure recognised by the European Commission for breast cancer screening is mammography.*

Mammographic examination should be administered as (a) part of an *organised, population-based screening programme*; (b) offered to all members of a given target group; (c) of a given age range; (d) by personalised invitation (by letter generally); and (e) at designed centres. **It is strongly recommended for women between 50 and 69 years, every 2 years.** In Italy, in 2012, the Ministry of Health widened the extension, leaving the choice to regions, to the **70–74** and **45–49** age brackets. The **European Commission Initiative on Breast Cancer ECIBC** indications about the frequency of invitation were updated in June 2022. The recommendation of the **Guidelines Development Group GDC** [6] are as follows: (a) for women belonging to the youngest bracket (45–49) could be every 2 or 3 years, because there is rather little evidence that a higher frequency is useful; (b) from 50 to 69 every 2 years; and (c) from 70 to 74 every 3 years. The recommendations include women who have an average risk of developing breast cancer. Therefore, an Italian guideline on the subject was published (August 2022) and included in *the National Guideline System SNLG* [7], in adolopment *to* the recommendations of the European guidelines. **Adolopment** refers to the *adoption* of the recommendations, in which case the direction and strength of the recommendation itself are not changed, and the *adaptation* of the recommendations, in which direction and strength are instead changed. It results in:

1. A conditional recommendation against mammography screening for women at average risk, between 40 and 44 years of age
2. A conditional recommendation in favour of mammography screening offered to the average risk population, between 45 and 49 years of age, every 2 or 3 years, rather than annually
3. A strong recommendation against mammography screening between the ages of 50 and 69 once a year or every three; recommended every 2 years
4. A conditional recommendation in favour of mammography screening offered to women between 70 and 74 years of age; the suggested frequency is 3 years
5. Strong recommendation against mammography screening offered to women aged 70–74, annually

The region of Tuscany covers the whole range in the provision, 45–74, currently having an annual call for the 45–49 bracket, and a biannual call up to 74. In the UK, for example, breast cancer screening is currently routinely offered to women aged from 50 to 71, every 3 years. It was previously offered from 47 to 73 years, until 2020. In America, the *US Preventive Services Task Force (USPSTF)* recommendations, issued on 9 May 2023, indicate a net, albeit moderate benefit of biannual mammography frequency from ages 40 to 74, compared to annual frequency, considering women at average risk [8].

*Mammography must be performed in centres with specific and stringent requirements* [9–12]. In recent years, there has been a lot of talk about the need to raise the quality of organisations involved in the diagnosis and treatment of breast cancer. The aim was to create *networks of dedicated centres (breast units)*, as actually requested for many years at the European level. The *European Breast Cancer Council* manifesto even speaks of the creation of *universal breast units,* i.e., following supra-national criteria based on the most up-to-date scientific evidence [13]. A **breast unit** is defined as the place where breast cancer is diagnosed and treated. It must be able to provide many services, from genetics to prevention. A group of healthcare specialists, referred to as the **breast team,** works there, including the radiologist, the radiographer, the nurse, the surgeon and the pathologist. See Table 6.1. A key aspect of breast units concerns the so-called *critical mass*: breast cancer centres must be large enough to handle at least 150 new primary breast cancer cases per year and treat at least 50 cases of metastatic cancer (see below). These numbers are necessary to ensure and maintain the necessary *expertise* of each team member and also to make the centre (economically) viable. The literature shows that survival is closely related to the number of cases treated per year by the centre and that it is significantly higher in dedicated centres.

**Multidisciplinary meetings (MDMs) are very important,** in Italy called **GOM** (Chap. 5). During that, professionals compare and discuss not only cases but also different professional working aspects [12, 14]. In Table 6.1, some of the specialist positions working in a breast unit, their activity and dedicated time are provided. The network is crucial: in the United States, women with or without health insurance receive mammographic screening services through a set of independent providers supported by public and private funds. This is a highly heterogeneous system, which does not allow for an in-depth study of data relating to first diagnosis and outcomes.

**Table 6.1** Some of the specialist positions working in a breast unit: activities and dedicated time [9, 10, 12, 15, 16]

| Position | Activities | Dedicated time |
|---|---|---|
| Radiologist/who reports | Must reads at least 1000 examinations per year (5000 for those reading screening), according to EUSOMA [15]; do at least 200 ultrasound scans and 50 breast MRI examinations, plus at least 50 interventional procedures. Courses, audits, MDM (GOM, Chap. 5) | She/he must devote at least 50% of her/his working time to breast imaging |
| Breast radiographer (mammographer) | Must perform at least 1000 mammograms per year; initial training of at least 40 documented hours per week in an accredited centre. Refresher training courses every 3 years. Must participate regularly in audits, courses and MDMs; follow quality control protocols; monitor delivered doses | The indications are various: from at least 30% of the work devoted to senology out of the total (two out of six shifts), to 3–4 shifts (50–65%) |
| Breast nurse | Must monitor and record at least 50 primary and 25 metastatic cancer cases per year | Devoted 100% of her/his working time |
| Breast/plastic surgeon | Must have at least 50 patients undergoing surgery for primary breast cancer per year | Must devote at least 50% of her/his working time to the breast |
| Patologist/laboratory technician senology specialists | Must report/attend to at least 50 primary tumour resections per year and at least 100 pre-surgical samples per year; at least 25 surgical samples of metastatic breast cancer; follow national/European quality protocols and be familiar with national/European quality standards and guidelines | She/he must devote at least 50% of her/his working time to neoplastic breast disease |

ECIBC [6, 12] suggests a number of mammographic examinations to be read in screening, that is between 3500 and 11.000, to maintain and improve the reader's performance. It is more difficult to indicate the minimum number for clinical mammographies, and opinions are divided in Europe: the Royal College of Radiology (UK) suggests at least 500/year [16].

Evidence from European, Canadian, Australian and New Zealand literature confirms that implementing population-based (organised) screening programmes reduces the number of cases of advanced breast cancer and the relative risk of dying from this disease. This is why *in Italy mammography screening is an essential level of care (LEA)*. In other words, a service that must be guaranteed to citizens, without remuneration (they are funded by the stability law).

The examination performed by the breast radiographer, in accordance with strict criteria for the production of quality examinations (see Chap. 11), is read by the breast radiologists with *double-reading mode*. This means that the same examination is read in the blind procedure (independently) by two specialists. The tests are then sorted into two categories, *negative* and *sus-*

*pected* [12]. The negative response arrives by letter. In the case of **suspected lesions**, the readers ask for further investigations through which they arrive at a diagnosis. In some centres, there is also a third one, called *reviewer*. The diagnosis must in any case be confirmed by instrumental examinations. *Screening mammography is therefore not a true diagnostic examination, since it does not allow an immediate diagnosis to be made.*

It is possible to recall the patient after 1 year, not two, even if just one of the two readers asks so. It is the so-called early intermediate recall or **early recall.** The rate of early recalls is high in Italy, but not recommended by the European Commission EC [12].

## 6.4    Assessing a Suspicious Finding in the Breast Screening Realm

Diagnostic examinations requested by the radiologist following mammography screening have the purpose of verifying the nature of an abnormality found on the images. They are also called in-depth examinations, recalls, callbacks or level 2 examinations. The term *diagnostic mammography* is also used to differentiate this second level from the first (which is the screening test). The right balance between recall rate and *detection rate* depends on the target population and the characteristics of the programme. **Detection rate** could be defined as the proportion of cancers detected divided by the number screened. A project called *Recall and Detection of Breast Cancer in Screening* (ROCS) [17] is in place to examine this complex relationship. See Chap. 13.

## 6.5   Features of a Screening Test [18, 19]

The test chosen for screening must be highly sensitive, widely available and ideally inexpensive. Its high clinical validity or **sensitivity** must be balanced by a high **specificity**; i.e., the test must have a high capacity to limit negative effects such as overdiagnosis, interval cancers and false negatives. *In order to achieve mortality reduction with a screening programme and to limit its negative consequences, it is essential that a very high proportion of the target population participate.*

In order to quantify the value of a diagnostic test such as mammography, it is necessary to know its *accuracy*, *sensitivity* and *specificity*. See Table 6.2.

**Table 6.2**  Characteristics of a diagnostic test

| Accuracy No. Correct diagnoses | TP + TN/ TN + FP + FN + TN |
|---|---|
| Sensitivity No. True positive/Total diseased | TP/TP + FN |
| Specificity No. True negative/Total non-diseased | TN/TN + FP |
| PPV Positive Predictive Value | TP/FP + TP |
| NPV Negative Predictive Value | TN/FN + TN |

TP true positive, TN true negative, FP false positive, FN false negative

**Accuracy of a Diagnostic Test**: This refers to the ability to provide answers corresponding to reality, that is the number of correct diagnoses out of the total population examined

**Sensitivity**: It indicates the ability to recognise the greatest number of affected persons (the true positives) out of the total diseased population tested

**Specificity**: It expresses the ability to recognise the greatest number of healthy (true negatives), out of the total non-diseased population

In order to measure them, an optimal reference standard, or **gold standard**, is required.

*True positives* (VPs) are those persons whose examinations were indicated by the reader as "suspected for malignancy" and are such at the end of the diagnostic process. *False negatives* (FNs) are those people whose tests were classified as suspicious, but turned out to be negative at the end of the diagnostic process. The positive predictive value PPV and the negative predictive value NPV also express the probability of a positive or negative test (Table 6.2).

## 6.6   Limitations of Mammography as a Screening Test and Justification of the Dose Delivered: Minimum and Maximum Frequency of Testing

Although mammography is still considered the *gold standard for* the diagnosis of breast cancer, it has limitations, such as in *dense breasts* (see Chaps. 2 and 3). Mammographic density decreases the examination sensitivity to a sometimes considerable extent. An improvement in this sense for this subgroup of women could be achieved by the use of breast ultrasound and/or *tomosynthesis* (Chap. 20). The latter avoids, or rather minimises, *overlapping or summation* effects, by studying the tissues in a tomographic-like manner.

Obviously, **the dose delivered must also be taken into account. It must be justified** like any other radiological examination, *particularly for* *screening, as the subjects involved are assumed to be healthy. Therefore, it is even more important that the benefit in terms of reduced mortality from early diagnosis is counterbalanced by the risk related to the use of ionising radiation* (Chap. 21). To not overlooked, in screening there is a benefit both personal than for the community.

In addition to the dose delivered in the single examination, there is the frequency of execution over time to be considered. There are different positions on this subject. As stated above, the latest ECIBC indications point to the fact that there is no scientific evidence to recommend mammography once a year for women aged 45–49. There is instead convergence on *the minimum frequency of the screening mammography, which should not be less than 12 months. This is specifically for radiation protection reasons.* This is unless there is a reason for urgency: but in the case it is not screening anymore. *The maximum time interval, at least according to current knowledge, should not exceed 3 years,* depending on the subject's age and risk.

## 6.7    Recall Rate for Reasons Correlated to the Radiographer's Performance [12, 20–23]

One of the most important quality indicators of the mammography programme is the *rate of repeat examinations,* also called *technical* or *inadequate* recalls (see Chap. 12). They are recalls related to the performance of the radiographer, mainly due to incomplete documentation of the tissue, or the presence of artefacts impairing the reading of the images (Chap. 17). This again emphasises the responsibility of the operator, the breast radiographer, in terms of acquiring and maintaining the necessary specific skills and competencies. The images produced must be of high diagnostic value [23], and she/he must know how to evaluate them appropriately.

## 6.8    Personalised, Selective and Opportunistic Breast Screening

The mono-strategic approach, i.e. mammography alone, at a fixed constant frequency, for the entire target population should perhaps be abandoned in favour of a **personalised approach.** This is because the population is characterised by very high morphological and risk heterogeneity. In the personalised approach, all information useful for true risk assessment is taken into account, by appropriately adjusting the time interval between mammograms, for example, or offering different imaging modalities. It is also called *tailored screening* [24–26]. It should lead to an increase in effectiveness and a reduction in overdiagnosis and consequently to a decrease in false positives. Such an approach is, at least to date, difficult to implement.

*Selective screening* is a screening procedure offered to a specific subgroup of the population, based on its exposure to one or more recognised risk factors. This is a highly effective model, and people exposed to risk would participate in large numbers with a very favourable effect on the diagnostic process. There are currently no tests that can identify these subgroups, other than those carrying mutations that induce a medium to high risk of developing the disease, such as the *BRCA carriers* (Chap. 4) [16, 27].

Mammographic density could be considered in a risk-adapted screening; currently, there is no recommendation about it from ECIBC [28]. Many ongoing clinical trials are studying the additional value of ultrasound, DBT (Chap. 20) and MRI (Chap. 22) for breast cancer early diagnosis in women with extremely dense breast. However, a high rate of false-positive results is reported with these supplemental investigations [28, 29].

*Opportunistic screening* refers to undergoing the examination on a voluntary (individual or "opportunistic") basis, either by the user, voluntarily, or on the advice of the general practitioner (GP). In this case, the benefit of the screening will affect the individual, not the population.

## 6.9 Clinical and Follow-Up Mammography

Screening mammography is directed at women who do not have symptoms or signs of breast pathology. The term *clinical mammography* refers to the examination that is performed on symptomatic patients, outside the screening examination. It is a term used also within it, as a second-level or in-depth examination, when suspicious findings have been detected. In this case, we speak more precisely of *diagnostic mammography*.

The term **follow-up** is generally used to make reference to the set of examinations carried out after diagnosis and removal of a tumour, for surveillance purposes. It is determined by the fact that the incidence, which assesses the number of new cases of the studied disease in a given time interval, may vary (Chap. 1). It therefore requires at least two investigations spaced out in time. Conventionally, follow-up mammography means yearly examinations for the first 5 years after breast-conserving surgery. Surveillance includes both mammography and US. This is in addition to a series of standard laboratory and imaging tests specifically chosen for the individual case [30, 31].

## References

1. Cheung S, et al. Review of sojourn time calculation models used in breast cancer screening. https://warwick.ac.uk/fac/sci/statistics/crism/research/17-04/17-04w.pdf.
2. Deandrea S. Sovradiagnosi: il caso esemplare dello screening mammografico. Recenti Progressi in Medicina. 2020;111(5), il Pensiero Scientifico Editore.
3. Clift AK, et al. The current status of risk stratified breast screening. Br J Cancer. 2022;126:533–50. https://doi.org/10.1038/s41416-021-01550-3.
4. Mantellini P. Implementation of cancer screening programmes. ISPRO. https://www.salute.gov.it/imgs/C_17_notizie_6179_1_file.pdf. EU4H-2023-JA-06.
5. Paci E, Puliti D. Come cambia l'epidemiologia del tumore della mammella in Italia I risultati del progetto IMPATTO dei programmi di screening mammografico. ISPO; 2011.
6. ECIBC's Guidelines Development Group about organised mammography screening programme. https://healthcare-quality.jrc.ec.europa.eu/en/ecibc/european-breast-cancer-guidelines.
7. CTS, SOCIETA' SCIENTIFICHE e PANEL DI ESPERTI. Screening e diagnosi del tumore della mammella (Adolopment LG Europee)—Raccomandazioni fascia di età e intervalli. Roma: SNLG Istituto Superiore di Sanità; 2022.
8. Draft recommendation statement embargoed: May 9, 2023, at 11 AM ET screening for breast cancer: U.S. Preventive Service Task Force Draft Recommendation Statement. https://www.acr.org/-/media/ACR/Files/Advocacy/Screening-for-Breast-Cancer-Draft-RS_EMBARGOED-MAY-9-11AM-ET.pdf.
9. Biganzoli, L., et al., The requirements of a specialist breast centre, Breast 51 (2020) 65–84, produced by EUSOMA and endorsed by ECCO as part of Essential Requirements for Quality Cancer Care (ERQCC) programme, and ESMO. https://doi.org/10.1016/j.breast.2020.02.003
10. Breve Guida agli orientamenti Europei per la garanzia di qualità nello screening e nella diagnosi del tumore del seno III ristampa 2011 traduzione in italiano. Europa Donna. https://europadonna.it/wp-content/uploads/2016/05/ED-Guida-orientamenti-europei-screening-2011.pdfEnglishversion, https://www.europadonna.org/pdf/ED-shortguide-ENG-6th-priting-web.-OK.pdf.
11. Massa I, et al. The challenge of sustainability in healthcare systems: frequency and cost of inappropriate patterns of breast cancer care (the E.Pic.A study). Breast. 2017;34:103–7. https://doi.org/10.1016/j.breast.2017.05.007.
12. Janusch-Roi A, et al. European Commission Initiative on breast cancer-manual for breast cancer services—European quality assurance scheme for breast cancer services, EUR 30750 EN. Luxembourg: Publications Office of the European Union; 2021. isbn:978-92-76-39192-0. https://doi.org/10.2760/155701. JRC125431.
13. Cardoso F, et al. European cancer conference manifesto on breast centres/units. Eur J Cancer. 2017;72:244–50. https://doi.org/10.1016/j.ejca.2016.10.023.
14. Blackwood O, Deb R. Multidisciplinary team approach in breast cancer care: benefits and challenges. Indian J Pathol Microbiol. 2020;63(Supplement):S105–12. https://doi.org/10.4103/IJPM.IJPM_885_19.
15. Michalopoulou E, et al. A survey by the European Society of Breast Imaging on radiologists' preferences regarding quality assurance measures of image interpretation in screening and diagnostic mammography. Eur Radiol. 2023;33:8103. https://doi.org/10.1007/s00330-023-09973-7.
16. The Royal College of Radiology. Guidance on screening and symptomatic breast imaging, 4th ed. 2019. https://www.rcr.ac.uk/publication/guidance-screening-and-symptomatic-breast-imaging-fourth-edition.
17. Sechopoulos I, et al. Evaluation of reader performance during interpretation of breast can-

cer screening: the recall and detection of beast cancer in screening (ROCS) trial study design. Eur Radiol. 2022;32:7463–9. https://doi.org/10.1007/s00330-022-08820-5.

18. World Health Organization Regional Office for Europe. Screening programmes: a short guide. Increase effectiveness, maximize benefits and minimize harm. WHO; 2020. isbn:978-92-890-5478-2.

19. Šimundić AM. Measures of diagnostic accuracy: basic definitions. https://www.ncbi.nlm.nih.gov/pmc/articles/PMC4975285/pdf/ejifcc-19-203.pdf.

20. Giordano L, et al. Indicatori e standard per la valutazione di processi dei programmi di screening del cancro della mammella E&P anno. 2006;30(2) Supplemento 1 ONS GISMA. https://win.gisma.it/pubblicazioni/documenti/ManualeIndicatori.pdf.

21. Martaindale S, et al. Analysis of technical repeat studies in screening mammography. J Breast Imaging. 2023;5:416–24. https://doi.org/10.1093/jbiwbad039.

22. Rouette J, et al. Evaluation of the quality of mammography breast positioning: a quality improvement study. CMAJ Open. 2021;9:E607. https://doi.org/10.9778/cmajo.20200211.

23. Taplin SH, et al. Screening mammography: clinical image quality and the risk of interval breast cancer. AJR Am J Roentgenol. 2002;178:797–803. 0361-803X/02/1784-797.

24. Paci E, et al. Tailored breast screening trial (TBST). Epidemiol Prev. 2013;37(4–5):317–27. https://pubmed.ncbi.nlm.nih.gov/24293498/.

25. European Commission on Breast Cancer Guidelines Development Group. European guidelines on breast cancer screening and diagnosis—Should tailored screening with digital breast tomosynthesis in addition to digital mammography vs. digital mammography alone be used for early detection of breast cancer in asymptomatic women with high mammographic breast density in organized screening programmes? European Commission; 2020.

26. Roux A, et al. Study protocol comparing the ethical, psychological and socio-economic impact of personalised breast cancer screening to that of standard screening in the "My Personal Breast Screening" (MyPeBS) randomized clinical trial. BMC Cancer. 2022;22(1):507. https://doi.org/10.1186/s12885-022-09484-6.

27. Clift AK. The current status of risk-stratified breast screening. BJC. 2022;126:533–50. https://doi.org/10.1038/s41416-021-01550-3.

28. O'Driscoll J, et al. A scoping review of programme specific mammographic density related guidelines and practices within breast screening programmes. Eur J Radiol Open. 2023;11:100510. https://doi.org/10.1016/j.ejro.2023.100510.

29. Yuan W-H, et al. Supplemental breast cancer-screening screening ultrasonography in women with dense breasts: a systematic review and meta-analysis. Br J Cancer. 2020;123(4):673–88. https://doi.org/10.1038/s41416-020-0928-1.

30. AIOM Linee guida neoplasie della mammella, edizione 2021, in collaborazione con AIRO, ANISC, SIAPEC-IAP, SICO, SIMG, SIRM. https://www.aiom.it/wp-content/uploads/2021/11/2021_LG_AIOM_Neoplasie_Mammella_11112021.pdf.pdf.

31. Cardoso F, et al. Early breast cancer: ESMO clinical practice guidelines for diagnosis, treatment and follow-up. Ann Oncol. 2019;30:1194–220. https://doi.org/10.1093/annonc/mdz173.

# Part II

# Technical Quality

# The Mammographic Unit and the Image Receptors

**7**

## 7.1 Introduction to Image Formation, Contrast and Spatial Resolution [1–4]

The image formation of an object in diagnostic radiology involves the use of **radiation**, defined as the emission or simple transport of energy in the form of electromagnetic waves or particles. The radiation can travel in space or other media along straight-line trajectories, with the ability to pass through objects. When the radiation hits an object, an interaction takes place. A transfer of energy is noted, to a greater or less extent, to the target encountered. Thanks to the ability of radiation to pass through the object, and the fact that it has a rectilinear path, the surviving fraction of the radiation that emerges from it and reaches a suitable detector contains information that can be used to image the object.

The radiation used in mammography is **X-rays.**

When a uniform beam of X-rays strikes the patient, it interacts with the tissue, producing a variable transmitted (outgoing) X-ray flux. The variation depends on the type of interactions that occurred along the taken path. That is to say, the X-ray image is obtained by irradiating an object with a uniform X-ray beam, which is modified by the attenuation characteristics of the object being studied. It is produced by (1) the *primary beam,* which does not interact with the target, and passes through it without changing direction and with-

out releasing energy; (2) the photons that are completely absorbed or "removed" from the beam. For this reason, *the radiographic image is the negative of the object being radiographed.* The differential attenuation of the radiographic/mammographic images is expressed in terms of its *radiopacity* and *radiolucency.*

**Radiopacity** is the relative ability of matter to block the transmission of radiant energy. It appears as an absence or scarcity of signal on the image, and it is expressed by the white colour.

**Radiolucency** is the ability of matter to be permeable to X-rays and appears on the image as a high signal, expressed by the black colour.

*The radiographic image is the 2D representation of the different attenuation capacities of the 3D object irradiated by the X-ray beam.*

**Contrast** expresses the spatial variation in the energy of the X-ray beam emerging from the patient. It is due to the difference between the attenuation capacities of the traversed tissue, by density, atomic number Z and thickness. Contrast is defined as (a) the ability to recognise shapes and structures of interest, which are intended to be differentiated from the rest of the image called *background*; (b) the system's ability to detect small variations in the intensity of the radiation incident on the image detector and display them. One cause of contrast degradation in bio-medical imaging is **noise**. Another cause is *scattered radiation*. Table 7.1 summarises the comparison between contrast and spatial resolution.

**Table 7.1** Definition of contrast and spatial resolution

| | |
|---|---|
| Contrast resolution | Is the smallest change in exposure (= amount of charge produced by X-rays in a mass of air; see Chap. 21) that can be perceived. It depends on the pixel depth |
| Spatial resolution | Is the ability of an imaging system to see two neighboring structures as separate. The ability to accurately distinguish the edges of an object<br>It is lost mainly due to (a) the size of the focal spot (= source of the beam), which is not point-like, (b) the dimensions of the pixel, (c) the movement of the patient |

## 7.2 The Mammographic Imaging System: The Prerequisites for a Dedicated Equipment [5, 6]

The imaging system in mammography must produce images that have high **spatial resolution SR** and **contrast**, while maintaining an acceptable **dose** (Chap. 21). This is not an easy task, because it requires to:

1. (a) Effectively document *microcalcifications* of an average size of around 100 μ (1 micron μ = 10⁻⁶ m) with which the tumour may manifest. They are characterised by high contrast. (b) Accurately assess the morphology of a lesion, particularly the *edges* (Chaps. 5 and 13). The resolving power should include objects of 50 μ.
2. Effectively document areas of breast tissue with very low contrast between them, to highlight (a) any thickening in the texture of the healthy tissue and (b) architectural *distortions* (Chap. 13). High-contrast resolution is required for both.

The organ under study, the breast, is made up of relatively radiolucent soft tissues, with very similar densities and atomic numbers. Their abilities to attenuate the beam are poorly differentiated, resulting in poor contrast between the various healthy tissues and between healthy and pathological tissues.

To increase tissue relative differences, and therefore contrast, mammographic units work at low-voltage values and with a *low-energy spectrum of the X-ray beam.* Low energy is meant a low penetration capacity. See Sect. 7.4. The spectrum must be of low energy also because of the relative radiolucency and thickness of the breast. The intensity of the beam is proportional to the voltage squared. Therefore, in order to keep it low, it is necessary to increase the exposure time, with an increase in (a) the dose delivered; (b) the risk of patient motion artefacts; and (c) edge blurring. These technical difficulties are addressed by using a (1) high-frequency generator at as constant a potential as possible; (2) **source-to-image distance (SID)** at 60–65 centimetres (cm), smaller than those used in conventional radiological imaging. The aim is to compensate for low intensity and *small/very small focal spots* (see below). The image receptor or *detector* is also optimised.

To summarise, **the contrast depends on the acquisition protocol, which must be such to emphasise the very low intrinsic contrast of the object, the breast.** Therefore, it is easy to understand that the mammographic system must be highly specialised. This not only concerns the geometric parameters but also the characteristics of the beam that impacts the matter. The desired aim, in mammography as well as in general radiology, is to privilege the *photoelectric effect* and reduce the *Compton effect.* It should also be considered that the breast is an organ that presents subjective differences, in size and composition, and undergoes significant changes throughout the life of the women.

## 7.3 On the Mammographic Unit: An Overview of Basic Physical Principles and the Most Important Constituent Elements [7–9]

The mammographic unit is a highly specialised radiological device. The X-ray tube and detector are mounted on an assembly that can be easily rotated, so that images of the breast can be acquired from different angles. The purpose of the mammographic machine is to provide an X-ray source that is as point-like as possible without risking damage due to the heat produced by the beam generation. The main aim is a high-quality final image, ready for reporting.

The tube and detector, the latter inserted in a support plane, can also be lowered and raised jointly, depending on the patient's height and the mammographic projection.

The **compression device** (paddle) is made of plastic and is intended to compress the breast onto the supporting plane.

Integrated in the detector is the **automatic exposure control (AEC)**. See below.

The X-ray production takes place inside the X-ray tube, as in conventional radiological practice. Electrons endowed with high kinetic energy are extracted from the cathode (focus) and collide on the anode.

*The X-ray beam produced has a particular geometry with respect to general radiology. Its central axis, which joins the focal spot, i.e. the source, and the detector, is not located in the centre of the field of view. It represents the innermost limit of it, which corresponds to the patient's chest wall.* This is because it is essential to include as much as possible of the deep tissues in the image. *In addition, the beam is halved. This is made to avoid undue tissue exposure, since half of the beam inside the central axis would not be used to produce image anyway* (Fig. 7.1).

The acceleration of electrons towards the anode for the formation of the X-ray beam is achieved by applying a high voltage. In digital mammography, this is much lower than that used in general radiology. To avoid beam filtration, the emission window is made of beryllium, which has a low atomic number Z.

The **cathode filament**, or **focus**, is the negative electrode of the tube. From it, the electron beam is extracted and collides on the **anode**, the positive electrode (also called **target**), to produce the X-ray beam. The cathode is very small, to produce very small *focal spots*. The impact area of the electron beam is highly collimated and is indeed small, and it constitutes the **focal spot**. There are generally two cathode filaments of different sizes. The material they are made of is one with a high melting point, like tungsten. It is brought to the necessary temperature only during exposure. During the rest of the time when the mammographic unit is on, it is kept at a lower temperature, on standby mode. The distance between anode and cathode is smaller compared to conventional radiological tubes, around 0.7 cm.

The anode is rotating and disc-shaped. The material from which it is made must have characteristics such as high X-ray production, high melting point and high heat dissipation capacity. Rhenium-tungsten and molybdenum alloys are

**Fig. 7.1** Beam central axis in radiology and mammography, and beam halving. Bordered in red is the area of tissue that would be lost if conventional geometry were used in mammography

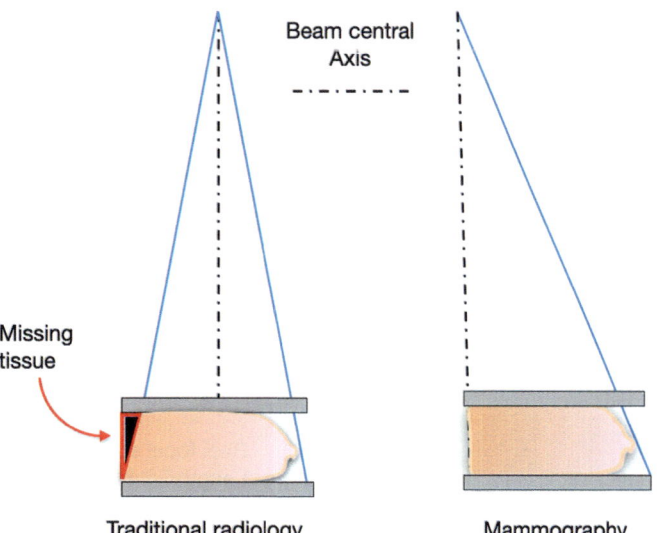

mainly used. Graphite anode bases can also be encountered. *The area struck by the electron beam in full-field digital mammography (FFDM) is generally tungsten (W); rhodium (Rh) is generally used as a filter.* Other typical anode materials are rhodium (Rh) and molybdenum (Mo). In terms of filters, aluminium (Al) and silver (Ag) are used, the latter for thicker breasts. The anode takes the form of a track laid on the circumference of the disc. The tracks are usually two, made of different materials. The *focal spot* ranges from 0.3 mm$^2$ for contact examinations, to an ultra-thin 0.1 mm$^2$ for magnification examinations (Chap. 13). *The size of the focal spot is not measured at the anode. What is measured is its projection along the central axis of the X-ray beam, called the optical, effective or apparent focal spot. This is thus defined as the projection of the real focal spot towards the detector* (Fig. 7.2). The size of the effective focal spot is one of the parameters that can be selected by the operator, depending on the desired spatial resolution. The two focal spots, real and effective, are different because the anode is angled relative to the cathode, in order to obtain a sufficiently large area (the real focal spot) to reduce the risk of melting. At the same time, a smaller effective focal spot is obtained, to improve the spatial resolution of the image. The smaller the **anode angle**, the better the dissipative capacity and the smaller the effective focal spot, but the **heel effect** (see below) is larger.

The extension of the beam is limited by the presence of the anode itself, and the photons produced within it are attenuated or even absorbed. Thus, it is not possible to cover a wide **field of view (FOV)**, given the small source-to-image distance used in mammography. To avoid the narrowing of the FOV (which must reach 24 × 30 cm for large breasts), the **anode angle** needed was calculated to be approximately 16°. Added to the tube angle, it sums up to a total angle of **22°**.

The size of the effective focal spot also changes along the FOV or, rather, the length of the effective spot is larger on the cathode side and decreases proceeding towards the anode. This is the so-called *line focus principle*, which should be taken into account when assessing the spatial resolution of the image along that direction. See Fig. 7.3.

*The line focus principle represents the change in length of the effective focal spot along the cathode-anode axis. More precisely, it represents the decrease in its length proceeding from the cathode to the anode, due to the angle of the latter. This leads to a parallel increase in spatial resolution SR (by a decrease in the effective focal spot), proceeding in the same direction.*

*Bi-Angular Design*: This term means that the small and large cathode filaments use different anode angles for the beam production, as shown in Fig. 7.4.

The **heel effect or anode effect** refers to the **variation in intensity of the produced X-ray beam, whereby the intensity is maximum on**

**Fig. 7.2**  Anode angle, real and effective focal spot

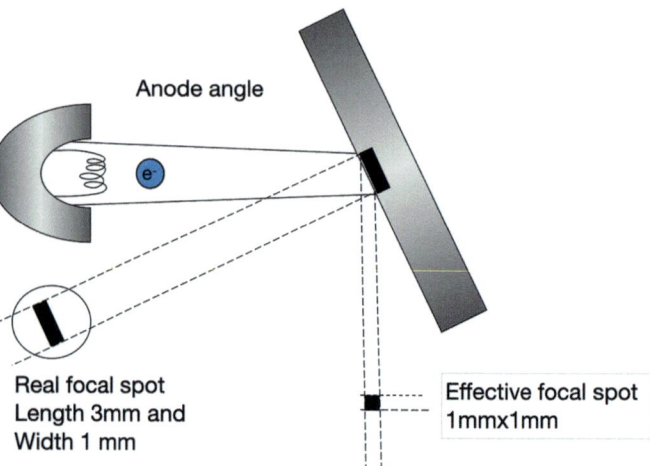

Anode angle

Real focal spot
Length 3mm and
Width 1 mm

Effective focal spot
1mmx1mm

**Fig. 7.3** The line focus principle: decrease in effective focal spot length and thus increase in SR from cathode to anode

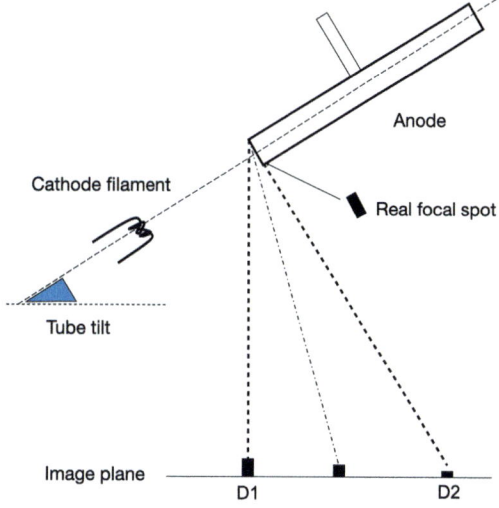

**Fig. 7.4** Bi-angular focus design: focal spots at different angles

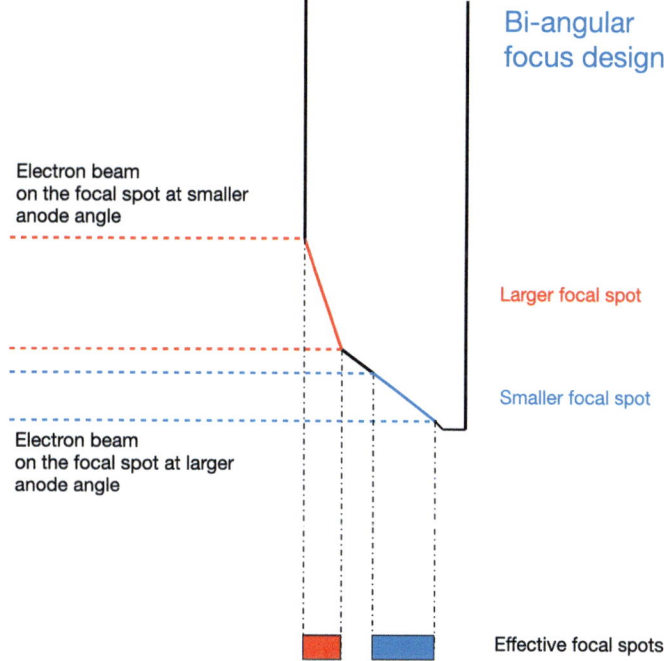

**the cathode side and minimum on the anode side.** The variation along the cathode-anode axis can be reflected on the image plane. This is due to the absorption by the anode of those photons that have a low emission angle and therefore travel a longer path within the anode itself (being attenuated). It depends not only on the anode angle but also on the detector size and the source-to-image distance (SID). In mammography, it is exploited to compensate for the varying thickness of the breast along the posterior-anterior axis (thorax-nipple), so that the posterior side corresponds to the cathode, where the beam intensity is higher (greater penetration).

*In contrast to what happens in conventional X-ray tubes, the decrease in beam intensity in mammography is from the outermost part of the field, towards the anode side.*

**Filtration**: In diagnostic radiology, its purpose is to attenuate the part of the X-ray spectrum that is least likely to penetrate the patient and reach the detector. Furthermore, it is a system that allows for spectral and spatial modification of beam distribution, depending on the desired results. X-rays pass through various materials before exiting the tube: (a) the anode where they are produced; (b) the glass envelope containing the two electrodes, (c) the tube window; (d) the oil contained (not in mammography); and (e) the housing window. This is the **inherent filtration**. Then, there is the so-called **additional filtration** for eliminating the low-energy component of the spectrum. Filtration effects are summarised in Table 7.2.

The attenuation of the beam is measured by the **linear attenuation coefficient**, which expresses the fraction of incident photons that will be attenuated per unit of thickness of the traversed medium. The **half-value layer (HVL)** is the material thickness, in millimetres, that reduces the intensity of the incident beam to half its initial value. It is used to measure the attenuation undergone by the beam and is based on the fact that photons of different energies have different penetrability. See Chap. 21.

**Anti-Scatter Grid**: It is placed between patient and detector. One of the most widely used grids in mammography is the *high transmission cellular (HTC) grid*, built from intersecting strips of radio-opaque lamellae. It is capable of removing the diffuse or scatter radiation (Sect. 7.3.2 and Chap. 21) in two directions and a smaller percentage of the primary beam than a linear grid. The latter consists of parallel radio-opaque and radio-lucent lamellae.

**Table 7.2** Filtration effects

| |
|---|
| Filtration removes the low-energy component of the spectrum: |
|     – That component would be responsible for the delivery of an improper dose |
|     – Its elimination increases the average energy of the beam, increasing its quality or penetrability |
|     – It decreases the entrance dose for the same dose measured at the detector |
| Filtration reduces quantity, improves quality: The beam is attenuated, but more penetrating |

**Collimators**: These consist of two opposing pairs of movable metal diaphragms, which can be moved closer together or farther apart to achieve the desired beam size. Thus, the delimitation of the area in which the image is produced is obtained.

**Automatic Exposure Control (AEC)**: In digital mammography, this ensures the modulation of technical factors according to the characteristics of the breast. It exerts control over the delivered dose, stopping it once a sufficient *pixel value* has been reached. The **pixel value (PV)** is equivalent to the *optical density* in the analogue system, i.e. the signal intensity value associated with that pixel. In direct digital systems, a very low-dose, non-displayable pre-image is acquired and analysed in real time at each individual examination. The aim is the optimisation of the beam production parameters; the breast density and thickness are also examined. This is why the waiting time during exposure can be very long for the digital mammography system, with which, however, the image is always optimal, unlike in the analogue one. This is true even when greatly varying the **delivered dose**. Therefore, it is essential to closely monitor the dose, through the parameter **average glandular dose (AGD)**. On average, it should not exceed 2.5 mGy per projection, as recommended in Italy and other European countries (see Chap. 21).

### 7.3.1 The X-Ray Beam Production Parameters and the Spectrum

The *tube current* is defined as the number of electrons travelling between the two electrodes and is measured in milliamperes (mA). The typical current in a mammographic unit is between 25 and 100 mA. The voltage, which is measured in kV, is between 25 and 35 kV. The **tube current** (i.e. the flow of electrons) is proportional to the current in the cathode, which in turn determines the number of electrons emitted. In a mammographic unit, this is between 25 mA for a small focus examination and 100 mA for larger focus. The **kilovolt (kV)** is the unit of measurement of the **voltage** or the **potential difference** applied between the two electrodes. It expresses the potential or energy with which electrons are accelerated, and it indicates the average energy of all incident electrons. It is also the most common unit by which the energy of the X-ray beam produced is measured. The maximum value of applied voltage is denoted by the term **kilovoltage peak (kVp)**. **Exposure Time**: This is defined as the time during which the electrons are produced and varies depending on the used diagnostic modality. It is measured in seconds. The exposure time controls the energy flow of the X-ray beam. *The kilovoltage peak kVp, the tube current in mA and the exposure duration in seconds, mAs, are parameters that can be adjusted by the operator, depending on the examination to be performed and the patient's anatomy.*

Another key parameter is the distance between source and detector or image (SID). Since the voltage value varies between a minimum value and a maximum value, equal to the chosen kVp, the electrons that reach the anode will not all have the same energy. Thus, the same will apply to the X-ray photons produced. Interactions with the anode occur within a very small penetration depth, with subsequent loss of energy until they come to a stop. For the most part, their kinetic energy is transformed into thermal energy.

It should be considered that the voltage used for the mammographic unit tube is low, so the X-ray production efficiency is even lower than the already very low efficiency of a traditional radiological tube.

The effects on the image of the operator-modifiable parameters are presented in Table 7.3.

The process that is most likely to occur in X-ray production is *bremsstrahlung*, translated as **braking radiation**, which is poly-chromatic (i.e. poly-energetic) and continuous. Another possible process leads to the production of **characteristic radiation**. See also Chap. 20 on CESM. *In mammography, the useful X-ray component is precisely the characteristic radiation.*

**X-Beam Spectrum**: It visualises the intensity distribution of a radiation frequency, as a function of its energy. The spectrum of characteristic radiation is discrete, and it is represented by lines (which depend on the element constituting the anode). It is important to select the most suitable

**Table 7.3** Operator-modifiable parameters. Effects on the image

| kVp | An increase in kVp is associated with a **decrease in low-contrast resolution**; all else being equal, exposure is proportional to $kVp^2$. Changing the kVp changes the maximum energy of the generated photons |
|---|---|
| mA | An increase in mA corresponds to an **improvement (decrease) in noise and in low-contrast resolution**, thus affecting **SNR** (Chap. 8). All else being equal, exposure is proportional to mA. Changing the ma changes the number of generated photons |

**Table 7.4** Factors that affect the spectrum

| Beam quality | This represents the penetration power or maximum energy of the emitted X-ray beam. It is mainly determined by the kilovoltage peak (kVp) and the filtration used. It plays a role in image contrast |
|---|---|
| Beam quantity | This indicates the number of X photons and is mainly influenced by mAs and the source-to-image distance SID, according to the inverse square law (Chap. 21 and Annex 2) |

spectrum for each acquisition method. Beam quality and quantity are defined in Table 7.4.

*The optimisation of spectrum in mammography is also achieved through the selection of the anode filter combination. The W/Rh combination appears to have the best performance in terms of SR, SNR and DQE compared to other combinations* [10].

These features allow the use of a lower dose for the same *contrast-to-noise ratio (CNR)* (see below). *Detective quantum efficiency (DQE) is* the efficiency with which X-radiation is converted in image production: see Chap. 8 about it.

## 7.3.2   A Brief Overview on the Interaction of X-Rays with Matter and Influence on Image Contrast: The CNR [7–11]

The X-photons that are transmitted (outgoing) from the patient *without any interaction* constitute the **primary radiation**. The attenuation of the X-rays from the incident beam can occur for

1. Coherent scattering or classical scattering
2. Compton effect or incoherent scattering
3. Photoelectric effect

(1) The *diffusion or scattering of photons* plays no role in image formation, but contributes, albeit very minimally in mammography, to the increase in background noise; (2) the *Compton effect* is the dominant interaction of X-rays in soft tissues in the energy range used in radiology and must be taken into account for environmental radiation protection; and (3) the *photoelectric effect* is also of fundamental importance: it is highly dependent on the atomic number Z. Thus, it plays a key role in X-ray imaging, regarding in particular the contrast between tissues that have precisely small differences in Z. The energy dependence is also important: it is the low energies that contribute most to the radiographic image contrast (see also Chap. 21).

Another type of X-ray attenuation is the *pair production* that will be discussed in Chap. 20, regarding molecular imaging (MBI) of the breast.

*The attenuation of X-rays by the target (the patient) occurs selectively and differentially because it is related to the different probabilities for the photoelectric and the Compton effects to occur.*

The different attenuation experienced by the beam in passing through the object, i.e. the tissues *different linear attenuation coefficients,* is evaluated into the digital system by means of the *pixel value*, in terms of *radiopacity and radiolucency* (Sect. 7.1). Ideally, only the primary beam would contribute to the formation of the image, with the achievement of the maximum achievable contrast, exclusively through the photoelectric effect. In reality, there is, as mentioned, an amount of scattered radiation that degrades the contrast. In other words, signal that is not representative of the anatomy, the **noise**, is introduced. This is why we speak of **contrast-to-noise ratio** (**CNR**), particularly important in the digital imaging system. See Chap. 8.

## 7.4  Compression from a Physical Perspective [11]

Compression is of fundamental importance in mammography as it improves all technical quality parameters, as outlined in Table 7.5.

The force exerted is in **decanewtons (daN)**, and it is measured with a dynamometer. The **Newton** is the unit of compression measurement in the SI International System: 10 N corresponds to approximately 1 kg of mass force. The *kilogram force (kgf)* is an engineering force measurement that corresponds to the force exerted by a one kilogram mass on the Earth's surface, subjected to a gravity acceleration of approximately 10 m/s$^2$. Therefore, 1 daN is used as an approximation of 1 kgf.

1 kgf = 10 N = 1 daN.

The *compression paddles* used for standard examinations in mammography are generally two, measuring 18 × 24 cm and 24 × 30 cm. They are to be chosen according to breast size; see Chap. 16. On the topic of compression; see also Chap. 11 and the two lessons on the YouTube channel of the author, @cristinapoggi7579 (2021) at the links:

**Table 7.5** Technical quality parameters influenced by compression in mammography

| |
|---|
| Improve the contrast by reducing scattering (the same reason why low-energy beams are used: scattering increases as the beam energy increases) |
| Reduces anatomical noise or summation or masking artifact, given by the overlapping of structures, in the transformation from 3D object to 2D image |
| Reduces the likelihood of patient movement (a likely phenomenon given the long exposure times) |
| Decreases the dose required to obtain a good image, all other factors being equal |
| Provides a uniform thickness of the breast, allowing the reporter to attribute a change in density to a lesion rather than to a change in thickness |

- https://youtu.be/LxSuhj8Gbqk
- https://youtu.be/aHAxFZFCHQ8

## 7.5   FFDM Full-Field Digital Mammography Vs. SFM Screen Film Mammography

Compared with the **screen-film (SF)** analogue mammography **system**, the **full-field digital mammography (FFDM)** has several advantages. Among them, (1) lower dose delivered under the same conditions, due to the use of more penetrating beams and to other inherent characteristics; (2) the reduction in repeated projections due to the elimination of the possibility of wrong exposure. This fact is determined by the *dynamic range*, which is very wide in the direct digital system. See Chap. 8.

*Dynamic range refers to the relationship between signal intensity shown (density) and relative exposure, which is linear and very wide in the FFDM system.* It is about 1000 to 1 compared with 40 to 1 in the SF system. This means that obtaining an acceptable image in the FFDM system is possible with a very wide exposure parameter range. The dynamic range is recorded as a number of grey shades on the image. Their high number compared to that of the SF system allows all areas of the breast to be visualised to the fullest. Although the spatial resolution was certainly much higher in the analogue system, the loss in resolution of the digital one is compensated by the *data processing* (Chap. 8). Various *post-processing* operations of the acquired images are possible. Moreover, the implementation of *tomosynthesis techniques* (Chap. 20) can be achieved, as well as digital archiving and presentation as **soft copy** on a high-resolution monitor. The workstations display monitor in the senology department has a resolution of at least 5 Megapixels (MP or Mpx). The term means one million pixels (Chaps. 8 and 23). The digital image can still be printed (**hard copy**).

## 7.6   The FFDM Direct Conversion Detector

**Full-field digital mammography** is a mammographic system in which the X-ray film is replaced by a **solid-state receptor** (or detector). Its task is converting X-rays into an electrical signal and then into images for clinical use. It is also called **flat panel detector** [12, 13].

The first step is always the same: the patient is placed in front of a detector that records the intensity of the X-rays that pass the breast. Finally, as all with electronic detectors, an electrical signal, i.e. analogue, is produced. It varies continuously and depends on the quality of the radiation received.

Full-field detectors have an array of millions of pixels, called an **active matrix array (AMA)**, on which a layer of **amorphous selenium (a-Se)**, the *photoconductive material,* is applied. *Selenium is the ideal material for mammographic detectors because its X-ray absorption efficiency is almost 100 per cent. This allows the dose delivered to the patient to be lowered.* It has a very high intrinsic resolution, little noise and a well-established fabrication process, ensuring (a) high reproducibility and reliability and (b) high uniformity of response. The task of amorphous selenium is to directly capture and convert incident X-photons into electrical charge, more precisely, into *electron-hole pairs*. A hole is defined as the "missing" electron. The pair production is proportional to the intensity of the incident X-beam. An electric field is then generated that separates the charges from each other, preventing their recombination. The first ones are directed towards the surface (positively charged), and the second ones towards the negative electrodes of the pixels (Fig. 7.5). There is practically no lateral movement, since the direction is determined by the electric field gradient.

Each pixel is connected to an **electrode**, a **capacitor** to store the charge released during exposure and a **thin-film transistor (TFT).** The latter is a switch through which charge is passed from one

**Fig. 7.5** Simplified diagram of a direct conversion FFDM flat panel detector

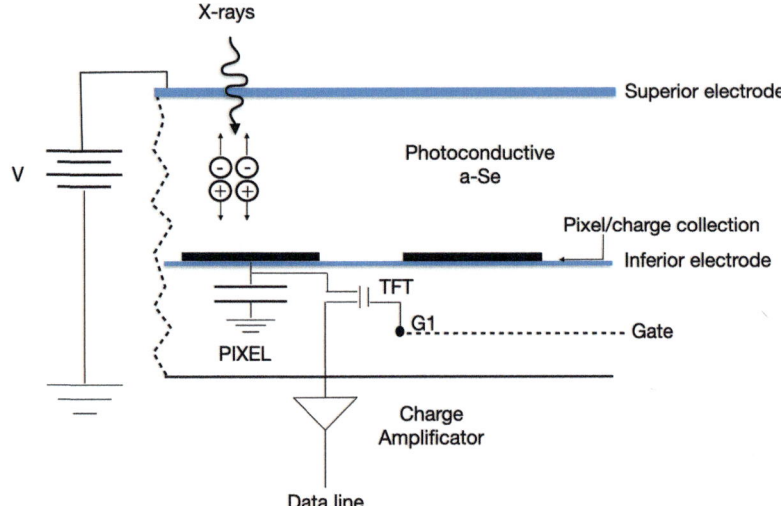

pixel to another along a line, called **data line**, until it reaches the detector's external electronics. At the end of the exposure, the charge stream (the analogue signal) is collected by computer systems and amplified and converted into a digital signal. Then, it is sent to the computer for image reconstruction. To note, the detector is mounted in the mammographic unit's support plane, so, it is never moved or rotated with respect to the X-ray beam, which is always perpendicular to it. This aspect is important, since it allows **flat-fielding calibration** (see Chap. 8, Quality Controls).

## 7.7 The Dimensions of Pixel, Detector and FOV [14]

The smallest detail that can be resolved in any digital system is a function of pixel size. The smaller the pixel, the smaller the detail that can be resolved, leading to higher spatial resolution. Theoretically, in the direct conversion digital detectors the pixel could be manufactured to be extremely small. In reality, there is a limitation that arises even before manufacture: the pixel too small cannot intercept a sufficient flow of photons. It is called *quantum limitation*. Furthermore, the smaller the pixels, the higher their number must be for the same covered area. The generated data grow proportionally to the number of pixels, and therefore, the cost for their storage and read-

ing also increases. The active matrix is characterised by:

- Pixel width
- Pixel collection width
- Pixel pitch (distance between the centres of the pixels)

*The pixel pitch and the dimensions of the pixel determine the maximum spatial resolution of the system.*

The important geometric aspects of the pixel include the so-called **fill factor**, which is the ratio of active area to the total area of the pixel. This indicates the presence of a larger or smaller micro-dead zone, which is not sensitive to photons. The **detector element (DEL) is the active or sensitive part that is capable of responding to radiation**. All improvements in spatial resolution result in a reduction in pixel size, but the fill factor decreases as spatial resolution increases (as pixel size decreases). This is because the reading electronics cannot be reduced in size, so the micro-dead zone increases proportionally to the sensitive part.

The voltage increases as a function of exposure, but in some cases, by accidental overexposure, for example, it can reach high values which can damage the detector. For this reason, there is an insulating layer that protects against artefacts caused by charges not produced by X-rays.

Another disadvantage of direct detectors is the need to apply a high voltage and the *dark current* that can result from it. By **dark current,** we mean a different response (output) by a certain number of pixels compared to others, for the same input signal. It translates into noise on the image.

A final element that needs to be considered is the size of the detector. This is larger than the *active area*, the one that is capable of producing the image, which must allow the study of larger breasts and require the "large" compressor (24 × 30 cm). *The use of the "small" compressor paddle, 18 × 24 cm, results in the automatic reduction of the active area, that is to say the FOV and light field reduction.* This means that one part of the detector does not produce an image. A portion of these inactivated areas contains the electronic readout circuits and is therefore never sensitive to X-photons, whichever compression paddle is chosen. This is precisely located in the innermost part of the detector, towards the patient. The other inactive areas resulting from the choice of the small compressor are located on the sides of the detector, performing CCs, and above and below in MLOs. This has an important impact on the positioning technique for the extension of the tissue documented in mammography (see Chaps. 9 and 11 about it).

## References

1. Carlsson CA, Carlsson GA. Basic physics of X-ray imaging, 2nd ed. Institutionene för medicine ouch vård Avdelninge för radiofysik Hälsouniversitetet, ISRN: LIU-RAD-R-008; 1996.
2. Seibert JA, et al. Imaging for nuclear medicine technologists. Part 2: X-ray interaction and image formation. J Nucl Med Technol. 2005;33(1):3–18.
3. Stewart BK. Chapter 1. Introduction to medical imaging. Chapter 2. Radiation and the atom. http://faculty.washington.edu/bstewart/mywebs/Rad_Atom_Inter_Dx_Rad_Imaging_Physics_Course-040506d.pdf.
4. Di Bartolomeo A. Principi alla base della formazione dell'immagine diagnostica in medicina nucleare Parte 2 anno Gennaio 2006 Istituto Nazionale di Fisica Nucleare sezione di Napoli.
5. Zamora D, Kalpana K. Basics of X-ray and mammography systems: techniques, filtration, and system configuration. University of Washington Medical Center, Department of Radiology. http://courses.washington.edu/radxphys/.
6. Zamora D. Introduction to radiography (lecture 3 of 3): geometry, contrast, scatter, and heel effect. http://courses.washington.edu/radxphys. ultimo accesso 9/2019.
7. Wilson CR. Review of the physics of mammography, PPT, AAPM. https://www.aap.org/meetings/amos2/pdf/41-10112-77849-656.pdf.
8. Jaffe MJ, Maidment ADA. Chapter 9: Mammography slide, on the IAEA publication. In: Lawinski CP, editor. Diagnostic radiology physics: a handbook for teachers and students, slide set prepared by IAEA. isbn:978-92-0-13101010-1.
9. Yaffe MJ. Detectors for digital mammography 2. In: Bick U, Dieckmann F, editors. Digital mammography, XIII. Springer; 2010. 219 p. isbn:978-3-540-78449-4.
10. Alkhalifah K, et al. Image quality and radiation dose for fibrofatty breast using target/filter combinations in two digital mammography systems. J Clin Imaging Sci. 2020;10:56. https://doi.org/10.25259/JCIS_30_2020.
11. Mercer CE. Practitioner variation of applied breast compression force in mammography. Thesis 2014. University of Salford, UK. https://salford-repository.worktribe.com/preview/1496464/PhD_Thesis_Claire_Mercer_Practitioner_variation_of_applied_breast_compression_force_in_mammography.pdf.
12. Rowlands JA, Nietzel U. Chapter 7. Image receptors. In: Maher KP, editor. Edyvean S. IAEA. isbn:978-92-0-131010-1.
13. Kuzmiak CM. Digital mammography, imaging of the breast-technical aspects and clinical implication. In: Tabar L, editor. InTech; 2012. isbn:978-953-51-0284-7.
14. Nett B. Digital X-ray imaging [Dels, Marie size, bit depth, dynamic range, sampling frequency]. How radiology works. https://howradiologyworks.com/digital-x-ray-sampling.

## Further Reading

Bushberg JT. et al. The essential physics of medical imaging, 3rd ed. Lippincott & Wilkins; 2012. isbn:978-0-7817-8057-5.

Dance DR, et al. Diagnostic radiology physics a handbook for teachers and students. IAEA; 2014. isbn:978-92-131010-1.

Hogg P, et al. Digital mammography a holistic approach. Springer; 2015. isbn:978-3-319-04831-4.

# The Digital Image and Its Processing: Quality Controls in Mammography: An Overview

**8**

## 8.1 Introduction

Although digital imaging has many advantages over analogue imaging, it also requires a lot of **quality controls**.

The purpose of checking the overall image quality is to identify all deviations from what has been objectively indicated as the *optimal performance*. This applies to all areas, including equipment, the clinical practice and the necessary training of the staff. With regard to mammography, all stages of the production chain are tested, from acquisition to processing and visualisation. The first two stages deal with *technical quality*, and the third stage deals with *clinical quality*.

## 8.2 The Conversion of the Signal from Analogue to Digital [1, 2]

All image detectors or receptors produce an electrical signal, analogue. This is to say, one that varies continuously over time can take infinite values within a certain range, which depends on the amount of radiation received. The signal must be converted, in order to be processed, into a digital output signal. This signal again represents the amount of charge corresponding to the number of X photons absorbed by the pixel. **Analogue-to-digital conversion** deals with the transformation of certain parameters of an electrical signal, while keeping the amount of information it possesses unchanged (as far as possible). The charge is represented by a digital value that is stored in the image matrix, the ***pixel value***. The digital signal is discrete; it goes from one constant level to another. **The digital signal is a sequence of voltage pulses**, in which only two representations are possible: 1, positive, where the signal is present, and 0, negative, where it is not present. These are the **BITS** or **binary data**. **Sampling** (i.e. **an interval detection of**) the analogue signal with a certain frequency is ultimately done. The higher the frequency, the more points are detected over time, and the better the representation of the input signal will be. That is to say, the more similar to the original, the object will be reproduced. The signal is then examined by applying the *Fourier transform*. This mathematical operator allows to obtain the frequency information of a complex signal through its decomposition into a sum of simpler waves, each associated with a known frequency (and a phase). We speak of *spatial frequencies*. Each of them represents the spatial location of the pixel, according to its x and y coordinates. In this way, the signal goes from the so-called *time domain* to the *frequency domain*. This makes sense because many mathematical operations are faster in the second. Spatial frequencies express the spatial variation of the object to be reproduced (in lines per millimetre). They therefore describe its shape and dimen-

C. Poggi, *Breast Imaging Techniques for Radiographers*,
https://doi.org/10.1007/978-3-031-63314-0_8

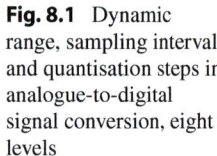

**Fig. 8.1** Dynamic range, sampling interval and quantisation steps in analogue-to-digital signal conversion, eight levels

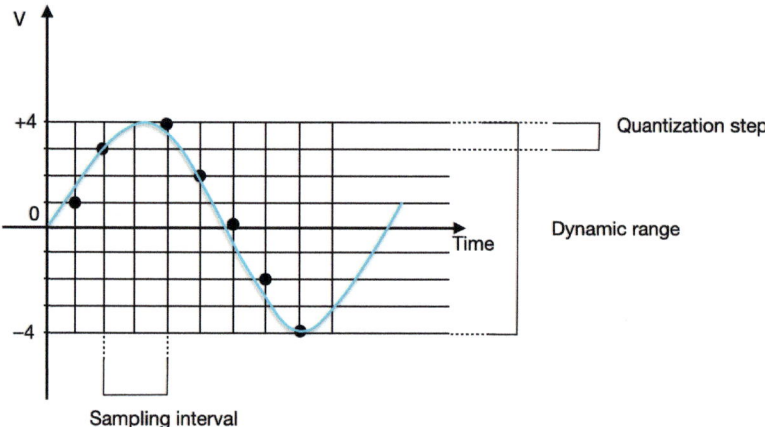

sions. A high frequency indicates a sudden change (edge).

*Any object (the analogue signal) can thus be described in the frequency domain as a sum of spatial frequencies*. More precisely, there are a few low spatial frequencies that contain a large part of the signal and can effectively describe the shape of the object and many high spatial frequencies that describe its edges.

To obtain the image, it will then be necessary to apply the inverse Fourier transform.

Digitalisation is performed by the **analogue-to-digital converters (ADCs)**. In addition to sampling, there is also the process of **quantisation:** the amplitude of the signal is made discrete; i.e., a unique value is given to each sample of the signal (which contains a given range). The number of bits used to encode each sample, or quantisation bits, is important, as is the higher sampling rate, for the quality of the image produced.

**Dynamic range** can be defined as the ratio between the minimum and maximum exposure of the X-rays reaching the detector (Fig. 8.1). This range is linear in direct digital imaging (see also Chap. 7).

## 8.3    The Digital Image Displayed

The amplitude value of the signal is transformed into an intensity or grey value. All levels of grey in biomedical imaging are referred to by the term **tone scale or greyscale**. Brightness, or rather *luminance* (see Chap. 24), does not go from black to white by smooth graduations, but by small increments (hence the term "scale"). This is expressed by the quantisation operation and the number of bits chosen to encode each level.

The image stored in a digital processor is a two-dimensional series of numbers, which are arranged in a regular pattern in a grid called *"matrix"*. It consists of **pixels (picture elements or PELs)** (see Chap. 7). Each pixel takes on a value in the available greyscale range L (0, L−1):

$$L = 2^b$$

where L represents the levels and b represents the bits used to encode each pixel. b is also called *pixel depth* and is measured in *bits per pixel (bpp)*.

*The pixel depth therefore determines the amount of information available (in terms of grey shades) for each pixel in the image.* For pixel encoding, the greater the number of **bpp,** the greater the range of visible shades of grey, and thus, the better the representation of the object. In biomedical imaging, 12 to 16 bpp is generally used; the average size of a mammographic examination and DBT is shown in Table 8.1.

Within each pixel, a digital pixel value (PV) is stored, related to the amplitude of the analogue signal at that point. It will be translated into light intensity or grey shade once the inverse Fourier transform is applied. The number of bits used to represent each level of grey, or pixel depth, expresses the *contrast resolution* of the image (Chap. 7).

**Table 8.1** Pixel depth (bpp) and image size in FFDM and DBT examination

| Depth in bbp | Between 12 and 16 bbp |
|---|---|
| Image size in megabyte | For four projections, considering FOV of 18 × 24 or 24 × 30 cm, SR between 50 and 70 microns: FFDM: 100–200 MB; DBT (two projections): 1 GB (data storage depends also on PACS vendor configuration, image format and compression ratio) [3] |

## 8.4  The Quality of the Digital Image Displayed [4–11]

The image can be described, among other parameters, in terms of *spatial resolution*, *contrast resolution*, **noise**, **detective quantum efficiency (DQE)** and the presence or absence of **artefacts** (Chap. 17).

### 8.4.1  Spatial Resolution of the Acquired and Displayed Image

Spatial resolution (SR) indicates how small a detail can be resolved. It is controlled by the size of the matrix, i.e. the pixel size and the pixel pitch (Chap. 7). The SR of an electronic image is generally measured in **dots per inch** or **points per inch (ppi).** It is a measure of density. Recalling the concept in the SF system, we also speak of line pairs per millimetre (lp/mm). In the FFDM system, the value is equal to or below 10 lp/mm, while in the SF system it was as high as 20. Image processing compensates for the lower resolution, as already stated. Furthermore, it depends on how many pixels are used to display the image on *workstation monitors* (see below).

Theoretically, the size of the pixel of the acquired image identifies the limit of the resolution power, in the sense that we should not be able to see an object that is smaller than the pixel size. In reality, it is not only the size of the object that matters, but also its contrast. If the amplitude of its signal is high enough, it can influence the greyscale in such a way that it is detectable, even when it is smaller than a pixel. This is exactly what happens with *microcalcifications,* which can be an impor-

tant indication of breast cancer; they are very small but characterised by high contrast and thus generally well detectable (Chap. 13).

An important aspect to consider in mammography with regard to technical quality, is that the geometrical characteristic of the tube are such that the *effective focal spot* (Chap. 7) is different in size along the cathode-anode axis. Thus, the spatial resolution is worse towards the cathode, corresponding to the deep (thoracic) breast tissues, with the focal spot being larger and better towards the anode (the nipple). This concept is called the *line focus principle* (Chap. 7), and it is important, especially in acquisition with magnification (Chap. 13). A drop in spatial resolution might also be due to the patient's movement and is referred to as *kinetic blurring.* Given the long exposure times, this is not a rare phenomenon in mammography. The concept of unsharpness is very broad, depending on various parameters, such as the size of the focal spot, which is not point-like. *Geometric unsharpness* is defined as the representation of the object with a more or less extensive peripheral shadow (penumbra). See also Appendix 2. The object-image distance (OID) also matters. Adequate compression brings the object closer to the receptor plane, so that edge blurring is more contained. However, kinetic blurring in mammography is an extremely significant phenomenon, so a blurred image is always to be considered inadequate. The mammography needs to be repeated, even if the blurring affects only a small area out of the total.

### 8.4.2  Contrast Resolution (See Also Chap. 7)

Contrast expresses the smallest variation in exposure that can be perceived. More simply, the ability of the imaging system to distinguish very small differences in grey and to detect them above the noise is the greatest deterrent to digital image quality. It depends on the pixel depth and is limited by the exposure range and quantisation. To assess the impact of scattered radiation, which contributes to image noise, the so-called **scatter-to-primary ratio (SPR)** is considered. The reduction of scattered radiation is a fundamental requirement in mammography as well, even though its impact is low if compared to almost all radiological examinations.

For the image to have sufficient contrast for diagnostic purposes, there must be a high signal and little noise. Thus, **contrast can be measured by measuring the signal-to-noise ratio (SNR).**

$$SNR = C \sqrt{AQ}.$$

where $C$ stands for contrast, $A$ for area and $Q$ for the number of photons per area.

This means that, *when dealing with a small object size, the more the noise increases, the greater the probability of not detecting it*.

The minimum dose required to perceive an object against the background increases according to (1) the inverse of the object size raised to the fourth power and (2) the inverse of the difference between the linear coefficients squared (Chaps. 7 and 21).

Therefore, *for the same dose and contrast, there will be a minimum object size that can be visualised*. This aspect is crucial for mammographic imaging. In addition to the *high-contrast resolution*, for the study of soft tissue, the *low-contrast resolution*, defined as the ability to distinguish structures that have little signal difference between them (Chap. 7), is also important.

### 8.4.3 Noise

There are various types of noise. *Electronic noise* is added to the signal but is not the result of the photon revelation event, so it is disturbing. It can be decreased, but not substantially. *Structured noise* derives from the fact that multiple elements are used for signal detection. They cannot be perfectly in tune with each other, as they would be in an ideal world. This kind of noise is also inherent in the system, but since it has periodic fluctuations, special calibrations can be made. They are called **flat-field corrections,** can help reduce its impact and are made at specific time intervals depending on the type of device (see below). **Anatomical noise** comes from the fact that mammography is not a 3D imaging modality, so the

problem arising from the tissue overlap is unavoidable. However, anatomical noise can be abated, although not completely, by *tomosynthesis DBT* (Chap. 20). *Quantum noise* results from the fact that X-rays are used for image formation, and it is given by the statistical fluctuation of photons absorbed in different areas of the detector.

Noise is measured by the **signal-to-noise ratio (SNR).** It can be said that *SNR is by far the most significant parameter for measuring the ability to detect an object*, also called *"conspicuity"*. It is measured with the *contrast-detail curves (CDCs)*, which practically combine the concepts of spatial resolution and contrast.

### 8.4.4 Detective Quantum Efficiency (DQE)

*DQE represents the measure of the efficiency with which SNR is preserved in the image in the conversion from the incident radiation to the image viewed on the display monitor.*

In an ideal world, this would be 100%, or 1 (total transfer), because this would mean no information is lost. This indicates maximum efficiency of the system. High DQE systems provide higher quality images at a lower dose: this is because DQE also measures the percentage of photons absorbed out of the total of those reaching the detector. DQE is expressed as the ratio of output SNR to input SNR, both squared. Having a high DQE, and the fact that the beam in digital mammography is more penetrating than that used in the analogue system, allows for a reduction of the compression value required compared with the SF. DQE is high for a-Se detectors, generally used in FFDM, and depends on:

1. Exposure.
2. The **modulation transfer function (MTF): MTF** measures the detector's ability to transfer features related to the object's spatial frequencies to the image. In an ideal world, this would also be 1 (total transfer).
3. The detector material.
4. The quality of the radiation.

See also Chap. 7.

Note that MTF decreases as spatial frequencies increase. A low MTF, and thus a poor transfer of high spatial frequencies, results in a blurred image.

## 8.5 Digital Image Processing (DIP) or Digital Signal Processing (DSP)

The image that is acquired is the *raw image*. In the image DICOM format, the raw image is called the **processing image**. It needs to be processed with specific algorithms in order to be visualised, and to form what is called the **presentation** image. This dual aspect is typical of digital radiology, where the acquisition and display phases are separate and thus optimised separately.

### 8.5.1 Pre-processing

The pre-processing phase is done automatically. Thus, among the different operations, a *flat fielding or uniformity correction procedure* is applied. Signal variations/distortions are compensated for, also taking into account, the *dark current* (Chap. 7). The signal must truly correspond to the characteristics of the breast tissues the beam has passed through. There is a **flat-field mask** used for correcting the raw image, whose quality must be monitored (see below). *Edge equalisation* is also part of these pre-processing operations: in the case of a very dense breast, there would be a saturation of the signal at the edge, due to the abrupt thickness change (high gradient). Compensation is therefore needed, through the application of a correction algorithm (histogram based).

### 8.5.2 Post-processing

Many post-processing operations can be performed, the main purpose being to change the input pixel values in order to improve the perceived diagnostic quality of the displayed image.

One of the most important advantages of digital mammography is, in fact, its wide dynamic range. In order to exploit this to the full and to obtain the best possible contrast resolution, the most suitable greyscale must first be identified.

**Windowing/Levelling W/L**: The most well-known operation performed on the image for presentation is windowing and level variation, which allows the tonal scale or dynamic range *window width (WW)* to be contracted or enlarged to the full range available. It should also be centred on the level of interest, w*indow level (WL)*. WW and WL are synonymous with contrast and brightness, respectively, and can be manually adjusted.

In mammography, this is a rarely performed operation, once the WW and WL that are considered optimal have been chosen by the operator.

**Lookup Table (LUT)**: It indicates how the monitor hardware (the video card) transforms p-values into luminance (grey) values. You can choose between different LUTs for displaying the image. This is a reference histogram: a series of mathematical equations is used in post-processing to correct the grey values of the image (all the dynamic range), with other values. This is called *remapping*, and the aim is to improve the image in a diagnostic sense (Fig. 8.2). Generally, more intermediate shades of grey are used, relegating the very whites and very blacks to a few values.

A *Grayscale Standard Display Function (GSDF)* was introduced: it mathematically describes how pixel values of digital images should be converted to luminance, in DICOM format. See Chap. 23.

**Smoothing**: This results from the application of a low-pass filter to the image, i.e. a filter that only (or rather mainly) allows the low frequencies of the image to pass. It (a) improves SNR; (b) worsens SR; (c) reduces noise; (d) smoothes out edges; and (e) degrades image detail.

**Edge Enhancement**: This results from the application of high-pass filters: it improves SR but increases noise (high spatial frequencies of the object pass through).

**Image Inversion**: This inverts the normal radiographic representation from a dark to a light base, whereby dense structures are outlined in

**Fig. 8.2** Dynamic range and LUT

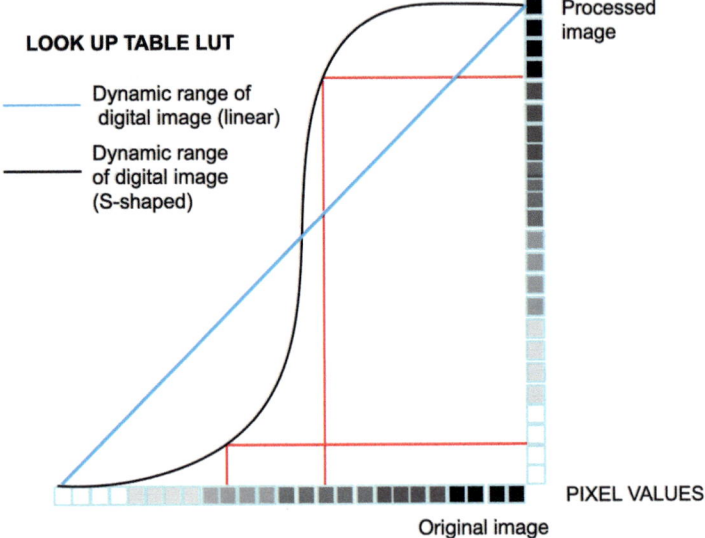

dark tones. It is widely used in mammography, for a better perception of microcalcifications, distortions and tissue consolidation (Chap. 13).

There are other types of operations, which usually do not produce another image, but rather yield numerical or graphical information of the same. These include the measurement of angles or distances, which are very useful in mammography for (a) planning interventional procedures, for example the distance between a lesion and the nipple, or between a lesion and the pectoralis muscle, or between one lesion and another (Chap. 5); and (b) stereotaxis, measuring lesion-skin distance, to establish the best needle entry approach for sampling (Chap. 18).

Regarding the measurement of lesion size on the mammographic image, it should be noted that the congruence with the lesion size measured on the surgical specimen is high [12].

**Electronic Magnification or Zooming**: It allows all or part of the mammographic image to be enlarged. The result in terms of resolution is worse than with real magnification acquisition, but it can be useful for the radiographer, especially for the reasons mentioned below:

1. To evaluate the presence or absence of an area affected by kinetic blurring.
2. To better locate the lesion on which to focus in a *second-level* examination (recall or call

back). In this case, it is to be subsequently restored to 1:1 to obtain the exact spatial information (Chaps. 13 and 25).

## 8.6    Technical Quality Controls (QCs)

Technical quality controls (QCs) refer to a series of planned and systematic actions aimed at verifying the reliability of the mammographic system, which must comply with the standards established at the European level. Italy is part of a working group on technical quality control in mammography within the *European Federation of Organisations for Medical Physics (EFOMP)* [13], which collaborates with *American Association of Physicist in Medicine (AAPM)*. The QCs that are carried out by both medical physicists (MPs) and radiographers are mainly *constancy checks*, in which certain parameters are measured over time [14].

*Quality controls carried out on the equipment must be regularly updated and follow guidelines that have been published by regulatory bodies.* It should be noted that guidelines for QC in mammography do not evolve as fast as technology; some tests that were once considered important are omitted in many new publications [14].

In Italy, the quality reference manual of each individual company, whether public or private, if involved in dose delivery for medical purposes, must contain all the items mentioned in Annex XXVIII of Legislative Decree *101/2020,* part 1, drafted by MPs themselves, in transposition of the *2013/59 EURATOM* Regulation (Chap. 21).

### 8.6.1  Acquisition

The acquisition represents the first point in the mammography production chain whose quality must be verified. There are various tests dedicated to this task, some to be performed by a radiographer and some by a medical physicist. The parameters to be evaluated are essentially the following: *exposure, spatial resolution, contrast* and *noise.*

### 8.6.2  Exposure QC

In mammography, the exposure data useful for obtaining a high-quality image are in such a narrow range that the use of an *automatic exposure control (AEC)* is mandatory. Currently, this function is no longer performed, as it used to be, by actual phototimers, i.e. ionisation chambers. Instead, it is the entire detector that evaluates when the exposure produces a *pixel value* that is sufficient to stop radiation emission (Chap. 7).

These checks are generally the responsibility of medical physicists.

### 8.6.3  Display, Noise, Contrast and Dose Delivery Monitoring QC

Image quality (IQ) control aims to verify the constancy of the acquisition system and the display chain, independently of the AEC. It is a qualitative test; the quantitative analysis is done by MPs. It involves the use of an anthropomorphic model (phantom), which includes objects that simulate various types of real breast lesions, with different sizes and contrasts. The QC test is always per-

formed with the same parameters and the same compression force, and the visible objects are recorded on the resulting image. On the acquired image, it is also possible to draw a *region of interest (ROI)* of a predetermined size, from which information can be obtained about (a) the noise (the standard deviation); (b) the mean value of the signal; and (c) the dose delivered, both entrance and averaged glandular (Chap. 21). The image acquired should then be compared to a baseline image and assessed for the presence of artefacts or inhomogeneities (also using the digital mag lens). Especially under observation is the mAs value, which should not exceed ±10% of the value reported in the baseline image, with the same acquisition parameters.

*Frequency: Generally weekly.*

### 8.6.4  Flat-Field Calibration: Image Receptor Uniformity

This is usually performed with a plexiglass phantom, acquiring images with a series of different exposure parameters, kV, mAs and anode/filter combinations. It is then observed whether the image exhibits uniform brightness or the presence of *bad pixels.* These are pixels with anomalous signal, either much lower or much higher than the surrounding ones. See also Chap. 17. It is an accept/reject method. What is desired is that the flat-field mask applied to the raw image remained unchanged, i.e. effective, over time. It is a uniformity test.

*Frequency: This depends on the different mammographic machines and manufacturing companies, according to the request of the mammographic unit, but can be done monthly.* A quality detector uniformity study including five ROIs, placed on the four corners of the image and in the centre of it, gives data on the mean value of the pixel and should be done on a weekly basis.

The new machines generally have a simplified procedure (*"usability"*; see Chap. 23), with a reduction of the parametric conditions to be evaluated. ***The appropriateness of the performance, i.e. the quality of the mammographic image produced, both technical and clinical, must be*** *monitored over time and improved when needed.* Quality control alone represents only a part of the verification process.

## 8.7    Hints on Biomedical Image Management and Interoperability

Due to the large amount of data generated by a hospital, coordination of their collection, management, visualisation and transfer through integrated information systems has become necessary. These include the **radiological information system (RIS)** and the **picture archiving and communication system (PACS)**. PACS is an integrated system of software and hardware dedicated to archiving, transmission and presentation of biomedical images. Its components are the *image acquisition computers*, such as the one associated with the mammographic machine, and the archiving, display and processing devices, the *workstations*. The **monitor displays of the workstations in mammography,** on which the reader reports, must have a resolution of at least **5 megapixels (MP)**. It is worth mentioning that the *American College of Radiology (ACR)* recommends 12 MP. For traditional radiology, monitors with a resolution between 2 and 5 MP are usually considered sufficient (see also Chap. 24). One megapixel corresponds to one million pixels and indicates the graphic display resolution, which depends on the number (and size) of sensitive display elements present on the monitor. Images are received and transmitted in the standard **Digital Imaging and Communications in Medicine (DICOM)** format. All images must be DICOM-compatible (conformance statement) in order to be exchangeable and archivable [15]. The DICOM standard, in addition to the image itself, contains an alphanumeric **header,** in which information useful for encoding the image is stored in the form of **TAGS**. It is also called meta-information. Among the recorded tags, we can also find *dose information* (Chap. 21).

A key aspect to mention with regard to health care is the so-called *interoperability.* We could define it in a very simple manner, as the integra-tion between systems to better coordinate the management of patient data, considering all aspects. This is a complex concept that starts with the creation of standards, such as DICOM for images. **The Integrating the Healthcare Enterprise (IHE)** is an ongoing initiative that has been running for many years, promoting multivendor integration, precisely based on standards. IHE profiles ensure that the images contain all the information needed for subsequent processing. For example, they allow up to eight images to be displayed on the workstation for comparison with a previous examination, but also 1:1 images (at zero magnification, full size), for preparation for a biopsy or a preoperative planning. On the other hand, the so-called *"hanging protocols",* which are the display preferences for combinations of laterality and orientation, are part of the modality-specific DICOM standard (see also Chap. 16). The **Health Level Seven (HL7)** aims at facilitating the transfer of healthcare data between different systems in a healthcare facility. It has recently proposed a new integration standard called **Fast Healthcare Interoperability Resources (FHIR)**. It consists of a *repository* into which all data pertaining to each individual patient can be stored, in a standardised format, and thus easily usable and exchangeable, throughout the diagnostic or clinical treatment pathway.

All integration profiles use **information technology (IT)**, which is increasingly important, for the need of privacy and data protection [16]. In light of the progressive implementation of **artificial intelligence (AI), machine learning (ML)** and **deep learning (DL)**, it must be emphasised that any data used as part of imaging modalities must necessarily be appropriately encrypted, secured and anonymised [17].

See Chap. 24 for an overview of the topic of AI.

## References

1. Woods G. Digital image fundamentals PPT. https://www.corsi.univr.it/documenti/OccorrenzaIns/matdid/matdid950092.pdf.
2. Kulkarni SR. Chapter 5. Sampling and quantization, lecture notes for ELE20 intro-

duction to electrical signal and systems 1999-2002. https://studylib.net/doc/18246916/chapter-5%2D%2Dsampling-and-quantization.

3. Siemens Healthineers. 3D mammography. https://cdn0.scrvt.com/39b415fb07de4d965 6c7b516d8e2d907/1800000005714266/54b 8c8374eea/Mammography-Site-Readiness-brochure_1800000005714266.pdf.

4. Boone JM. Image quality parameters and their measurement PPT. Brighton: ICMP; 2013.

5. Nishikawa RM. The fundamentals of MTF, wiener spectra, and DQE, Kurt Rossmann Laboratories for Radiologic Image Research Department of Radiology. The University of Chicago.

6. Samei E. Performance of digital radiographic detectors: quantification and assessment methods; factors affecting sharpness and noise, advances in digital radiography: RSNA Categorical Course in Diagnostic Radiology Physics; 2003. pp. 37–47.

7. Guidelines for Quality Control Testing for Digital CR DR mammography, version 4.0; 2018, RAZCR, ABS 37-000-029-863.

8. Digital mammography 2018 quality control manual, revised 2nd ed. ACR, Radiologic technologist's section; 2020.

9. ACR–AAPM–SIIM practice parameter for determinants of image quality in mammography, revised 2022 (Resolution 46). https://www.acr.org/-/media/ACR/Files/Practice-Parameters/dig-mamo.pdf.

10. Gennaro G, et al. Quality controls in digital mammography protocol of the EFOMP Mammo Working Group. Phys Med. 2018;48:55–64. https://doi.org/10.1016/j.ejmp.2018.03.016.

11. Perry N, et al. European guidelines for quality assurance in breast cancer screening and diagnosis, 4th ed. Supplement; 2013. isbn:978-92-79-32970-9.

12. De Oliveira Pereira R, et al. Evaluation of the accuracy of mammography, ultrasound and magnetic resonance imaging in suspect breast lesions. Clinics. 2020;75:e1804. https://doi.org/10.6061/clinics/2020/e1805.

13. Gennaro G, et al. Chapter 2b. Quality control in digital mammography: "keep it simple". European protocol for the quality control of the physical and technical aspects of mammography screening, Digital mammography, PPT, EFOMP MAMMO WG; 2013.

14. IAEA Human Health Series No. 47. Handbook of basic quality control test for diagnostic radiology. AAPM, EFOMP, ISRRT; 2023. isbn:978-92-0-130422-3.

15. Ciconi A. Illuminazione delle workstation di refertazione radiodiagnostica, Applicazione di un sistema di illuminazione innovativo. Università di Pisa, tesi di laurea magistrale in Ingegneria edile; 2012-2013. https://core.ac.uk/download/pdf/19203764.pdf.

16. Galfione P. Interoperabilità: il Sacro Gral della Sanità. Sanità Digitale; 2021. healthcare-digitale.it.

17. Walsh G, et al. Responsible AI practice and AI education are central to AI implementation: a rapid review for all medical imaging professional in Europe. BJR Open. 2023;5:20230033. https://doi.org/10.1259/bjro.20230033.

## Further Reading

Dance DR, et al. Diagnostic radiology physics a handbook for teachers and students. IAEA; 2014. isbn:978-92-131010-1.

# Part III

# Clinical Quality

# Standard Mammography Examination Technique

**9**

## 9.1 Introduction

Teaching mammography is more difficult than teaching other radiology examinations. There are many reasons for this: (1) there is a limited knowledge of breast anatomy and how the various portions appear in the different projections in mammography; (2) there is definitely a lack of clarity in cause-effect, i.e. between specific movement and result on the image; (3) the theoretical knowledge acquired during studies is usually insufficient to know how to solve a problem that arises during positioning. Problems practically always arise, given the extreme variability of the breast and of the patient's cooperation. In fact, there has always been a talk of the science of imaging, emphasising the extreme complexity of the mammography system, which is certainly undeniable, but of the "art" of positioning. This suggests that there is no real scientific basis and that positioning cannot therefore be taught scientifically. The opinion advocated in this text is the opposite. Just as it is essential that examinations be reproducible in radiology, so too should it be in the breast department. Mammography is certainly a specialist imaging test, but still a radiological one. *Reproducibility* means the possibility for all radiographers to carry out the examination in the same way. More exactly, radiographers should have in mind a clear procedure of what must be obtained at each step, for any patient. It reduces the repetition of projections, improves efficiency, and allows better comparison between exams, which is the cornerstone of the diagnosis in this imaging methodology. Furthermore, it improves teaching, because if you have an execution procedure in mind (a *mind map*), it is easier to say how to perform it. Even more precisely, thinking about a series of procedural points in sequence, i.e. breaking down the exam into steps, each with a clear purpose, allows you to easily identify the areas of difficulty. For each of them, specific solutions can be provided. It is a systemic approach that is all the more valid the more complex the examination is, and the more it is related to contextual factors.

Actually, in mammography, there are also problems of *consistency*, which can be defined as the ability of the same radiographer to conduct the exams while maintaining the same level of performance. Both reproducibility and consistency are significant challenges, but they must be a goal to strive for. Unfortunately, there is no comprehensive information on the topic of positioning, and the specific literature for radiographers is not sufficient, at least in the opinion of the writer. Undoubtedly, there are many variables to consider, but let us begin by reiterating that even in mammography, as in radiology, anatomical points of reference must be used. They have to be visible and palpable. Besides, there are also points of reference on the mammographic unit. Both must guide the mammographer in positioning, allowing a gradual improvement in her/his performance, indeed, in a scientific way.

## 9.2 Basis of Positioning: The Poggi Method

Three parameters have to be considered: (1) the area to be documented; (2) the pectoral muscle; and (3) the *posterior nipple line (PNL)*. This was suggested by the colleague Louise Miller, *RT, (R)(M)(ARRT)*, specialised in mammography, involved in training in this field for many years.

The first fundamental step is to bring the breast to a position such that the PNL, 2D transposition of the median axial plane, is parallel to the receptor plane. In practical terms, it means that the breast must be lifted by "opening" the inframammary fold IMF. Advantage must be taken of the fact that the breast is a mobile organ and therefore more or less easily detachable from the chest. This must be coupled with a thorough knowledge of the anatomy of the organ and therefore of the perimeter of the area to be documented and also on how and how much the pectoral muscle should and can be documented. Material on the pectoral muscle topic is available on the author's YouTube channel and on Facebook; see links below and at the back of the book.

*A fundamental point of reference to be taken into account, in addition to the said three parameters, is certainly the position of the nipple.* It is variable and mobile in reality, fixed and decisive for the extension of the tissue acquired, on the image. It is also the point from which the distance of a lesion is measured, in depth (see Chaps. 13 and 25). Another important point of reference, this time on the mammographic unit, is the *top right corner of the detector* (see Fig. 27.5). This indicates the posterior, deep limit of the axillary tissues to be shown on the MLO projection. It should also be noted that positioning the breast for its effective documentation actually means positioning the entire body of the patient. See Table 9.1. The standard examination is composed of two projections: cranio-caudal (CC) and mediolateral oblique (MLO).

**Table 9.1** Aspects to consider when positioning the patient for the mammography examination: orientation and distances

| |
|---|
| 1 Positioning to be given to the patient in relation to the detector |
| 2 The radiographer orientation with respect to the patient |
| 3 The right height to bring the detector to |
| 4 The distance at which to hold the patient from the detector |
| 5 The posture to be adopted by the patient, from head to toe |

### 9.2.1 Subdivision of the Breast

The breast has two fixed and two movable parts. The lateral and inferior aspects are movable, whereas the other two—medial and superior—are fixed (see also Chap. 3).

*Mammography always consists, whatever projections are involved, in lifting the movable side towards the fixed one, aiming for perfect parallelism between the two planes.*

The parts are identified by subdividing the breast according to the median axial plane passing through the nipple, into the upper and lower parts, according to the median sagittal plane, always passing through the nipple, into the lateral and medial parts. They must be parallel to each other in positioning, for various reasons: (1) the condition of the nipple in profile is obtained in both projections (if the quadrants are of equal size); (2) in CCs more deep tissues will be included; (3) also in MLOs, the parallelism between the medial and lateral planes will allow more deep tissue to be included, in particular the lower deep portion called *posterior inferior quadrant POSTINFQ* (above and anteriorly the *inframammary fold IMF*). See below, *first and second acquisition parameters*, and also Chaps. 25, 26, 27 and Annex 1. For compression paddle size selection and pre-examination procedure, see Chap. 16.

## 9.3  Cranio-Caudal (CC) Projection Positioning: First Step and First Acquisition Geometry Parameter [1–7]

It is good practice to ask the patient in front of the detector, before starting the exam, to relax both shoulders, assuming a relaxed position of the entire torso, arms hanging along the sides.

As far as the patient-detector distance is concerned, it is approximately equal to the palm of the open hand (fingers parallel to the plane of the detector). This means that the patient must lean slightly when the breast is brought onto the detector. This movement should stretch out the skin folds that can form in the IMF. Posture is very important: the patient should not bend forward at the waist, but only lean slightly forward, thorax and hips on the same line. This is to prevent the lower deep tissues from moving away. Thorax and hips must always be in the same line (see Chap. 25).

**To position the breast for the CC projection, the breast radiographer must be on the medial side of the patient** and perpendicular to her. Whenever possible, the patient is placed in front of the detector with the nipple at 12 o'clock (Fig. 9.1). First, the radiographer places her/his hand perpendicular to the patient's thorax, lifting the breast with a cupped hand, until the median axial plane is parallel to the image plane. The fifth finger must be placed in the IMF, well into the depth. The shoulders should be girded, and the one under examination slightly lowered (Fig. 9.2). The detector must therefore be raised up to approximately touch the radiographer's hand. The breast must then be brought forward, without rotations, until all of them is resting on the detector.

The breast is brought forward until the fifth finger is on the detector. This makes sure that the lower deep tissues, including IMF, and therefore the pectoralis muscle are included in the image (Tabar® school). In the Poggi method, it is recommended to bring the lower deep tissues further forward, lifting the breast again and pulling it anteriorly. The skin folds in contact with the inner profile of the detector must be eliminated. The tissue is therefore smoothed downwards. This operation leads the patient to move her hips backwards: *it is a movement that must be carefully controlled.* The breast should now be in the desired position, with the median axial plane parallel to the image plane, and all on the detector, deep planes included. ***First acquisition geometry parameter to be satisfied: bring the axial plane in parallel with the detector. The upper quadrants must be parallel to the lower ones and to the detector. The nipple is in profile.***

**Key Point 1**  *The patient is in front of the detector, nipple at 12 o'clock, at a distance from the detector*

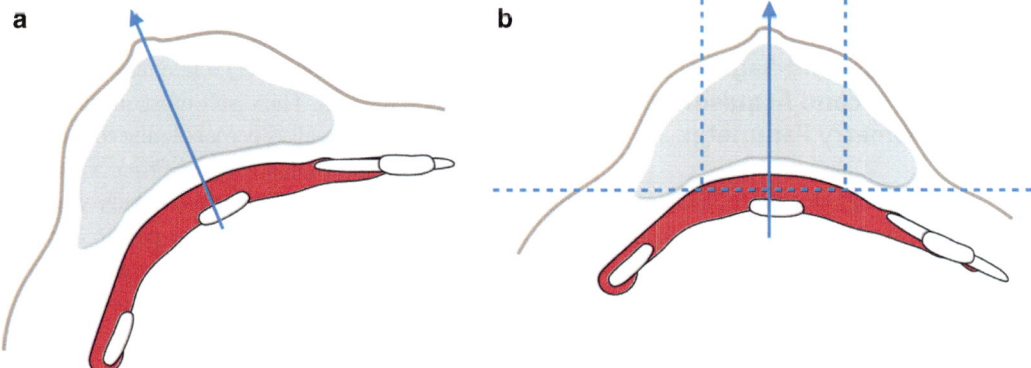

**Fig. 9.1** (**a**) Natural position of the breast on the chest, (**b**) Positioning of the breast in the mammography examination, with the nipple on the midline, coinciding with the mid-sagittal plane; the chest wall is perpendicular to the median sagittal plane (second acquisition geometry parameter) and to the sagittal planes passing through the IQ and OQ quadrants. "Two train-track theory"; see text

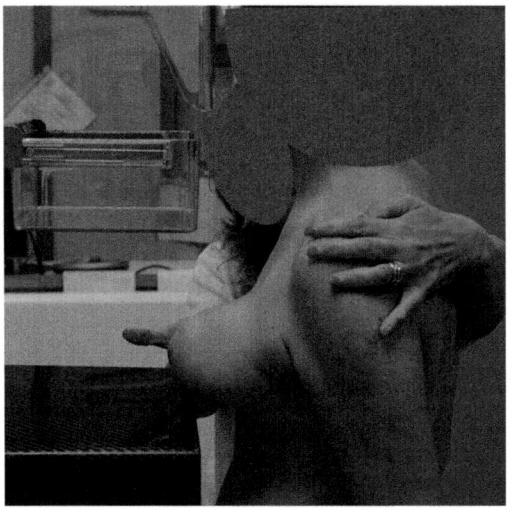

**Fig. 9.2** Correct height of the detector. Lowering the ipsilateral shoulder. CC projection

*equal to the palm of the hand. Her hips are brought back, if necessary, so that they are on the same line as the thorax. The patient's shoulders are girded, and the ipsilateral shoulder is lowered. The breast is lifted until the median axial plane is parallel to the sensory plane. The fifth finger of the radiographer's hand is in the fold (well deep). The detector is brought to the height of the mammographer's hand; the breast is placed on the detector and brought forward until our fifth finger is on it. The lower tissues are lifted and brought forward again.*

### 9.3.1 Nipple on the Midline, Coinciding or Not with the Mid-Sagittal Plane: The Second Acquisition Geometry Parameter

The breast is naturally positioned on the chest with a certain obliquity, directed laterally, with respect to the mid-sagittal plane of the body (sternal line); see Fig. 9.1a. They are although infinite anatomical variations. To perform the CC correctly, it is important that the nipple points at 12 o'clock; i.e., it is located on the midline (which divides the breast into the medial and lateral quadrants). The midline coincides with the median sagittal plane of the breast (which divides the breast into two parts), Figs. 9.1b and 25.12. The nipple, as already stated, is an important anatomical point of reference for the evaluation of good positioning in mammography and for the localisation of a lesion. To obtain this geometry the patient must therefore be rotated (not the breast, but the trunk) medially, in an appropriate manner.

The midline corresponds exactly to the median sagittal plane of the breast, ONLY when the outer and inner quadrants are the same size.

If there is a significant difference, making the midline forcibly coincide with the mid-sagittal plane results in the failure to document a part of the *dominant quadrant* (the larger one).

**Second Acquisition Geometry Parameter: the chest wall must ALWAYS be in a plane perpendicular to the median axial and sagittal planes**. The nipple, in cases where the inner and outer quadrants are not the same size, will be shifted towards the smaller one (*this is the reason why the midline and mid-sagittal lines may not coincide*). The second parameter must be satisfied in any case.

Even more specifically, it can be said that the chest wall must be perpendicular to the sagittal planes passing through the outer and inner quadrants, as it appears in Fig. 9.1b. Thus, the breast is brought forward as if on **"two train tracks,"** i.e. without any rotation, external or internal.

In order to pass from condition a to b in Fig. 9.1, two options are possible: (1) position the patient with straight feet (at 0° with respect to the detector), preferably slightly separated from each other to ensure a better balance, and then rotate the torso appropriately; (2) rotate the whole body, including the feet. The result must still be one in which the chest wall is perpendicular to the sagittal plane, as shown in the figure. From experience, I recommend the first option, which does not require corrections of the torso posture. In fact, generally in the second option the patient tends to rotate too much medially, as if performing a CC for outer quadrants, which requires correction in order not to miss the inner ones. See Chap. 10. The fulfilment of the acquisition geometry, but especially of the correct stretching, can be assessed considering the *sign of the arch* drawn by the glandular tissue; see Chap. 26 about it.

### 9.3.2   Nipple in Profile

*The nipple must be in profile or on the axis*, which means that the X-ray beam is tangent to it, projecting *out* of the breast tissue. This is an important criterion, as not only does the nipple not obliterate a part of the tissue, but a greater extension of deep tissue can be documented. This is thanks to the parallelism between the two planes; i.e., there was no rotation in any direction. For the correction, we need to know that *the nipple points towards the missing tissue*, so if it points downwards (inferiorly directed rotation), inferior tissue will be missed. More deep inferior breast tissue must be collected, lifting and bringing the breast further forward. If the nipple points upwards (superiorly directed rotation), it is usually sufficient to lower the detector. *The condition of the nipple in profile (first acquisition geometry parameter) should only be respected if the upper and lower quadrants are approximately the same size.* In the case, for example, that the upper part is dominant, and therefore, the nipple is turned inferiorly in a natural way, placing it in profile would mean sacrificing the documentation of a portion of upper tissue. It must be remembered that *the first quality criterion to meet is that of the maximum tissue inclusion.* Taking CC projections in these people will result in the nipple overlapping the glandular tissue [3]. See Chaps. 11, 26, 27 and Annex 1. Summarising, to fulfil the condition of the nipple in profile in general, it is necessary to have the complete inclusion of the upper and lower deep tissues, i.e. the parallelism between them, according to the first acquisition geometry parameter. A correct tissue stretching out and an adequate compression are also necessarily included.

### 9.3.3   Positioning the Patient for the CC Projection: Second Step

As described, the ipsilateral shoulder is lowered approaching the patient to the detector. This is an important action to better document the outer quadrants, bringing the breast well forward. The patient is asked to turn her head medially, as much as possible, until her ear is centrally placed on the facial screen, with her chin slightly up.

Given her position, the patient must absolutely not wear voluminous glasses or earrings, and her hair must be pulled away or tied up, so that no artefacts are created on the image. The arm of the side under examination is preferably extended along her side. Alternatively, it may be useful to bend the elbow and bring the arm forward, with the hand under the detector. This is as long as the patient does not stiffen her arm and shoulder. This position can help to minimise the skin folds of the axillary lobe and gives security to people with balance problems (also feet apart). The breast is brought forward, up to include our fifth finger, making the midline coincide with the mid-sagittal plane, if the anatomy requires it (inner and outer quadrants of the same size). No rotation needs to be performed to include all outer quadrants, which can be entirely studied in the MLO projection. Inner and outer quadrants must be carried forward, as if they were on "train tracks" (Fig. 9.1). Complete documentation of the outer quadrants by lateromedial rotation (medially displacing the nipple) would inevitably lead to the sacrifice of the inner quadrants.

To be sure of the complete and correct documentation of the inner quadrants, a quality criterion of primary importance in the CC projection (Chap. 11 and Annex 1), it may also be useful to bring the other breast on the detector. This is then moved away by the patient herself. Second, it is useful to push the contralateral shoulder forward. In this way, the second acquisition geometry parameter is more easily met. Finally, the breast is stretched anteriorly very carefully so as not to deform the breast by manipulation, until the intermammary cleft appears, when the patient's anatomy allows it.

**Key Point 2** *The patient is asked to turn her head medially, while bringing her breast forward on the detector. She is asked to place the ear on the facial screen, keeping her chin up. This allows very deep tissues to be brought forward. Ipsilateral arm along the side.*

*Very useful for assessing the correct geometry and the correct height of the detector is the "tent sign" (Poggi method). In it, an almost identical flaring appears in depth, at the lateral and medial extremities, indicating that the attachment of the breast to the thorax wall is documented* (see skin envelope, Chap. 25). The *tent sign* yields valuable indications on how much the ipsilateral shoulder should be lowered and on the correct height of the detector. However, this verification is not always possible, depending on the anatomy of the patient. Furthermore, verification of the parallelism between the two upper and lower planes and the perpendicularity of the chest wall to the mid-sagittal plane can be made on the acquired image, by observing the *thickness of the subcutaneous fat* (Chap. 3). It *must be the same throughout the perimeter* (Fig. 12.1). However, this check is possible in a low percentage of cases, as the thickness of this area is very variable and sometimes too small to be assessed with certainty.

Another important consideration to be made is that *the correct acquisition geometry of the breast cannot be achieved without correctly positioning the rest of the body*, head-neck, thorax and hips.

This aspect further explains how challenging is in the correct execution of the mammography examination and how many factors affect the final iconographic result.

### 9.3.4   OQ Inclusion in CC Projection

A high-quality mammography involves documenting the OQ as completely as possible. The position of the patient, including the thorax and the head, must be such as to allow to get as deep tissue as possible. *The essential task of the CC is to always include the inner quadrant completely*, given that it is not effectively documented in the MLO projection. *The outer quadrant should be included as far as possible, without ever sacrificing the medial tissues.* It is very useful to observe the position of the nipple. If the dimensions of the two quadrants—inner and outer—are equal, the midline must coincide with

the mid-sagittal plane (Chap. 26). If the nipple appears to be turned sideways, and this is not the case in the actual anatomy, it will result in ineffective documentation of the outer quadrants. The nipple should be brought back to the midline, ensuring that as much deep internal tissue as possible has been included, before acquisition. In other words, the mistake of improperly bringing the OQs forward, sometimes associated with an ipsilateral shoulder pushed too low, must not be made. This creates the **breast** called "**ogival**" in this text, which is not real but "constructed" (Chap. 17). This is an error that must be corrected because it induces a false displacement of the internal structures, anteriorly and laterally, as well as an incomplete documentation of the inner quadrant.

There is a significant percentage of women in whom the outer quadrant develops far towards the axilla, partially hiding from frontal view: see Chap. 26 for this topic.

### 9.3.5   IQ and Intermammary Cleft Inclusion in CC Projection

For the documentation of the portion of postero-medial tissue, facing the intermammary cleft, the patient's sternum must touch the detector.

It is important to also bring the other breast on the detector. It must then be carefully moved away by the patient herself. In fact, if the gesture is abrupt or exaggerated, tissue which must be documented can instead be moved away. *The patient is also asked to bring the contralateral shoulder forward.* This helps to document the deep IQ, obviously keeping the nipple in the midline. In other words, the breast should not be rotated mediolaterally. Actually, any rotation that takes the chest wall away from the perpendicularity with the median sagittal plane is wrong for standard acquisitions. In case of a suspected finding in the deep medial area, the patient can be asked to turn her head laterally (see Chap. 10).

The correct and adequate stretching out of the breast, and above all bringing the contralateral shoulder forward, mostly lead to the documentation of the intermammary cleft.

This criterion is not contemplated in the European Guidelines, even if it is increasingly cited in the literature. Assessing the quality of the CC projection is indeed extremely difficult, even more than that of the MLO projection, and *the presence of the intermammary cleft on the image is a good indicator of effective inner quadrant deep tissue documentation.*

### 9.3.6 Deep Tissue Inclusion in the CC Projection (Pectoralis Muscle)

Failure to include the deep tissues, the retromammary space, and the pectoralis major muscle behind is often due to poor positioning and compression. However, sometimes, it is made difficult by the patient's particular anatomy, or it is (often) the height of the detector that is not correct. Another parameter to be evaluated is the patient's posture: if she bends forward with straight hips or pulls her hips back, the loss of the lower deep tissues is certain.

The pectoralis major muscle appearing on the CC projection results from the inclusion of all deep tissues: it is therefore essential that the height of the detector and the posture of the patient are such as to bring them onto the image plane. *The height of the detector is approximately equal to the hand of the radiographer who lifts the breast until the median axial plane is parallel to the image plane. However, the height of the detector must be chosen with the patient having the thorax and hips aligned.* Otherwise, the height will be wrong (see also Chap. 26). In order to bring the *lower deep tissues* onto the detector, the breast must be raised further and brought forward onto the detector, firmly. Particular attention should be paid to the chest wall, which should be perpendicular to the mid-sagittal plane. The formation of the *tent sign* also helps: it is only noticeable when the height of the detector is correct.

It should also be noted that the two breasts in the same woman can have different shapes, sizes, and even positions on the chest. This requires great care in choosing the height of the detector *for every single projection.*

### 9.3.7 Stretching and Compression in CC Projection

As much decision as that used to bring the lower deep tissue forward must be made in bringing the *upper deep tissues* forward. *The stretching out, which must include the whole breast, is in the posteroanterior direction.* At most, slightly mediolateral, a useful procedure for bringing the inner quadrant forward, but not recommended in this text. The posteroanterior stretching is also called **neutral**, because it aims to avoid any manipulation that causes artefactuality. The tissue is to spread out effectively, in order to avoid, again as far as possible, the summation artefact (Chaps. 3 and 17). *The breast must be manipulated as little as possible, for the mammography to faithfully reproduce the original object.* To the stretching made with the hand should be added, whenever possible, a pressure exerted by the arm surrounding the patient's shoulders, always directed forward.

Using one's own body to position the patient is always a winning strategy. However, using one's own body should only be implemented by those who are truly experts, and when the physicality of the radiographer, and the patient's collaboration, make it effective.

It is necessary to check that no skin folds have formed, especially on the lateral aspect. During the descent of the compression paddle, the skin is kept well stretched in this area. If necessary, gently smooth the upper tissue with the compression paddle already in position (*first stage of the compression process*, see Table 11.2). The contralateral breast should be moved away by the patient, generally in a superior and posterior direction. Preferably not downwards, even if this choice is necessarily related to the design of the available mammography machine and the patient's anatomy.

It is important to check that this manoeuvre is not accompanied by a backward movement of the hemithorax opposite the side under examination. This would in fact result in: (1) the removal of the inner quadrants; (2) the formation of the "ogival breast."

Attention should also be paid to the *skin folds not visible* in the IMF. Before ending the compression (*second stage*, see Table 11.2), especially for large and ptotic breasts, smooth the lower part of the chest vertically in the lower direction, below the fold. It is useful to ask the patient to move her hips back a little. This smoothes out very well the folds affecting the lower tissues that can form in the IMF and at the extremities of the breast.

To avoid folds in the IMF, and not only there, always in the case of large and ptotic breasts, it may be useful for the radiographer to lift the breast to be brought on the detector with the back of the hand rather than the palm. The hand is then rotated clockwise, until the breast is collected in the palm. This technique is very effective for the elimination of the skin folds, as well as for bringing the deep tissues well forward, and it is proposed by my colleague Vincenzo Mazzalupo (breast radiographer), who works at the *Institute for the Study, Prevention and Network Oncology (ISPRO)*, Florence.

See also Chap. 17.

The distance of the patient from the detector must also be checked. If it is greater than the palm of the hand, skin folds can be created more easily, and balance is more difficult to maintain for the patient. In addition, ***it should be Checked that the patient does not bend her knees or does not stand on her toes during positioning. The detector height would not be correct***, and the patient would be more likely to move during acquisition.

Compression is applied, warning the patient (see also Chap. 23).

**Key Point 3** *Verifying that the patient's sternum is in contact with the detector. The other breast should be carefully moved away by the patient herself, usually backwards and upwards. It is anyway to be evaluated the best strategy to eliminate the skin folds for each case. The patient is asked to bring forward the contralateral shoulder.*

**Key Point 4** *A firm forward stretching is performed, eliminating the skin folds of the lateral extremity of the breast during the descent of the compressor paddle. Anteriorly directed pressure*

*is added whenever possible, exerted by the arm around the patient's shoulders.*

**Key Point 5** *The skin folds in the IMF are smoothed out, with a slight vertical movement on the abdomen, in an inferior (downward) direction. Then, the breast is compressed effectively.*

## 9.4  Positioning for the Mediolateral Oblique MLO Projection: First Step

The patient is positioned in front of the mammography machine, with the whole body, including the feet, to form an angle of about 45°-50° with it. This is according to Professor Tabar's school (Tabar, L., *MD medical Doctor, FACR, Fellow of the American College of Radiology*, internationally renowned breast radiologist). The iliac crest looks approximately at the bottom right corner of the detector (Fig. 27.5) in mammographic machines without *shift* (Chap. 11). The height of the detector must be adjusted according to the patient's anatomy (length of the torso, superior and inferior dimensions of the breast). It must be always confirmed by verifying the centring of the organ in the available FOV. While two to three centimetres are sufficient for the inframammary fold, the rest of the active area (Chap. 7) is to be dedicated to the breast, the axillary tail and fossa.

The patient is asked to raise the arm of the side under examination, and to rest it loosely, i.e. in a relaxed way, on the upper profile of the detector. Arm and shoulder must be on the same plane: this is a useful criterion to understand if the height of the detector is correct (see below). The radiographer is behind the patient, and the distance between the patient and the detector is always approximately equal to the palm of the open hand (with fingers parallel to the profile of the detector). At this point, the breast under examination should be collected with both hands. The right hand brings the left breast forward, just above the inframammary fold (Fig. 9.3). The right hand pushes the deep lateral tissues from behind to the front to be collected in the other

**Fig. 9.3** Pinch grip, four fingers behind, and first finger in front, MLO view. Also, note the other hand of the radiographer, immediately in front of the armpit. Also seen from behind. The patient is guided without rotations and forward inclinations on the detector, until the arm and breast are resting on it

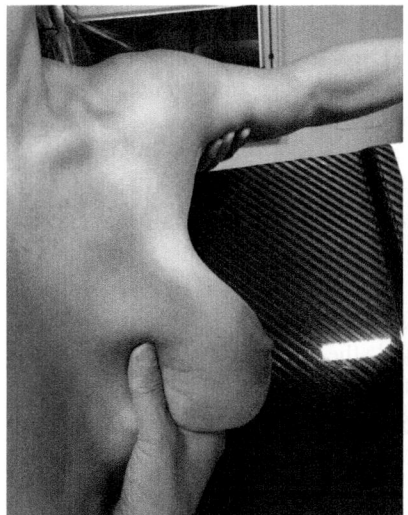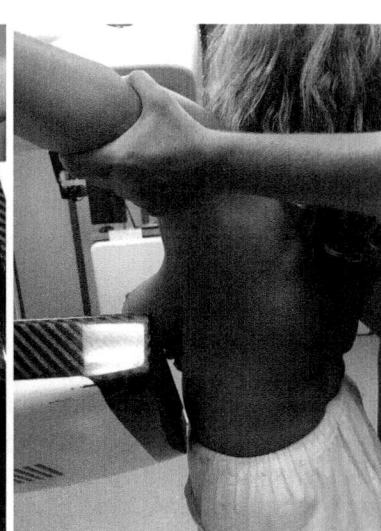

hand, together with the medial. Vice versa for the right breast.

**Key Point 1** *The patient is in front of the detector, at about 45–50° with respect to it, nipple pointing towards the lower third, iliac crest facing the bottom right corner. The radiographer is behind her. See also Chap. 23.*

**Key Point 2** *Both hands should be used to position the breast. The right hand for the left breast brings the breast forward, just above the inframammary fold. The left hand for the left breast pushes the tissues forward from behind, so that they are then collected in the right hand (and vice versa).*

One hand then moves from behind the patient's thorax to her arm, guiding her towards the detector, while the other remains on the breast, with a **pinch grip.** In this grip, the thumb is on the medial quadrants, and the four fingers are on the lateral ones (see Fig. 9.3). The arm should be grasped firmly, immediately in front of the axilla. The patient is guided forward towards the detector, asking her not to rotate her trunk, and not to move her feet. In this way, the deep lateral tissues are brought onto the detector and therefore will be documented on the image. It may be useful to

ask the patient to lean slightly towards the detector, as if she were to lie down on it. This manoeuvre makes it easier to obtain parallelism between the lateral and medial aspects of the breast. However, the patient must not bend over at the waist; this action easily brings the upper tissues onto the detector, but pulls back the central and lower ones.

**Key Point 3** *Once the breast under examination has been collected, the hand that pushed the deep lateral tissues forward moves around the patient's arm, immediately in front of the armpit. The patient torso posture is to be maintained, so as to bring all the deep lateral, superior (axillary), central and inferior tissues onto the detector. The radiographer holds the breast with a "pinch grip."*

According to Professor Tabar's school, the pinch grip should be maintained throughout the positioning. However, it is not easy to do, for many reasons, mainly those related to the different heights of the radiographer and the patient, given the same mammographic unit. If the grip on the breast has to be released, it must still be "recovered" later.

**Key Point 4** *During the movement towards the detector, the posture of the patient should be monitored (no bowing or rotations).*

### 9.4.1   Positioning for MLO Projection: Second Step

We then move on to the arrangement of the patient's shoulder and arm, which are resting on the upper profile of the detector, with the *two-rotation manoeuvre* according to the *Poggi method*. This is an important step, as it makes feasible to effectively document the upper deep tissues.

**First Rotation**: In order to be sure to show upper deep tissues, including if possible the latissimus dorsi, the arm is raised by rotating it anteriorly (internally) and superiorly (upwards) (Fig. 9.4a). The rotation is easily achieved by supinating the patient's hand.

**Second Rotation**: Keeping the shoulder in position, a firm external (posterior) and upper (superior) rotation of the arm is carried out (Fig. 9.4b). This is to be followed by a forward extension of the arm, using both hands. That is to say, hands surround the arm, with joined fingers, bringing it again forward and downwards (see Fig. 9.4c, d).

The two rotations do not cancel each other out, since the position of the shoulder remains unchanged. The second aims to minimise the folds that can form in the soft tissues of the axillary extension.

If these movements are well performed, the *top right corner of the detector* (see Fig. 27.5 in Chap. 27) will be free, i.e. not covered by the posterior tissues of the axilla. The skin folds at this level will be distended, cancelled or minimised.

The patient's hand does not grip the handle: in this text, it is recommended to hold it with the palm directed towards the patient, to prepare for better relaxation of the pectoral muscle. The elbow is flexed and pushed down (Fig. 9.4d)

**Key Point 5** *To bring the deep tissues of the axilla on the detector (possibly also the latissimus dorsi), an upper and anterior rotation of the arm is performed. To eliminate the skin fold in the axilla and in the axillary extension, a second posterior and superior rotation of the arm is carried out, without modifying the position of the shoulder. The top right corner of the detector is free. Shoulder and arm should be relaxed. The arm is extended forward and down, elbow flexed (Fig. 9.5).*

*Documentation of the latissimus dorsi in the top right corner of the MLO image is strongly recommended in this text. It makes sure that the entire axilla fossa in the anteroposterior direction has been included.* This is because the latissimus is the only part of the posterior axillary wall that may be visible in mammography, and the anterior one is represented by the pectoralis major.

**Reference Point on the Mammographic Unit: The Top Right Corner of the Detector Must be Free.** This gives assurance that the upper deep lateral tissues have been included (Fig. 9.4b).

**Key Point 6** *The elbow must be pushed firmly downwards. It must be well outside the upper profile of the detector (Figs. 9.4b, d and 9.5).*

### 9.4.2   Positioning the Patient's Arm in Relation to the Detector Height, MLO Projection

The height of the detector should be such that the arm and shoulder are approximately in the same plane. If the detector is too high, i.e. the patient is too low with respect to the detector (Fig. 9.6b), the lower tissues and deep planes are lost. Furthermore, a higher compression value is needed to secure the breast and prevent it from falling, increasing the patient's discomfort and the likelihood that she will move. Too low a detector, patient too high (Fig. 9.6a) leads to the loss of upper tissues, as well as deep planes.

There is another important consideration to be done about the height of the detector: not all mammography units are equipped with a *shifting compression paddle* (see also Chap. 11).

To obtain the correct documentation of the breast in mammographic units not equipped with this device, it is necessary to raise the detector to include the upper portion of the breast.

This leads to increased discomfort for the patient that must be explained by the need to document the axillary tissues, including the lymph nodes.

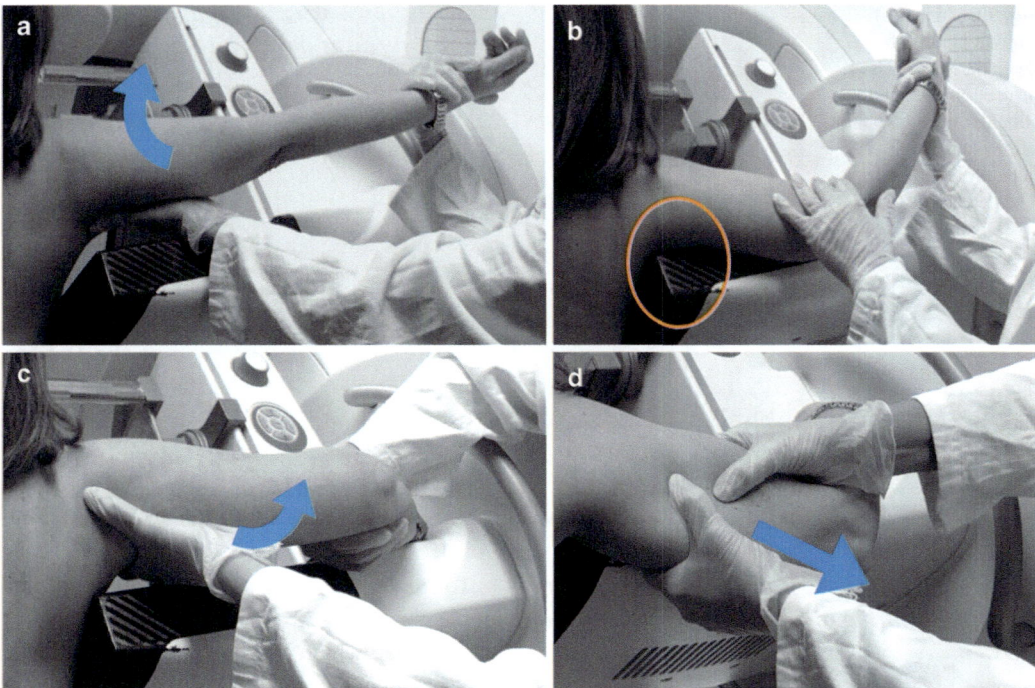

**Fig. 9.4** Two rotations—Poggi method: (**a**) Internal and upper rotation of the arm to include deep axillary tissues (supination of the patient's hand). (**b**) The arm is placed on the detector, relaxed. (**c**) External and upper rotation of the arm to stretch the skin folds out in the upper part of the breast. (**d**) Forward stretching of the arm and pushing downward of the elbow. Note the inclusion of deep axillary tissues obtained with the first manoeuvre, (orange circle in **b**), which must remain unchanged during the second one

**Fig. 9.5** (**a** and **b**) Top right corner of the detector free. Elbow and had relaxed, not gripping the handle. Shoulder and arm on the same plane (see below)

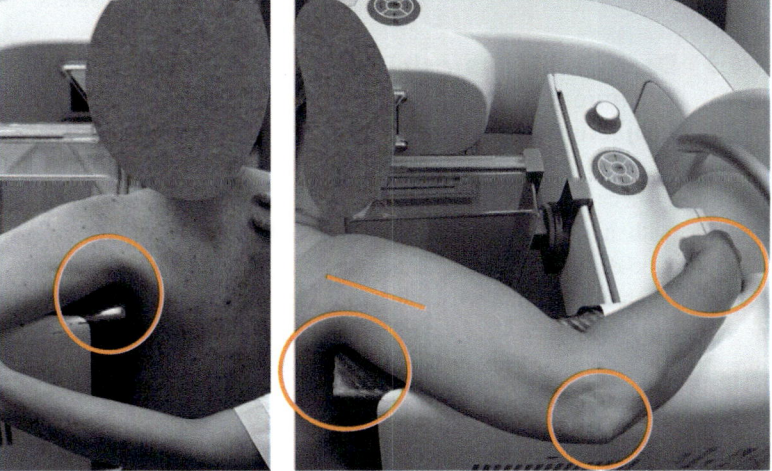

Not only that, the incorrect height of the detector can lead to an inadequate documentation of the pectoralis major muscle in terms of width. Breast radiographers accustomed to working without the shifting paddle generally carry out an initial correction, moving the patient towards the bottom part of the detector.

**Fig. 9.6** (**a** and **b**) Correct height of detector, MLO projection: arm and shoulder must be on the same plane. (**a**) The detector is too low; (**b**) The detector is too high

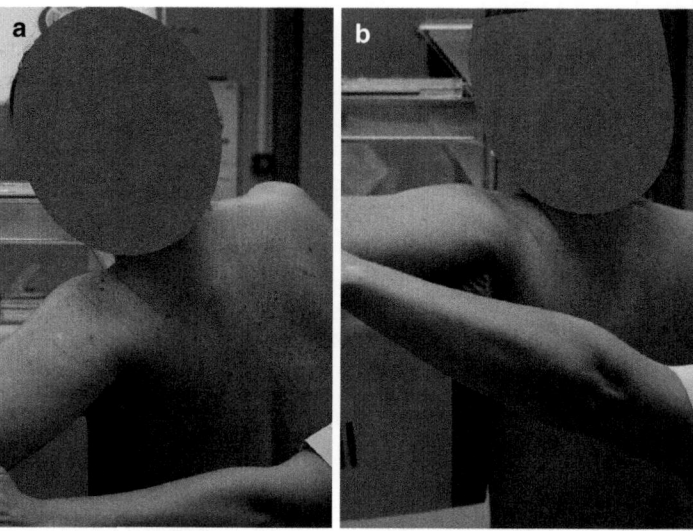

*Before acquisition, it is always necessary to assess the centring of the breast in the available FOV.*

**Key Point 7** *The patient's arm and hand must be relaxed as much as possible to avoid stiffening of the pectoral muscle. This is because it would lead to (1) a worse documentation of its width; (2) the formation of skin folds; and (3) generally, the worsening of the pain felt by the patient.*

### 9.4.3  Deep Medial (Sternal) Tissue Documentation in MLO Projection

Since the patient has been brought forward on the detector with a medial direction (45–50° with respect to the detector), the nipple will be facing medially. To bring the nipple back in profile, it is necessary to rotate the patient laterally, i.e. in the direction of the detector. This allows: (1) the deeper medial tissues to be included, showing the correct length of the pectoralis muscle; (2) obtaining the correct projection of the nipple (in profile).

It is observed that *if the nipple is still slightly medial after hip rotation, there is no need to rotate the more laterally. The divergence of the beam "corrects" it automatically. On the contrary, a slightly lateral position of the nipple is emphasised.*

To correct the lateral pointing nipple: since the nipple points towards the missing tissue, the deep lateral tissue which may be "trapped" out of the FOV must be advanced further onto the detector. The very medial pointing nipple requires further lateral rotation of the patient to include more medial deep tissue.

In summary, what we want to achieve with the steps listed so far in the MLO projection is to bring onto the detector and, therefore, document, medial and lateral tissues: upper, central and lower.

Attention again is to be paid to the patient's posture. Thorax and hips must be aligned. If only the patient's arm and shoulder are brought forward correctly, and therefore excellent documentation of the upper deep tissue is obtained, but the patient brings her hips back, the lower deep tissue and the IMF will be missing. That is, the hips must be brought well forward, not just rotated laterally.

See also Chap. 26 and Fig. 9.7.

**Key Point 8** *The patient should be rotated laterally (towards the detector), so that the deeper medial (sternal) tissues are included in the image, and the nipple brought back into profile. This requires not only the lateral rotation of the hips but also their advancement for the complete documentation of the lower medial tissues. Thus, the patient is asked to rotate her feet towards the mammographic unit simultaneously with her hips.*

**Fig. 9.7** IMF and shoulder angle, elbow flexed, MLO view. The angle (in orange) documents the decisive lowering of the elbow—external—and the opening of the IMF (orange circle), which is better visible in the second photograph. Note the relative thorax-hip position (blue line)

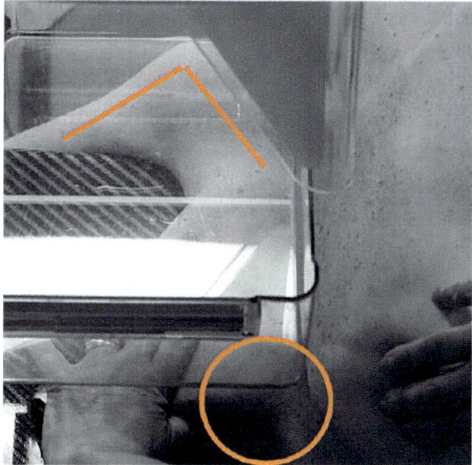
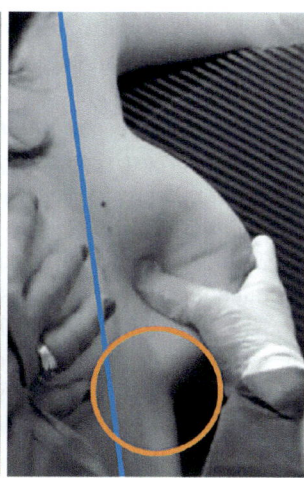

A question may spontaneously arise: What is the point of making the patient assume an initial medially directed position with respect to the detector, if it is then necessary to rotate laterally? The result of the two movements (medial entry, and subsequent lateral rotation) is not the same as that obtained with the patient facing the unit frontally, according to the experience of the writer. The first manoeuvre, i.e. the medial entry, allows to effectively document the deep lateral tissues. The second, i.e. the lateral rotation, leads to the documentation of the deep medial tissues. The aim is to bring them in parallel to each other. Although it may seem counter-intuitive, the result is better (larger tissue extension shown) than the one resulting from the single movement. The *ergonomic dimension* should certainly also be considered, a lot is achieved with relatively little effort. The ergonomics is covered in Chap. 23. It is certainly a key strength of the Tabar technique, which is fully assimilated here in the Poggi' method.

At this point, the *UP&OUT manoeuvre* is performed.

### 9.4.4   UP&OUT Manoeuvre

The breast is to be lifted. Since the grip on the breast has been released to adjust the patient's arm, the radiographer first moves in front of the medial side of the patient. The breast is to be lifted medially with respect to the detector, towards the radiographer, using the pinch grip, shown in Fig. 9.3.

It must then be brought firmly upwards, to rebalance the lateral and medial planes. In fact, we have to think that the lateral aspect, which is the one that touches the detector, is somehow fixed by the support. The medial part is free and slides naturally downwards. The breast is then stretched forward, decisively, "spreading" the tissue as best as possible. The mobile parts of the breast are brought towards the fixed ones, as already stated. This is what English speakers call the *UP&OUT* manoeuvre. It allows to get: (1) the documentation of the IMF, which is "opened"; (2) the documentation of the deep planes, especially the central and inferior ones, gaining also in length of the pectoral muscle; (3) the stretching ("opening") of the retromammary space, especially of the central and lower portions (see Fig. 17.8); and (4) the elimination of lower deep folds.

It is particularly **important to regain the pinch grip of the breast, so that the fingers do not cover the nipple. This is in order to monitor its position throughout the manoeuvre**. Understandably, the Up&OUT manoeuvre is easier for small and medium breasts due to their size, consistency and weight. It is a little more challenging for large and heavy breasts (see Chap. 23 on MSDs). It should be remembered that in the case of a patient with a lean chest it is easier to include the latissimus dorsi below the axillary level, which should be avoided. It leads to the formation of skin folds that force to projection to be repeated. Therefore, the chest is checked from behind, and the tissue facing the detector, i.e. the deep lateral, is rounded off, carefully (see also Chap. 17).

**Key Point 9** *The pinch grip is regained, lifting the breast with respect to the detector. The medial aspect is brought firmly upwards, to balance the two planes and obtain the desired geometry (first acquisition geometry parameter). The manoeuvre "opens" the IMF and brings the posterior inferior quadrant POSTINFQ onto the FOV. The hand holding the breast must never cover the nipple, in order to understand whether corrections are necessary for its documentation in profile.*

Moving the patient's shoulder upwards, which has already been partly obtained by pushing the elbow downwards, is very important. The aim is to reduce the thickness of this area and to ensure that the compression paddle reaches the anterior portion of the breast first with respect to the axillary extension, thus ensuring an optimal distribution of the gland that is mostly contained in the anterior part of the breast.

*The radiographer's hand then*—left for the left breast—*stretches the shoulder with an upward movement in order to "take it away" from the compression paddle.* In some patients, the shoulder distancing manoeuvre is decisive for optimal clinical quality. If the axillary thickness is greater than that of the breast, in fact, all the

compression is absorbed by the first area at the expense of the second, with:

1. Possible "dropping" of the breast and formation of the sagging breast or camel nose).
2. Possible kinetic blurring if the acquisition is simultaneous with the fall.
3. Obliteration of the IMF.
4. Missing the POSTINFQ documentation. See Chap. 17 and Fig. 11.3.

The compression is applied by alerting the patient and by making her move the contralateral breast away, outward and downward.

**Key Point 10** *The shoulder is moved away, pushing it upwards, and backwards. This is to decrease the thickness of the axillary area and obtain optimal compression of the gland, i.e. optimal distribution. The patient is asked to move the contralateral breast outwards and downwards.*

### 9.4.5   Checking the Anatomical Area to Be Included in MLO Projection

*The light field is turned on throughout the positioning.* If it turns off, switch it on again. It is very important to control the extent of the area we are about to acquire. The top right corner of the compression paddle is at the sternoclavicular joint; the upper side is under the clavicle; the medial side runs along the sternum; and the lower side is under the IMF, about two fingers below. Obviously, this last distance depends on the patient's anatomy and the compression paddle's dimensions, which must be chosen according to the dimensions of the breast to be documented (Chap. 16).

### 9.4.6   Inframammary Fold IMF Documentation, Free from Artefacts

The documentation of the IMF is one of the most difficult quality criteria to meet, especially

free from skin folds. This was highlighted in the preliminary phase of the **VMM** project (*Valutazione Miglioramento Monitoraggio della performance del tecnico senologo,* Evaluation, Improvement, Monitoring of the performance of the breast radiographer, Poggi C) in the Area Toscana Centro [8]. The data obtained confirm the international literature on the subject. The folds are of two types: (1) horizontal, originating from the medial side; (2) vertical, arising from the lateral side. The latter are the most common because they are the hidden ones (see Chap. 17 about it). The UP&OUT manoeuvre greatly helps fulfil this quality criterion, Figs. 9.7 and 11.3.

### 9.4.7 Pectoralis Major Muscle PM Correct Documentation by Length, Shape and Width, MLO Projection

Length. The muscle must be documented at least up to the PNL.

For the inclusion of deep tissues, it is important to:

1. Lift the breast with respect to the detector.
2. Stretch it rigorously in the UP&OUT manoeuvre.

To include the deep medial (sternal) tissues:

3. Make the patient rotate correctly towards the detector. This makes you get more PM in length.

Shape. Regarding the shape of the muscle, the height of the detector, the arm-shoulder positioning, and again the lifting of the breast are crucial.

It is important to verify that no "steps" have formed between the deep lateral tissue and the detector, leading to the formation of folds which will force retaking the projection. Therefore, the hand should check the space between the thorax and the detector, with a movement from top to bottom. Then, the tissue is smoothed posteriorly (out of the detector).

Width and Shape. For the correct axillary width, it is essential to guide the patient well forwards and bring the arm and shoulder further forward. The patient should not squeeze the handle, and the arm should be relaxed. The resulting degree of relaxation of the pectoral muscle greatly affects the shape and width of the pectoral muscle.

**Supplementary Material on YouTube channel @cristinapoggi7579**
There are four lessons on the pectoral muscle in CC and MLO projections (2021–2022):

1. CC projection, first part: https://youtu.be/TvYITfNNPKU
2. CC projection, second part: https://youtu.be/9kDcWmalQhY
3. MLO projection, first part: https://youtu.be/lREhJKwooTE
4. MLO projection, second part: https://youtu.be/fN-hRRJcCNE

### 9.4.8 Protection of Clavicle, Sternum and Ribs from Compression

The manoeuvre implemented to move the shoulder away (upwards) from the compression paddle has an additional purpose: protecting the clavicle.

The same attention should be given to the sternum or the first ribs, if these are protruding.

Not only the positioning techinque is important: so too is building a good radiographeer-patient relationship, validating, i.e. understanding, the discomfort expressed by the patient.

### 9.4.9 Variation in C-Arm Obliquity in MLO Projection

The British colleagues suggest varying the obliquity of the C-arm of detector from 40 to 60° depending on the size of the patient's torso. In several European countries, it is not customary to modify this parameter. In Italy, the obliquity chosen is 45° by default. However, varying the angle could help documenting a greater portion of the pectoral muscle. Varying the angle, so to have the compression parallel to the muscle, would also be less painful. The British mammographers suggest to ensure an obliquity of about 40° for patients with a short and wide chest and up to 60° for those with a long and slender chest. In case of short, broad-chested women with very large breast, decreasing the obliquity is certainly useful. Americans' colleagues suggest a variation from 30 to 70°. It would be especially useful in women with a wide and short chest (30°), precisely to facilitate the documentation of the IMF.

## 9.5    Steps to Carry Out in the Standard Examination and Correction of the Most Common Positioning Errors, Poggi Method

The subdivision into steps of the technique to carry out the examination by positioning is fundamental.

Complex processes require their division into steps, each of which is related to a visible result on the image, so as to achieve a better understanding of them and a better performance. Furthermore, the division in steps is also useful for an ergonomic study of the work of the breast radiographer, which is presented in Chap. 23.

See the following pages: Table 9.2 for positioning steps in sequence for the execution of CC projection; Table 9.3 for the most common errors in CC projection, where type of error, causes and corrections are explained; Table 9.4 for MLO projection positioning steps; and Table 9.5 for the most common errors in MLO projection.

Figure 9.8 presents an iconographic 3D sectional representation of the median sagittal plane with respect to the thoracic wall; Figs. 9.9a, b and 9.10 show the muscles involved in the MLO projection.

For a more comprehensive description of positioning, tissue extension and rotation errors, and their correction, see Chap. 17.

**Table 9.2** Step in sequence for the execution of the cranial-caudal CC projection, Poggi method

| 1 | The patient is asked to stay in front of the detector, with shoulders relaxed, and the posture of the patient should be corrected if necessary, aligning thorax and hips |
|---|---|
| 2 | Distance of the patient from the detector: The palm of the open hand, parallel to the detector |
| 3 | Radiographer on the medial side of the patient: The patient is embraced, reaching her ipsilateral shoulder, which is slightly lowered |
| 4 | The patient's posture is checked again, ensuring that her shoulders are relaxed and her head is turned medially |
| 5 | The breast of the side under examination is lifted until it is parallel to the detector (the axial plane parallel to the detector) |
| 6 | The detector is raised up to the height of the mammographer's hand that supports the breast |
| 7 | The nipple should point to 12 o'clock, on the midline, in the case of outer and inner quadrants of equal size. In this case, midline will correspond to the mid-sagittal plane. In the case of different outer and inner quadrants, the nipple will not point to 12 o'clock, and the midline will not coincide with the mid-sagittal plane |
| 8 | The patient is asked to turn her face as much medially (towards the radiographer) as possible until her ear rests on the facial screen with the chin slightly up, if possible |
| 9 | Check that the contralateral shoulder has not been brought too high (due to a conditioned reflex of the patient). The height of the two shoulders must not differ too much |
| 10 | The fifth finger of the radiographer's hand that supports the breast is located deep in the inframammary fold. The breast is brought forward until it is on the detector. The breast is lifted again and carried further forward |
| 11 | It is verified that the chest wall is perpendicular to the mid-sagittal plane; the sternum is in contact with the detector. The contralateral shoulder is advanced anteriorly |
| 12 | The nipple should be in profile if the superior and inferior Q are equal in size |
| 13 | Anteriorly directed pressure is applied with the arm around the patient's shoulders, to bring the upper deep tissues even further forward |
| 14 | The breast is firmly stretched forward, without giving a medial or lateral direction to the stretching ("neutral stretching"). Compression is begun to be applied |
| 15 | Any skin folds in the outer quadrant (bevelling upwards) and the inframammary fold (bevelling downwards) are eliminated |
| 16 | The compression ends according to the consistency of the breast (Tables 11.1 and 11.2) |

**Table 9.3** Most common errors in CC projection: type of error, causes and correction

| Type of error | Causes | Correction |
|---|---|---|
| Incomplete IQ | It is caused by the approach of the patient's trunk too obliquely medially or by a medially directed distension (not neutral) | • Before the acquisition, check that the patient's chest wall is perpendicular to the mid-sagittal plane passing through the breast<br>• It helps to bring the contralateral breast on the detector and then having it moved away by the patient<br>• It is advisable to make the patient bring the contralateral shoulder forward<br>• The sternum should come into contact with the detector<br>• Resolute stretching, anteriorly directed |
| Incomplete OQ | This mainly results from two causes:<br>1. The patient's torso is laterally oblique, and/or a laterally directed (nonneutral) breast stretching was performed<br>2. There is a significant percentage of patients who show a laterally extended OQ that have been partially lost (see Chap. 26) | 1. The chest wall should be perpendicular to the mid-sagittal plane of the breast; the extension must be neutral, i.e. directed forward<br>2. The missing part of OQ is brought forward on the detector, maintaining the aforementioned perpendicularity to the chest wall |
| The pectoral muscle is missing | It can be due to various causes:<br>1. Anatomical: The patient has a wide base of attachment of the breast to the chest in the superior-inferior and lateral-lateral directions, and/or a high consistency (poor elasticity)[a]: Both factors make it more difficult to reach the deep planes<br>2. Related to the use of the mammographic unit: The detector has not been brought to the correct height<br>3. Related only to the positioning: Technique: The radiographer has not brought the lower/upper deep planes onto the detector<br>4. Related to the patient's posture: Especially in the case of lordosis/hyperlordosis or kyphosis[a] | 1. No corrections can be made<br>2. The detector should be brought up to the height of the radiographer's hand supporting the breast, so that the median axial plane is parallel to the detector, when the patient's thorax and hips are aligned<br>3. Place the fifth finger in the IMF and bring the breast forward until the finger is on the detector: The lower deep tissues must be then brought forward again; firmly distend the upper quadrants forward to bring the upper deep tissue onto the detector. Patient's head is medial, with ear resting on screen and chin up<br>4. In the case of lordosis, the upper deep tissues are lost more easily, Chap. 26: It is necessary to rebalance thorax and hips, bringing them on the same line; in case of kyphosis, the patient's posture tends to cause lower deep tissue loss; again, thorax and hips must be rebalanced as much as possible, aligning them. |

(continued)

**Table 9.3** (continued)

| Type of error | Causes | Correction |
|---|---|---|
| The pectoralis muscle is not central (it is medial or lateral) and has no lunette shape (semi-elliptical) | 1. If the muscle is present laterally but not medially: The ipsilateral shoulder has been lowered too much and deep medial tissue has been lost due to imperfect perpendicularity of the torso with respect to the median axial and sagittal planes<br>2. If the muscle is present medially but not laterally: The deep external tissues have been lost due to imperfect perpendicularity of the trunk with respect to the mid-sagittal plane<br>3. If the muscle is laterally shifted and fan-shaped: The ipsilateral shoulder has been lowered too much, the patient lays on the detector as for MLO projection, and/or there was a medially directed breast rotation | 1. Before acquisition, check that the chest wall is perpendicular to the mid-sagittal plane of the breast and that the shoulders are approximately at the same height (only slightly lower than the ipsilateral one); correct the excessive rotation of the trunk and the stretching action, which has been directed medially<br>2. Before acquisition, check that the chest wall is perpendicular to the mid-sagittal plane of the breast: Correct the excessive rotation of the patient's trunk and the stretching action that has been directed laterally<br>3. The patient must be repositioned: The height of the shoulders must be realigned, the patient must not lean sideways, but stay straight; the stretching action must be neutral, forward, and not directed medially |
| The nipple is not in profile: It points downwards | There are two possible causes:<br>1. Incorrect positioning in case the upper and lower quadrants are the same size: Since the nipple points towards the missing tissue, lower deep tissue will be missing<br>2. A correct positioning in case the size of the upper quadrants is greater than the lower ones; the nipple that is not in profile indicates that the entire dominant (upper) quadrant has also been documented | 1. The breast must be repositioned, being lifted well, by pushing the fifth finger into the IMF and bringing the breast forward until the finger is on the detector, and then pulling the lower deep tissue forward again<br>2. No correction is required. The first and absolute duty of the mammographer is to document as much tissue as possible (without operating rotations in any direction) |
| The nipple is not in profile: It points upwards | This results from two causes:<br>1. Incorrect positioning technique in case the upper and lower quadrants are the same size: Since the nipple points towards the missing tissue, upper deep tissue will be missing<br>2. A correct positioning in case the size of the lower quadrants is greater than the upper ones; the nipple that is not in profile indicates that the entire dominant (lower) quadrant has also been documented | 1. To have the upper deep tissues on the detector, the upper quadrants must be stretched forward firmly, with the breast positioned correctly with the upper and lower quadrants parallel to each other, and parallel to the detector<br>2. No correction is required. The first and absolute duty of the mammographer is to document as much tissue as possible (without operating rotations in any direction) |
| The nipple points medially to the mid-sagittal plane[b] (midline and mid-sagittal plane do not coincide) | This results from two reasons:<br>1. The nipple is on the midline, naturally coincident with the mid-sagittal plane (OQ and IQ equal in size): If the nipple appears medially on the image acquired, it means that the patient has the trunk rotated medially or that a medial rotation has been applied on the breast (even if only for nonneutral distension)<br>2. If the nipple is naturally medial (dominant OQ), the nipple must appear medially on the image acquired, where it really is located (*mammography as photography*, Chap. 26) | 1. The patient's chest wall should be perpendicular to the mid-sagittal plane of the breast; the stretching must be neutral, i.e. no direction should be applied on it. Otherwise, this would deform and modify the breast with respect to reality<br>2. No correction should be made: Forcing the midline and mid-sagittal plane to coincide in this case will lead to the loss of the lateral tissue (of the dominant quadrant) |

(continued)

**Table 9.3** (continued)

| Type of error | Causes | Correction |
|---|---|---|
| The nipple points laterally to the mid-sagittal plane[b] (midline and mid-sagittal plane do not coincide) | This results from two reasons:<br>1. The nipple is in the midline, naturally coincident with the mid-sagittal plane (EQ and IQ equal in size); if the nipple appears laterally on the image acquired, it means that the patient has the trunk rotated laterally, or that a lateral rotation has been applied on the breast (even if only for nonneutral distension)<br>2. As the nipple is naturally lateral (dominant IQ), the nipple must appear on the image acquired laterally, where it really is located (*mammography as photography*, Chap. 26) | 1. The patient's chest wall should be perpendicular to the axial plane of the breast; the stretching must be neutral, i.e. no direction should be applied on it. Otherwise, this would deform and modify the breast with respect to reality<br>2. No correction should be made: Forcing the midline and mid-sagittal plane to coincide in this case will lead to the loss of the medial tissue (of the dominant quadrant) |

[a] Chapter 26
[b] Chapters 25 and 27

**Table 9.4** Steps in sequence for the execution of MLO projection, Poggi method

| | |
|---|---|
| 1 | Position the patient in front of the mammographic unit with the whole body, including the feet, to form an angle of 45–50° directed medially with respect to it |
| 2 | Detector height: The bottom right corner of the detector (Fig. 27.5) is at the height of the iliac crest of the patient. With a shifting compression paddle the lower part of the light field is considered |
| 3 | The radiographer checks the patient from behind. Patient is held at a distance from the detector equal to an open hand, parallel to the detector |
| 4 | She is asked to rest her arm on the upper profile of the detector. Shoulder and arm should be approximately on the same plane |
| 5 | The breast is collected with both hands. For example, for the left breast, the radiographer takes it with the right hand, while with the left hand she/he pushes forward the tissues (deep lateral), which are then picked up by the right hand |
| 6 | The left hand then moves from behind the patient's chest to her arm, just in front of the armpit. The patient is guided forward decisively, without rotation or inclination of the trunk, until she rests her shoulder on the detector. Shoulder and arm should be stretched further forward (as far as possible) |
| 7 | The radiographer releases the grip and moves behind the detector to adjust the patient's arm and shoulder |
| 8 | A first rotation of the arm, directed superiorly and anteriorly (i.e. inwards), is performed, the patient's hand in the supinate position |
| 9 | It is checked that the top right corner of the detector is free |
| 10 | Shoulder still, the second rotation is performed, directed superiorly and posteriorly directed |
| 11 | The arm is extended forward using the two hands together, pushing the flexed elbow downwards, which must protrude externally from the upper profile of the detector |
| 12 | The patient is asked to relax the entire upper limb as much as possible; the hand should not grip the handle |
| 13 | After returning to the medial side of the patient, the breast is collected with a pinch grip and the patient is asked to rotate her hips towards the detector (including her feet). The patient's posture is checked to ensure thorax and hips are on the same line |
| 14 | The shoulder is moved away from the FOV, pushing it upwards, and the patient is asked to move the contralateral breast away, externally and downwards |
| 15 | The breast is raised with respect to the detector ("detachment") to verify that there are no posterior "steps," producing skin folds in the deep lateral tissues, which must be smoothed with a posterior directed movement from behind the chest |
| 16 | The UP&OUT manoeuvre is performed: The breast must be brought up and stretched anteriorly. IMF should thus be documentable without horizontal skin folds |
| 17 | The deep lateral part of the IMF is smoothed out to avoid vertical folds in this area |
| 18 | It is checked that no shadows are cast on the area to be acquired (the chin, the other breast) |
| 19 | The compression is applied until the breast is fixed in place |
| 20 | The compression is terminated (Tables 11.1 and 11.2), and the acquisition is carried out |

**Table 9.5** Most common errors in MLO projection: type of error, causes and correction

| Type of error | Causes | Correction |
|---|---|---|
| The pectoral muscle is not shown up to PNL PNL: Posterior nipple line, see Chaps. 11 and 25 | Deep tissues, especially the medial ones, were not included; the UP&OUT manoeuvre has not been carried out correctly | The recommended positioning technique involves the entry of the patient medial to the detector, and then the rotation of the hips (and feet) laterally, UP to including the deep medial tissues; in addition to this, the UP&OUT manoeuvre must be performed, operating a firmly anteriorly directed stretching |
| The pectoral muscle is not wide at the axillary level | The possible causes are mainly three: 1. The patient's arm and shoulder were not brought forward well 2. The patient stiffened her pectoral muscle 3. There is functional deficit of the shoulder on the side under examination | 1. The steps from 6 to 9 described in Table 9.4 must be carried out for the execution of the exam 2. The patient is asked not to squeeze the handle and to relax as much as possible 3. It should not be corrected, but the problem must be noted for the radiologist to justify the production of low-quality mammograms (also with medico-legal value) |
| There are skin folds in the axilla/axillary extension | This results from two reasons: 1. The patient is very thin and/or very stiff; the distance between the upper tissues and the detector occasionally exceeds two fingers 2. The patient has a fairly loose skin envelope and/or a very thick axillary extension | 1. It is not easy to get a patient with a very slender chest to relax: The ©RAmoruso manoeuvre, where the forearm is dropped behind the detector, can be used. This manoeuvre is very effective in decreasing the tissue distance from the detector, but the width of the pectoral muscle which can be documented is smaller 2. Steps 10 to 13 are implemented; the elbow must be flexed and pushed well down. It may also be helpful to ask the patient to "lie down" on the machine. As both movements tend to make the breast rise on the FOV, it is necessary to check that the area covered by the light field is the desired one. |
| The inframammary fold, the INFPOSTQ is/are missing | The causes are mainly two: 1. The hips are held back with respect to the thorax, and therefore are out of the detector 2. The patient's anatomy is such that she does not have an inframammary fold that can be documented | 1. The hips must be rotated laterally and forward in order to have the IMF (and the POSTINFQ) onto the detector, and the UP&OUT manoeuvre must be performed correctly 2. There is no correction to be made |
| There are horizontal folds in the inframammary fold | The UP&OUT manoeuvre has not been performed correctly | Correction requires that the medial side of the breast be lifted well with respect to the lateral one, until the IMF is open. Compression should be continued until the breast is fixed in place |
| There are vertical folds in the inframammary fold | The causes are various: These are skin creases that form on the breast lateral side, which is the one that rests on the detector | To avoid lateral skin folds affecting the IMF, the tissues in this area can be smoothed out following a vertical downward direction |

**Table 9.5** (continued)

| Type of error | Causes | Correction |
|---|---|---|
| The breast has fallen | The main causes are two:<br>1. The thickness of the upper tissues is such that adequate compression cannot be applied on the anterior part of the breast, leading to its fall<br>2. Compression was stopped before the condition at which the breast was fixed is reached | 1. The steps to be performed are steps 10–13 described in Table 9.4 to decrease the thickness of the zone<br>2. Compression should be continued until the breast is fixed in place |
| There is no latissimus dorsi | 1. The axilla, of which the latissimus dorsi represents part of the posterior wall, has not been brought forward sufficiently<br>2. The patient's anatomy does not permit this | 1. Steps 6 to 9 described in Table 9.4 are to be followed; it is important to ask the patient to relax the arm<br>2. There is no correction to be made; the latissimus dorsi cannot always be documented |
| The retromammary space is not wide | This aspect can only be evaluated by comparing it with a previous examination of the patient, in which an actually larger retromammary space was demonstrated in both projections or in only one<br>1. The breast was not stretched adequately in the UP&OUT manoeuvre | 1. The only correction is to distend decisively upwards and forwards, exerting sufficient muscle strength, possibly sitting down for MLO projection (for work-related MSDs, see Chap. 23) |

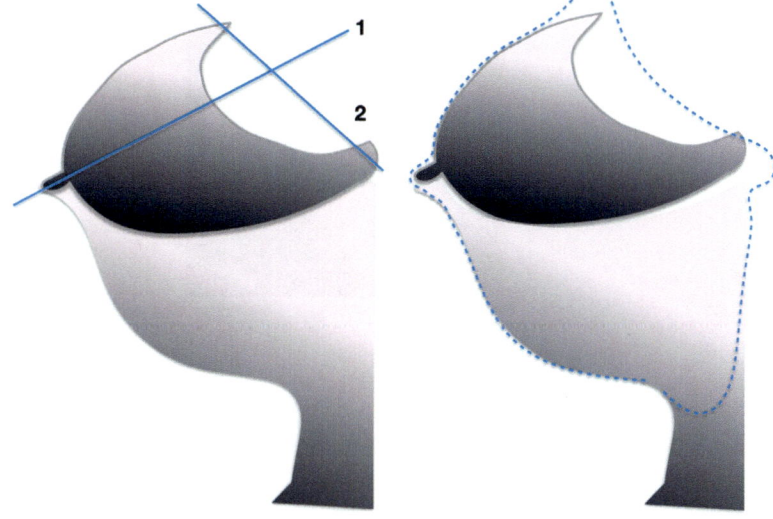

**Fig. 9.8** 3D sectional representation of the breast at the median axial plane for the correct positioning of the CC projection, according to the second acquisition geometry parameter (see text). Tissues to include, with the lateral and medial connections of the breast to the chest when possible (Chap. 26). (1) Median sagittal plane. (2) Chest wall

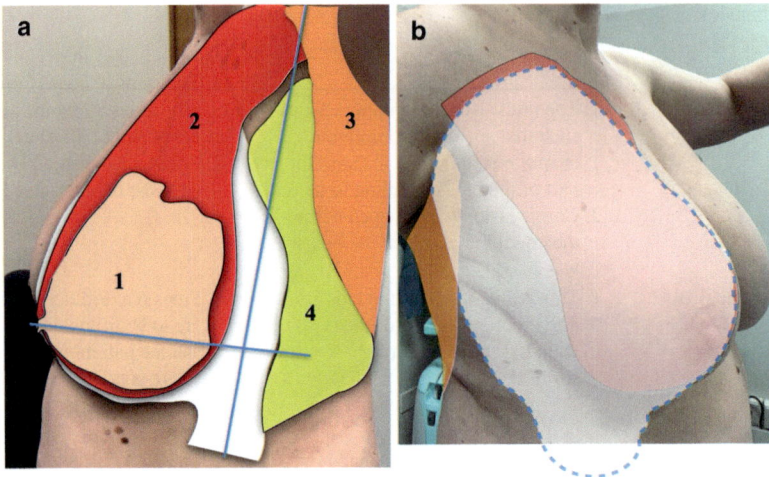

**Fig. 9.9** (**a**) Representation of the breast anatomy in a patient with the arm raised and the breast in a natural position. (1) Mammary gland, in pink; (2) Pectoralis major muscle, in red; (3) Latissimus dorsi muscle, in orange; (4) Serratus anterior muscle, in yellow, not visible on mammography. (**b**) In transparent white, the tissue area is to be documented in MLO projection, approximate delineation, for teaching purposes

**Fig. 9.10** Muscles involved in MLO projection; (**a**) pectoralis major and (**b**) latissimus dorsi; drawings by Silvia Bartolini

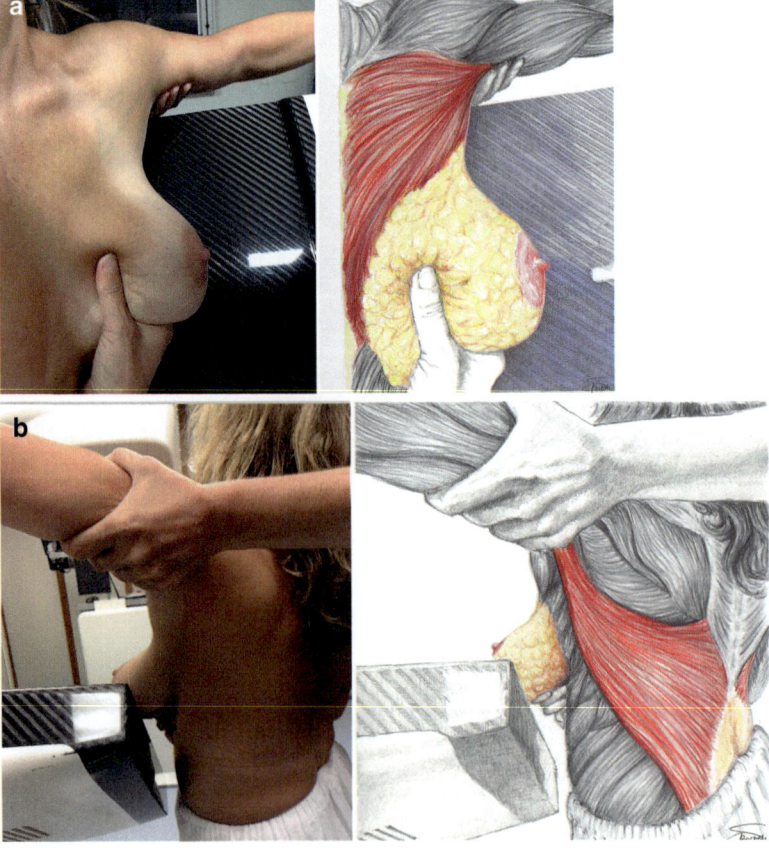

## 9.6 About the Standardisation of Positioning and Compression in Mammography: A Global Evaluation

It must be stated once again that a path that provides for *standardisation of positioning and compression* should be chosen. This is despite the huge difference between one patient and another in terms of anatomy, consistency and mobility of the breast, as well as emotional attitude and therefore degree of cooperation. It is a requirement for a common professional growth. An educational path that should be pointing to a single purpose, the production of high-quality mammograms. Quality that must be described by rules derived from international guidelines, according to evidence-based evaluations, correlating them, for example, to the detection rate (see Chap. 6). This holistic approach is therefore proposed to the radiographer working in senology, according to the method elaborated by the author:

1. **Visual Assessment of the Anatomy and Volume of the Breast to Be Mammographed.** The breast must not be "deformed" to follow the quality criteria. This is to say, CCs that always appear hemispherical, for examples, with outer and inner quadrants always the same size, with the nipple on the midline that always coincides with the mid-sagittal plane. In other words, it must be an accurate photography of the external anatomy, considering the satisfaction of the two acquisition geometry parameters stated. In the Poggi teaching method, this first step is indicated with the axiom "*Mammography as photography.*" The radiographer should always aim at the best possible correlation between anatomy and radiographic anatomy;

2. **Visual Assessment of the Size of the Chest's Base of Attachment to the Chest (Footprint), and Patient's Posture.** This allows the radiographer to understand which projection will be more difficult and what are the most common errors associated with it. See in Chap. 26 the project CATegorizzazione dell'ERrore per anatomia e postura, CATER, CATegorisation of the ERror for anatomy and

posture (Poggi, C.). This second step indicates the degree of ease with which the radiographer hypotheses how far she/he will be able to "detach" the breast from the chest, documenting the deep planes. This is referred to as "*Theory of anatomical relationships.*"

3. **Tactile Evaluation of the Consistency of the Breast.** *Skin envelope* is included in this evaluation: in addition to the breast size (thickness), the consistency of the skin evelope allows to choose the **appropriate compression value.** This is referred to as "*Evaluation of the compression and stretching resistance index.*" The hands of the breast radiographer must have the necessary competence to assess what can and should be obtained for each patient, as hypothesised in Step 2 and confirmed or not in Step 3.

*The adequacy of the compression exerted should be assessed according to the principles of the evidence-based practice (EBP)* (Chap. 24). It means that the appropriateness of the technical act is to be weighed up in relation to relevance and feasibility. Careful study should also address the correlation between iconography, quality criteria, *detection rate*, rate of recalls for inadequate and suspected findings that turned out to be *false positives* (Chaps. 6, 13 and 17) [9–12].

For radiographic anatomy of the breast, see Chap. 25. For the quality criteria, Annex 1. Poggi's teaching method is comprehensively described in the dedicated text cited above, which has not been published to date: "The technique for the execution of the mammography examination: the Poggi's Method." It is briefly presented in this text in Chap. 26. It also proposed a method of assessing clinical quality called POBMI INTEGRATO POGGI (POINT), summarised in Chap. 27.

## References

1. Dumky H, et al. The art of mammography with respect to positioning and compression-a Swedish perspective. J Radiol Nurs. 2018;37:41–8. https://doi.org/10.1016/j.jradnu.2017.11.006.
2. Sweeney R-J, et al. A review of mammographic positioning image quality criteria for the craniocaudal projection. Br J Radiol. 2018;91(1082):20170611.

3. Holen AS, et al. Visualization of the nipple in profile: does it really affect selected outcomes in organized mammographic screening? J Breast Imaging. 2021;3:427–37. https://doi.org/10.1093/jbi/wbab042.

4. Hofvind S. Quality assurance of mammograms in the Norwegian breast cancer screening program. EJR. 2009;1:22–9. https://doi.org/10.1016/j.ejradi.2008.11.002.

5. Manuale di tecnica mammografica capitolo sulla qualità clinica norvegese, aggiornato 2011, English version. https://www.kreftregisteret.no/Generelt/Rapporter/Mammografiprogrammet/Kvalitet/

6. Rinella D. Perfect positioning: the CC & MLO radiologycme.standford.edu/2008breast/handouts/Rinella_CC%20&%20MLO.pdf. Access June 2019

7. Miller LC. Mammography positioning basic and advanced. SBI. https://courseware.cutm.ac.in/wp-content/uploads/2020/06/Mammo-for-Techs-Positioning-pdf.pdf

8. Poggi C. VMM, Valutazione Miglioramento e Monitoraggio della performance del tecnico operante in senologia nell'Area Toscana Centro, Le buone pratiche organizzative delle Aziende Sanitarie Italiane, FEDERSANITA' ANCI, ed speciale Sanità 4.0, 2019.

9. Deandrea S, et al. Presence, characteristics and equity of access to breast cancer programs in 27 European countries in 2010 and 2014. Results from an international survey. Prev Med. 2016;91:250–63. https://doi.org/10.1016/j.ypmed.2016.08.021.

10. Peintinger F. National breast screening programs across Europe. Breast Care. 2019;14:354–7. https://doi.org/10.1159/000503715.

11. Eby PR, et al. The benefits of early detection: evidence from modern international mammography service screening programs. SBI. 2022;4:346–56. https://doi.org/10.1093/jbi/wbac041.

12. Tabar L, et al. Evaluation issues in the Swedish Two-County trial of breast cancer screening: an historical review. J Med Screen. 2017;24(1):27–33. https://doi.org/10.1177/0969141316631375.

## Further Reading

Andolina V, Lille' SL. Mammographic imaging a practical guide. 3rd ed. ED Wolters Kluwer Lippincott Williams& Wilkins. ISBN 978-60547-031-3

Hogg P, et al. Digital mammography a holistic approach. Springer; 2015. ISBN 978-3-319-04831-4 (E-book)

Miller LC. Mammography positioning guidebook CC, MLO, and commonly used additional views. 2nd ed. Mammography Educators; 2015.

Tabar L. Mammography positioning technique. Mammography Education Inc.; 2018.

van Landsveld-Verhoeven C. The right focus Manual on mammography positioning technique. LRCB; 2013. ISBN/EAN: 978-90-821079-1-3

# Patients Who Do Not Conform to the Standard Thorax Anatomy: The Lateral and the Additional CC for OQ and CC for IQ Projections

**10**

## 10.1 Introduction

Performing a high-quality mammographic examination is a very difficult task. It requires adhering to the quality criteria and satisfying the *acquisition geometry parameters* (Chap. 9). This takes specific professional skills provided by training done in qualified centres by professional trainers, experience and communication skills (*compliance;* see Chap. 24).

But it is still not enough: there are patients whose anatomy does not conform to the standard, or who have chronic or transient pathologies, making it even more difficult to perform this examination.

An anatomical standard is very difficult to delineate; however, we can consider a simple approach of four groups of "non-conforming to the standard thorax anatomy" patients [1–4]:

1. Women with large and very large breasts, with small attachment base or "footprint" on the chest (see also Chap. 26).
2. Women with small breasts and a wide base.
3. Women with a congenital malformation of the anterior part of the thorax, called *pectus excavatum* (hollow or sunken chest), in which there is a more or less prominent indentation of the sternum and proximal portion of the ribs.
4. Women with a congenital malformation of the anterior part of the thorax, called *pectus carinatum* (keel chest), in which the sternum protrudes forward more or less significantly. In some cases, only the manubrium of the sternum is keeled, while the body is sunken.

### 10.1.1 Women with Large Breasts and Small Chest Attachment Base

In this group, the breast's size on the anterior-posterior axis exceeds all other dimensions, sometimes by a large margin. The attachment base is medium or even small compared with the breast volume. The breast may have various degrees of ptosis, with high IMF. Positioning errors are understandably more common due to the heaviness of the breast. The ease with which skin folds form is due to an occasionally very important laxity of the skin envelope.

The greatest difficulty is in performing the MLO projection. Getting the correct UP&OUT position (see Chap. 9) can thus be complicated, due to the difficulty in lifting and stretching the breast. The IMF can therefore be affected by the presence of folds or by the abdomen itself. In the case of breasts larger than the maximum available FOV, additional CC and MLO projections can be acquired on the missing tissue. Generally, the projections are on the anterior and on the posteroinferior portions.

### 10.1.2 Women with Small Breasts and Wide Chest Attachment Base

The wide-based small breast is usually dense and on average more sensitive to compression. Unlike the first group, CC projection is much more difficult to perform than MLO projection. This is because the superior-inferior dimension can be truly significant in this group, even sometimes the lateromedial. The anteroposterior dimension can be almost non-existent. These are breasts with rather small mobility, sometimes also very little compressible, especially regarding CCs. This is also because of the skin envelope that is sometimes very thick and resistant to manipulation. In this group, it is also difficult to document the IMF that is sometimes very thin, or almost non-existent. The breast passes over the chest seamlessly.

### 10.1.3 Women with Congenital Malformation of the Thorax: The Pectus Excavatum

This malformation can be more or less severe. The nipples are medial to the breast mid-sagittal plane, sometimes very much so, which makes documenting the medial quadrants almost impossible. *CCs should be performed to document as much medial tissue as possible and MLOs for lateral tissue*. The opposite hemithorax can create an artefact that is difficult to eliminate in MLO projection (see Chap. 17). It may be helpful to perform an LM (see below) or bring the C-arm detector to an angle of about 55° for MLO positioning. The correction should be noted [4, 5].

### 10.1.4 Women with Pectus Carinatum

In this malformation, the nipples are lateralised, so that it may be necessary to add a projection for OQ (see below). In this group, however, the documentation of the medial aspect is really difficult. It may be helpful to bring the detector to 55° for

MLO projection, describing the reason for the different inclination of the tube from the standard for the interpreting reader.

## 10.2 Lateral Projection: Introduction

Lateral projection is performed with the tube at 90°. There are two lateral projections, the mediolateral ML and the lateromedial LM. This depends on the direction of the beam and, therefore, on the quadrants that rest on the detector. LM should be chosen in case the lesion is on the medial side, to ensure maximum spatial resolution [2, 4, 6–9].

### 10.2.1 ML Mediolateral Projection

In this projection, the lateral aspect of the breast rests on the detector, as it occurs in an oblique view. The detector height is at the level of the humeral head. The patient should be placed in front of the detector and set up for the ML projection, so that the sagittal plane is parallel to the detector. Regarding the arm-shoulder positioning, the steps for MLO which allow documenting the axillary fossa should not be followed. In fact, in the image the axillary tail should not be appeared angled, but straight. It implies that depth tissue will be lost, and the pectoral muscle will also be straight and barely noticeable. This projection is not intended for the study of deep planes, but for *triangulation* (Chap. 13). The nipple should always be in profile, the IMF well represented, while the retromammary space could be incomplete (Figs. 9.7, 9.10a and 10.1a, Table 10.1). *The portion that can be studied at its best, without any distortion, is the retroareolar area.*

### 10.2.2 LM Lateromedial Projection

The breast side resting on the detector is the medial one, which can therefore be better studied than the lateral one. The profile of the detector is

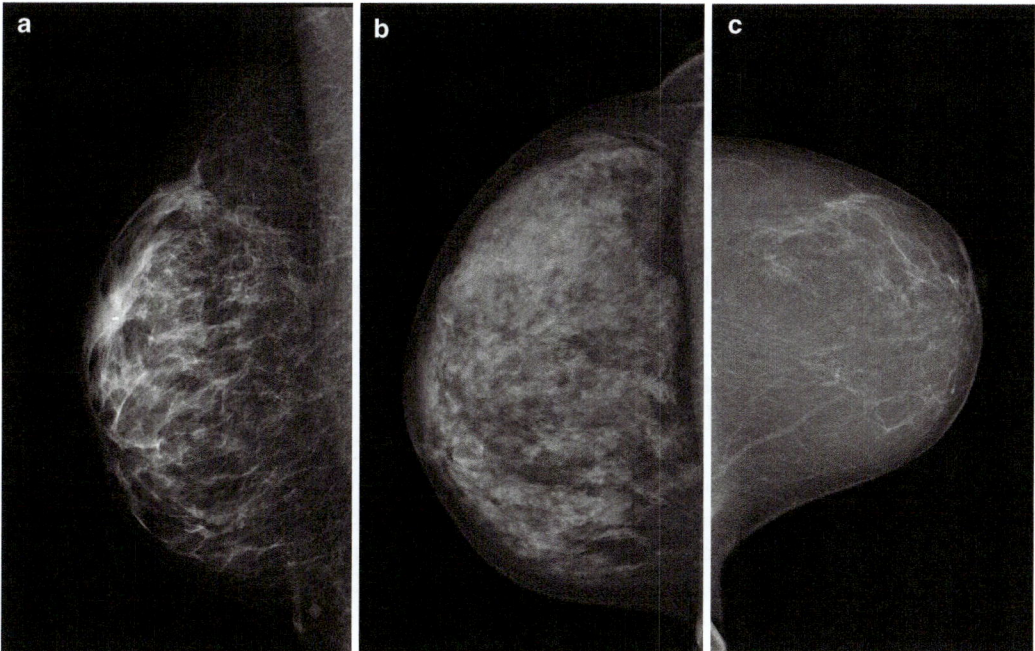

**Fig. 10.1** (**a**) ML; (**b**) CC for outer quadrants; (**c**) CC for inner quadrants

**Table 10.1** Steps for performing the mediolateral (ML) projection

1 The tube is brought to 90°; the height is about equal to that of the head of the humerus (to be evaluated for the presence or absence of a shift-compressor paddle; Chap. 11). The lateral side is to lie on the detector
2 Arm and shoulder are positioned only to avoid folds: The study of the axilla is not required in this projection
3 The patient's thorax is brought forward towards the detector, with the median sagittal plane parallel to it, hips aligned with the chest. More of the IMF should be seen in this projection than in MLO
4 The nipple must be in profile
5 The other breast (which is located in the lateral projection in the same plane as the one being examined) is carefully moved away; the breast is brought forward, stretched and compressed

**Table 10.2** Steps for performing the lateromedial (LM) projection

1 The tube is brought to 90°; the height is approximately equal to the patient's armpit: the medial side is to lie on the detector
2 The detector profile is placed on the inner side of the patient's sternal line (the patient is asked to step sideways towards the side being examined)
3 The ipsilateral arm is brought up and forward
4 The breast is brought forward, stretched firmly, and compressed

on the upper profile of the detector: lifting the ipsilateral arm upwards, elbow flexed, bringing it forward, and arranging and stretching appropriately the breast (Table 10.2).

### 10.2.3 Quality Criteria and Lateral Projection Purpose

*Due to the fact that the beam is not oblique, the lateral projection allows a better study of the anterior portion of the breast, and the lower tissue, particularly the IMF.*

Since it is set at 90° compared to the CC (performed at 0°), it is possible to *triangulate* the lesion

on the sternum, or, more precisely, it is not the centre of the detector that needs to be placed on the sternal line, but its inner profile. The patient, who is positioned facing the mammographic unit, is asked to take a small lateral step towards the side being examined. This causes the detector to press onto the other breast. To perform it correctly, some authors recommend resting the chin (see Chap. 13) (Fig. 10.1a). It is useful in the case of patients with congenital chest malformations and in patients with chemo-PORTs or pacemakers (PM), especially if recently inserted. However, this is not the projection to perform in order to see deeper tissues, as already mentioned. The MLO is actually able to include much more posterior tissue than the lateral. This is why it has been chosen as the default projection in the standard examination

## 10.3    CC for Outer Quadrants or xCCL Projection [4, 5, 10, 11]

The CC projection for outer quadrants (XCCL—eXaggerated cranio-caudal view or laterally extended CC) may be useful in case the outer quadrant has to be documented in its deepest portion. This is not always easily accessible in the standard CC projection due to the anatomy of the chest wall.

### 10.3.1  CC Positioning for OQ Documentation and Quality Criteria

It is a CC projection: preferably, the detector should be kept at 0°. The torso is rotated medially, so that the lateral portion of the breast and the axillary extension are brought forward. The nipple will then point medially. The patient will lower her ipsilateral shoulder, and her arm can be brought forward. In this case, this is also called the "Cleopatra projection", referring to Dicksee's 1896 painting "The Mirror". All the OQ must be documented, and therefore, the pectoralis muscle must be present, elongated but still lunette-shaped, in the central and lateral (not medial) part, as illustrated in Fig. 10.1b. *If the pectoralis muscle has a fan-like shape, it means that the projection has acquired obliquity.* This is often correlated with an excessive lowering of the shoulder on the side under examination, which must be corrected.

## 10.4    CC Positioning for Inner Quadrants Documentation and Quality Criteria [10, 11]

The CC projection for IQ is required in case the deepest portion of this quadrant, and/or the inter-mammary cleft, is to be documented. It is always performed at 0° like all CCs. The inner quadrant is brought forward as far as possible, so the patient's hemithorax (of the side under examination) is angled backwards. The contralateral arm is forward, holding the handle. It is useful to turn the patient's head laterally (instead of medially as in the standard CC). Regarding the quality criteria, the goal is to include the entire deepest portion of the inner quadrant and the intermammary cleft, for the portion pertaining to the side under examination (Fig. 10.1c).

## References

1. Peart O. Positioning challenges in mammography PPT. Radiol Techno. 2014;85(4):417–39M.
2. Miller LC. Mammography quality: the critical role of standardized positioning. San Diego, CA: FDA, Mammography Educators; 2015.
3. Borrelli C, et al. NHS breast screening programme guidance for breast screening mammographers. 3rd ed. Public Health England leads the NHS Screening Programmes PHE publications gateway number: 2017607; 2017.
4. Radiology Key Mammographic Technique and Image Evaluation Summary of Importance Points Routine breast Imaging and Special Imaging Situation. https://radiologykey.com/mammographic-technique-and-image-evaluation/
5. Miller LC. Mammography positioning basic and advanced. SBI. 2016. https://www.sbi-online.org/Portals
6. Bedene A, et al. Mediolateral oblique projection in mammography: Use a different angulation for patients with different thorax anatomy. J Health Sci. 2019;9(1):40–5. https://doi.org/10.17532/jhsci.2019.854.
7. Prasad S. Mammography positioning technique for lateral view (LM/ML). https://www.slideshare.net/SelinPrasad/mammography-positioning-technique-for-lateral-views-lmml

8. Spurr K, Poulos A. Mammography: current practice in Australia for the selection of Bucky angle in the mediolateral oblique view of the breast. EJR. 2010;1(4):115–23. https://doi.org/10.1016/j.ejradi.2010.02.001.

9. Rodríguez Suárez I, et al. Diagnostic mammography: how, why and when. EPPOS™ ECR; 2018. https://doi.org/10.1594/ecr2018/C-1972.

10. Kelly J. Supplementary mammographic projections, chapter. January 2015. (Downloaded from ResearchGate). https://doi.org/10.1007/978-3-319-04831-4_24

11. Derenburger D, Hadley R, Most commonly used additional views, part 1 variation of the Craniocaudal view. SBI 2020. https://mammographyeducation.com/wp-content/uploads/2020/10/Additional-Views-Part-1-SBI-newsletter.pdf

## Further Reading

Andolina V, Lille' SL. Mammographic imaging: a practical guide. 3rd ed. Wolters Kluwer Lippincott Williams& Wilkins. ISBN 978-60547-031-3

Miller LC. Mammography positioning guidebook CC, MLO, and commonly used additional views. 2nd ed. Mammography Educators.; 2015.

Tabar L, et al. Breast cancer the art and science of early detection with mammography. Thieme; 2005. ISBN 3-13-135371-6 (GTV)

Tabar L, Dean PB. Teaching atlas of mammography. 4th ed. Thieme; 2012. ISBN 978-3-13-640804-9

van Landsveld-Verhoeven C. The right focus Manual on mammography positioning technique. LRCB; 2013. ISBN/EAN: 978-90-821079-1-3

# 11 The Evaluation of Clinical Image Quality in Mammography

## 11.1 Introduction

*Clinical quality* concerns the last aspect of the quality control of the mammography production chain (from acquisition to visualisation). It is closely related to its diagnostic value, that is, the ease of interpretation by the reporter. This is part of the controls by which the iconography produced is evaluated, maintained, and, where necessary, improved. The clinical quality depends entirely on the work of the radiographer, and consequently, can vary greatly depending on her/his work performance. There are two parameters to assess: (1) the positioning technique, which must be strictly executed (2) the compression, which must be adequate. The objectives are to include as much of the tissue as possible in the image, because what is not documented cannot be read. Therefore, whatever findings were there, would not be diagnosed. The tissue must also be well spread out, and free of artefacts, not only of the occlusive type but also resulting from incorrect rotation and/or stretching (Chap. 17) [1–5].

All performance characteristics that can be defined, measured and controlled, are the subject of in-depth study. This is not so easy to do with clinical quality, as it is dependent on multiple factors [1, 6–8]. There are specific standards, or rather, *classification systems*, such as the *PGMI,* used in many European and non-European countries. It is the system included in the European Guidelines [9].

## 11.2 The PGMI and POBMI Evaluation Systems

**PGMI** [10–12]: P stands for perfect, i.e. fulfils all the quality criteria contained in this evaluation system; G stands for good, in which an important quality criterion is absent; M stands for mediocre, in which two or more criteria are not fulfilled, but the examination is nevertheless sufficient at a diagnostic level; I stands for inadequate, i.e. to be repeated. In the Emilia Romagna region, Italy, the PGMI has been adapted from 4 to 5 classes, thus moving to **POBMI**, with the addition of the OPTIMAL class [13]. Obtaining a perfect examination is admittedly difficult (but not impossible), in daily work practice [14]. Since December 2017, Emilia Romagna has adopted another system, the 6-class POGMIIR. See also Chaps. 13, 25, 27 and Annex 1.

## 11.3 PGMI Criteria

There are two lists of criteria, one general and one related to positioning, for the two projections. In terms of the first list, the criteria are:

1. To include the maximum amount of tissue that can be obtained.

   This is the most important criterion, and we are talking about the gland tissue, the retromammary space and the pectoral muscle;

2. Complete identification of the patient and the operator performing the exam [15].

   The identification of the patient in association with the images is the task of the radiographer, who is liable in a legal sense for this. The operator performing the examination must therefore also be identified unambiguously.

3. Correct exposure;
4. Correct compression;
5. Absence of movement;
6. Absence of artefacts;
7. Absence of skin folds;
8. Symmetry between the two sides.

The second list of criteria is associated with positioning for both projections, cranio-caudal CC and mediolateral oblique MLO (Annex 1).

### Quality Criteria of CC Projection (Fig. 11.1) [1, 2, 7, 16–20]

1. The deep portion of the IQ, the one looking towards the intermammary cleft, which cannot be sufficiently documented in the

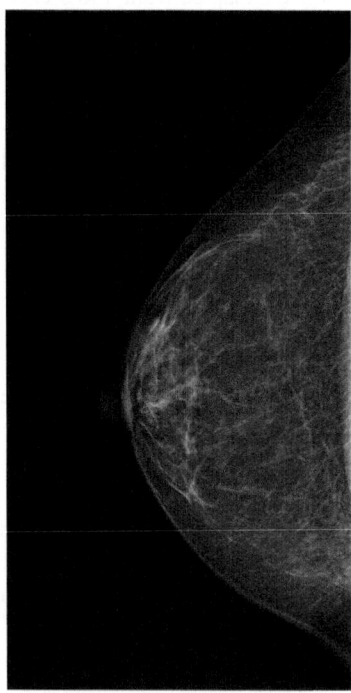

**Fig. 11.1** CC projection quality criteria

MLO projection, must be included. It is therefore the most important criterion of CCs;

2. The nipple should be in profile, or at least separated from the retro-areolar tissue;
3. It should also be on the midline (coinciding with the median sagittal plane, see also Chaps. 9 and 25);
4. The *PNL* (see below) should be about the same as that measured on a successful MLO, or at most a little shorter, but less than 1 cm.
5. If possible, the pectoralis major muscle should be visible: this makes sure of having included the deep planes, and the retromammary space, which may be the site of lesions. The pectoralis muscle represents (partially) the retromammary posterior wall (Chaps. 17, 25, 26 and Annex 1).

**The *PNL posterior nipple line*** is found by (1) drawing a line on the anterior edge of the pectoralis muscle, in the MLO projection; (2) then another line is drawn, perpendicular to the first, joining it to the nipple: this is the PNL. It is (3) measured, and (4) transferred to the CC projection (Chap. 25).

As far as MLO is concerned, it is essential that the pectoral muscle is depicted at least up to the PNL. This is generally achievable in up to 80% of cases. In the Australian publications (*Royal Australian and New Zealand College of Radiology, RANZCR*), the achievement of a straight line from the nipple parallel to the upper and lower edges of the image is cited as a criterion. However, this is met in less than 40% of cases [17, 18].

### MLO Projection Quality Criteria [1, 2, 7, 12, 17–20]

1. The pectoralis major muscle must be documented at least up to PNL;
2. The axillary portion of the muscle must be "wide," (European Guidelines)*;
3. The shape must be convex, straight is acceptable, but not concave (because it is associated with poor width);
4. The nipple should be in profile, as for CC projection;

5. The IMF must be present (not per se, because the possibility of finding lesions in this site is very low, but because it gives certainty of having included the POSTINFQ, which cannot be documented in the CC projection). It should be free of artefacts.

See Fig. 11.2.

*It might be useful to have the latissimus included, showing itself in the top right corner of the image, all else being equal* [AN, Author's Note].

**With regard to the above-mentioned criteria for both CC and MLO projections, it must be remembered that they are not to be complied with blindly, but always be related to the anatomy of each individual patient.** See Chaps. 9, 17, 25, 26 and 27. Any forcing in this direction leads to a loss of tissue acquired and of fidelity of reproduction, due to incorrect positioning.

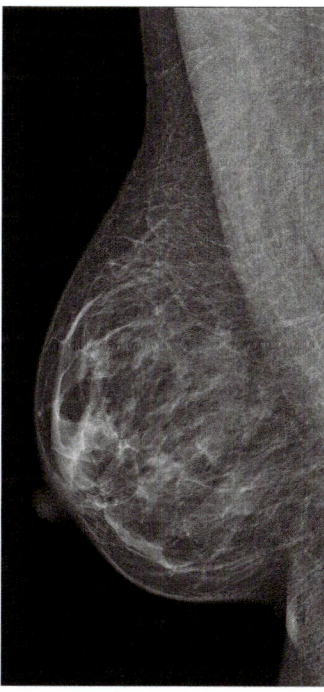

**Fig. 11.2** MLO quality criteria

## 11.3.1 Perimeter of the Area to Be Documented

The perimeter of the area we have to document is wider than one might think. The lateral side follows the median axillary line, the one in front of the latissimus dorsi (Chap. 3); the lower side is below the IMF; the medial side corresponds to the sternum, the superior side runs from the sternoclavicular joint, follows the subclavicular region and then passes into the axillary fossa [20].

## 11.3.2 On Compression

Compression was not born with mammography, we owe it to a radiologist in Uruguay, who first suggested the use of the compression paddle in 1949. It is fundamental in mammography, since it improves all parameters of technical quality (Chap. 7). *The positioning technique greatly impacts the distribution of compression.* Many studies have been made on this. Some Norwegian colleagues, Dustler et al. [21], found that compression has only in a proportion of cases out of the total number of patients, a useful effect on the anterior part of the breast. It is very important to effectively compress this portion, because this is where most of the mammary gland is. That is, in a significant percentage of patients, the compression is almost totally absorbed by the tissues close to the sternum, and by the axillary part, resulting in sub-optimal compression at the very front of the breast. *The compression should be distributed as evenly as possible*, although some patients have an anatomy that makes it difficult. First, the breast should be gathered with two hands, particularly in the oblique projection. This allows the breast to be more easily "detached" from the chest. Then, the stretching out: it should be carried out gently, but firmly. Arm and shoulder should be positioned to reduce the thickness at the axillary level (see Chap. 9). Communication skills are also very important, as they allow for a more effective cooperation from the patient (*compliance*, Chap. 24).

Another article, this time by Irish colleagues, O'Leary et al. [22], noted that P and B examinations (Perfect and Good) are associated with higher compressions than M and I examinations (Mediocre and Inadequate).

### 11.3.3 The Pain Associated with Compression

The level of discomfort reported by patients is extremely varied, and among other things is also difficult to assess, at least on a quantitative level. Certainly, it can be said that there are subgroups of women who feel pain when having their mammography, and surely among them are those who have undergone conservative surgery, usually combined with radiotherapy. Both treatments make the breast more difficult to compress (Chap. 5). There are also women who have extreme breast sensitivity, sometimes as a result of a negative personal or family history. However, at times, there are no apparent reasons to explain the pain. Pain in mammography is indeed a complex concept, in which physical, emotional and psychological factors are involved. Undoubtedly, the relationship that is established with the radiographer can play a great role, occasionally, even too much [23–26]. *The International Association for the Study of Pain (IASP) defines pain as an unpleasant sensation, both physical and emotional subjective, associated with tissue damage, actual or even just potential* [27]. The pain threshold, on the other hand, is defined as the minimum intensity of a stimulus perceived as painful. More interesting for the radiographer is the level of pain tolerance: It is defined as the maximum intensity that the subject "wants/can" endure, in a given situation. It could be very useful to enhance the patient's compliance, giving information on why one should compress, and why one should make certain movements.

### 11.3.4 Recommended Compression Values and European Trend

There are no recommended compression values in the European Guidelines, except in the technical quality control section [9], where the range

130–200 N (*Newton*) is mentioned. Compression in mammography is measured in Newton N, or in decanewton 10 N = 1 daN (see also Chap. 7). The radiographer's choice is based, as international studies have shown, primarily on the beliefs and convictions of the individual operator [28, 29]. However, this value tends to conform to the compression habits of the centre in which she/he works. In Europe, the average value is around 12–15 daN (120–150 N), but the minimum-maximum ranges are widely variable from one country to another. The Norwegians recommend a wide range, 11–18 daN [19, 30].

*The range 9–16 daN is proposed, with a mean value 12–13, therefore in line with the rest of Europe.* See Table 11.1. This is a range that should be applied to more than 85% of patients. As an aid to a more advanced standardisation, it is proposed in the project submitted to the Tuscany region, a subdivision into three ranges, considering the size of the breast, or better, the *contact area between breast and compression paddle* (see below).

When choosing the most appropriate compression value for the production of a quality image, many aspects are important: It is indeed a very complex operation because:

1. Breast tissues have different mechanical properties and therefore respond equally differently to increased compression;
2. The compression varies locally due to the uneven shape of the breast, not only in posterior-anterior direction;
3. The compression resistance of the tissues surrounding the breast (which must be included

**Table 11.1** Range of recommended compression values

| | |
|---|---|
| Minimum value: 80 N (8 daN); in the case of very small/thin breasts | |
| Maximum value: 180 N (18 daN); in the case of very large/very thick breasts, only in MLOs | |
| Range of average compression values: Between 10–16 daN | |
| **Small breast** | 8–11 daN, both for CC and MLO projections |
| **Medium breast** | 10–16 daN, both for CC and MLO projections |
| **Large breast** | 12–18 daN, both for CC and MLO projections |

in the mammogram), for thickness and consistency, varies;

4. The contact area with the compression paddle (and therefore the size of the breast), varies;
5. The patient compliance may vary, but an effective relationship should always be built between radiographer and patient, such that the appropriate compression value can be achieved for each case.

It should be added that the effect of compression on the detectability of lesions has not been studied in a statistically significant manner. Some studies indicate that too high values may worsen the sensitivity of mammography [31, 32]. On the other hand, it is well established scientifically that image quality is degraded by too low a compression (blurring, summation artefact), leading to an unjustified increase in the dose delivered [33]. Therefore, it would be of particular importance to know the minimum value sufficient, with the same breast consistency to make a contrast-to-noise ratio (CNR) useful for diagnostic purposes (Chaps. 7 and 8). The lower limit suggested in this text is 80 N (8 daN), using the 18 × 24 cm compression paddle. Below this value, compression would be considered as ineffective. The upper limit is indicated as 18 daN, with a 24 × 30 cm compression paddle. For a more general evaluation, differences in the compression calibration of different mammographic units should certainly be considered. *Standardisation must however absolutely pursued, in compression as well as in positioning*, to produce examinations that are easily comparable by the reader, performed on the same patient but by different radiographers [34, 35]. Also, and it should not be underestimated, to provide consistent quality of the images produced over time, even by the same radiographer. The fluctuation of performance is particularly important in this specialised branch of biomedical diagnostic imaging.

In recent years, there has been a trend in Europe towards decreasing compression values, associated with the use of *pressure*. *Pressure is defined as the ratio between the mechanical force exerted on the breast and the contact area provided.* It is actually not an easy task calculat-

ing the contact area, and several methods have been proposed. They are not routinely implemented in breast departments, at least at present. The use of pressure, measured in Pascals ($1 Pa = 1 N/m^2$), has been suggested by several scholars as a system that allows for easier standardisation of compression, thus reducing: (1) the potential variation in quality of the images produced; (2) the risk of over-compression of small breasts, compared to larger breasts.

Some authors have suggested **10 kPa as the ideal pressure value**, which corresponds to 75 mmHg (millimetres of mercury), the value of arterial pressure [36, 37]. The rationale behind this choice is that the reduction in thickness above this value would be poor.

What is ultimately meant by the term "**compression**"? One could say, first of all, that the breast is not compressible, at least not in the strict sense, understanding compression as volume reduction. What is done in mammography is to reduce the thickness. However, if we consider the breast as a system in its own right, a theory supported by the Dutch colleague De Groot [37], a very small reduction in volume during compression is indeed there. It is achieved by the viscous effusion of blood and lymph towards the central systems, i.e. from the breast towards the thorax. As soon as the compression is removed, of course, the breast regains its original volume, and this is referred to as "*elastic deformation.*" The compression process can be divided into two phases, again according to De Groot: with the first one, the thickness and volume are reduced, and with the second, the breast is immobilised. The two phases are crucial for both the technical and clinical quality of mammography. The first phase, which the author has further divided into two parts, should be carried out slowly. If it is too fast, there could be an opposite reaction to the compression known as *creep*. It is a minimal effect and perhaps does not really tangibly affect the reconstructed image. Modern direct digital mammography units are based on *Automatic Exposure Control* (AEC), Chap. 7, which in effect takes thickness into account. These systems are thus based on the gradual reduction of thickness, as a function of the equally gradual increase in compression. This certainly requires a suitably progressive action in compression, in the first phase, which therefore, should not be too fast. On the other hand, the last step, which requires the radiographer to move from the mammographic unit to the acquisition station after sufficient compression is achieved, must be fast, to reduce patient discomfort.

Standardisation of compression is still a goal to be achieved nationally and worldwide and also important from the point of view of the constancy of the patient's experience. The list of steps recommended is shown in Table 11.2.

### 11.3.5 The Maximum Compression Value

As for the maximum compression value chosen for certain types of large, thick breasts, the reason this is necessary is that you do not want the breast to fall. But why is it so important? There are sev-

eral reasons for this: (a) if the breast falls, the inframammary fold is partially obliterated, or lost; (b) if it falls, it means that the compression of the anterior part of the breast is insufficient; (c) if the breast is pulled forward and up, the Cooper's ligaments appear to be well distributed, and a lesion can be detected much better than in a *fallen breast*, Fig. 11.3. In some cases, remaining below 18 daN is not sufficient to achieve the result presented in the first part of Fig. 11.3. There are two possible solutions:

1. The MLO can be performed with a lower obliquity than the default obliquity, which is 45° in Italy. It can be changed to 35 or even 30°. The breast is "lying" on the detector and does not fall off. *Any change in angle must obviously be reported;*

2. If absolutely necessary, a kind of Eklund manoeuvre can be used, the one used for the mammographic documentation of breast implant-carriers (Chap. 14). This involves moving the implant backwards in order to be able to compress the tissue in front of it. In this case, it is the pectoral muscle that is moved away from the FOV. As a result, there is a decrease in the thickness and density of tissue included in the FOV, which allows an optimal image to be obtained in the recommended compression range. The problem associated with this solution is about radiation protection, and two projections must be added. This approach should be therefore discussed and agreed upon with the radiologists of the centre in which one works, as we do in Italy, for its *justification,* according to Italian Legislative Decree 101/2020, transposition of the 2013/59/EURATOM (see Chap. 21). It should be limited to cases that cannot otherwise be resolved. In a good mammography positioning technique, this problem is addressed, and various solutions are recommended in this text, Chap. 9.

Some mammographic units have a threshold of the maximum compression value that cannot be exceeded. Others display a warning pop-up window, but the recommended threshold can be exceeded. In the technical part of the European Guidelines for Mammography Screening, the

**Table 11.2** Compression procedure: recommended steps

| 1 First phase First part | CC projection: breast is compressed (decreasing its thickness) up to a maximum, for an average breast, of 7–8 daN; skin folds are adjusted at the level of the IMF and at the most lateral part of the OQ; MLO projection: compression must be steady, and not interrupted until the breast is locked in position (steps 1–3 without interruption) |
|---|---|
| 2 First phase Second part | Both projections: Compressing by evaluating the deformation of the breast, and therefore the response or resistance of the breast being studied, which also depends on the speed at which the compression paddle is lowered: this step must be completed slowly, up to the value considered adequate |
| 3 Second phase | Immobilisation phase: a few more N than already compressed (it should be considered that the compression paddle tends to rise in response to breast resistance) |
| 4 | The radiographer moves from the mammographic unit to the image acquisition station: this step must be carried out very fast, to limit the patient's discomfort |
| 5 | The radiographer acquires, using words of motivation. Release |

**Fig. 11.3** Breast in correct position and droopy, in relation to the tissue documented and Cooper's ligaments

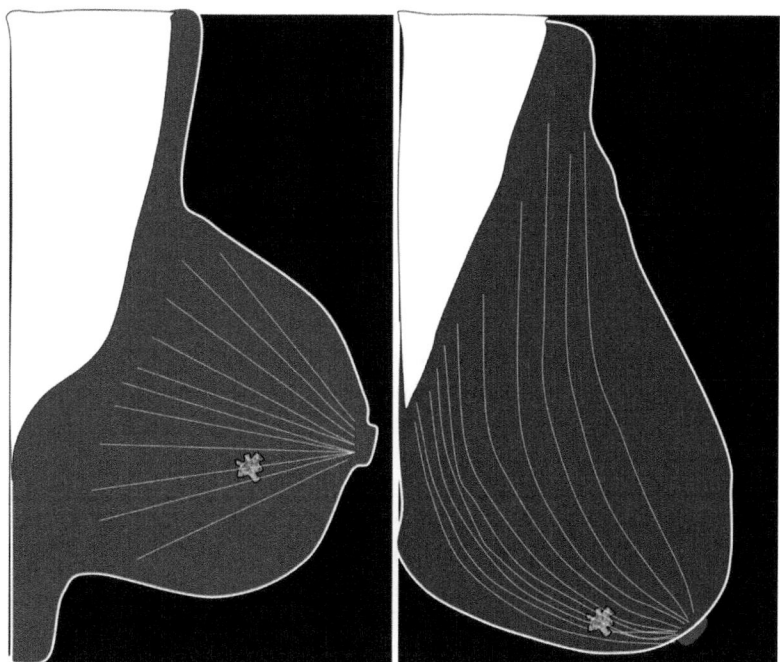

maximum value is 200 N, which can be understood as a limit not to go beyond, in the event of medico-legal disputes. Good positioning does not require such high values, however.

Interesting on the subject is a 2017 EPOS™ poster, by Ng et al. [38], which outlines the compression habits in mammography in many countries, internationally. Italian, Dutch, and particularly, Malaysian radiographers more frequently choose high compression values (compared to the global average).

**Supplementary Material on YouTube Channel @cristinapoggi7579**
For an in-depth discussion of compression in mammography, see the two lectures: Compression in mammography *Physics, chemistry anatomy and empathy of the process: Chaps. 1 and 2 (2021):*

- https://youtu.be/LxSuhj8Gbqk
- https://youtu.be/aHAxFZFCHQ8

### 11.3.6  Skin Folds in FFDM

The advent of the direct digital system led to a marked worsening of the presence of skin folds in the mammography image. *Since the dynamic range is infinitely wider than that of the analogue system, tissues of a considerable range of thickness and density can be visualised in the FOV.* As a result, skin folds can be seen very well, even the nipple, which was often out of range in the analogue system. This is also thanks to the application of the *skin edge filter.* Greater rigour in positioning is therefore required.

There are other problems related to the direct digital system: (a) the thickness of the detector has increased, and (b) the position of the face shields has changed, it has been moved a bit more towards the patient. This is true on average for all mammography machine manufacturers. Both make it more difficult to position the patient, particularly with regard to the inclusion of deeper tissues. See Chaps. 7 and 8 for technical quality, Chap. 23 for ergonomics in mammography and Chap. 26.

Another thing to be taken into account: there is only one detector, but there are usually two compression paddles, of different sizes, chosen according to the size of the breast. Changing the compressor delineates a so-called *active area,* i.e., one that can produce an image, which must exactly coincide with the light field. This area does not include the inner profile (the one towards the patient) of the detector. That is, there is a band of a certain width at this location, which is never active, because it is occupied by the electronics linking the mammographic unit and the radiographer's image acquisition workstation (Chap. 7). *Documenting the pectoral muscle in CC projection is then much more difficult than it was in the analogue system.* Of course, depth is also lost in the oblique projection. This non-active area differs depending on the manufacturer, averaging between 4 and 7 mm. Although all the manufacturing companies have been required to stay below 5 mm, not all of them have complied.

Furthermore, the active area is centred on the detector. When the small compression paddle, 18 × 24 cm, is used, the lateral and medial non-active area in the CC, and upper and lower in the MLO, becomes important (Chap. 7). In particular, the upper non-active area may force the patient's arm and shoulder to be positioned at an incorrect height in order to correctly centre the object in the FOV, for a good MLO projection. This problem is solved by a **compression paddle that shifts upwards**, associated with the activation of the upper area included by it.

For an evaluation of skin folds in mammography, and the strategies to correct them, see Chap. 17.

## References

1. Taylor K, et al. Mammographic image quality in relation to positioning of the breast: a multicentre international evaluation of the assessment systems currently used, to provide an evidence base for establishing a standardized methods of assessment. Radiography. 2017;23:343–9. https://doi.org/10.1016/j.radi.2017.03.004.
2. Dumky H, et al. The art of mammography with respect to positioning and compression-A Swedish perspective. J Radiol Nurs. 2018;37:41–8. https://doi.org/10.1016/j.jradnu.2017.11.006.
3. Huppe AI, et al. Mammography positioning standards in the digital era: is the status quo acceptable. AJR. 2017;209:1–7. https://doi.org/10.2214/AJR.16.17522.
4. Guertin M-H, et al. Clinical Image quality in daily practice of breast cancer mammography screening. Can Assoc Radiol J. 2014;65:199–206. https://doi.org/10.1016/j.carj.2014.02.001.
5. Borrelli C, et al. NHS breast screening programme. 4th ed. NHSBSP. Publication number 49, PHE publications gateway number 2016426; 2016.
6. Alukic' E, et al. The impact of subjective image quality evaluation in mammography. Radiography. 2023;29:526–32. https://www.sciencedirect.com/science/article/pii/S1078817423000585
7. Boyce M, et al. Comparing the use and interpretation of PGMI scoring to assess the technical quality of screening mammograms in the UK and Norway. Radiography. 2015;21(4):342–7.
8. Whelehan P, et al. Observer variability in accept/reject classification of clinical image quality in mammography. EPOS ™ ECR. 2015; https://doi.org/10.1594/ecr2015/C-2432.
9. Perry N, et al. European guidelines for quality assurance in breast cancer screening and diagnosis. European Communities; 2006. ISBN 92-79-01258-4
10. Gullien R, et al. Identifying the most common deviations in mediolateral-oblique (MLO) mammograms classified as "moderate" before and after implementation of improvement initiatives. EPOS ™ ECR; 2010. https://doi.org/10.1594/ecr2010/B-059.
11. Gullien R, et al. PGMI score of baseline mammograms before interval cancers in a population-based screening program. EPOS ™ ECR; 2016. https://doi.org/10.1594/ecr2016/C-0675.
12. Spurr K, et al. Mammography image quality: model for predicting compliance with posterior nipple line criterion. EJR. 2011;80:713–8. https://doi.org/10.1016/j.ejrad.2010.06.026.
13. Galli V, et al. Il Protocollo di valutazione della qualità tecnica dell'esame mammografia Contributi 95. Regione Emilia Romagna; 2017.
14. Galli V, et al. An Image quality review programme in a population-based mammography screening service. J Med Radiat Sci. 2021;68:253–9. https://doi.org/10.1002/jmrs.487.
15. ACR Clinical Image Testing: Mammography (Revised 3-3-2023). https://accreditationsupport.acr.org/support/solutions/articles/11000065937-clinical-image-testing-mammography-revised-3-3-2023
16. Sweeney R-J, et al. A review of mammographic positioning image quality criteria for the craniocaudal projection. Br J Radiol. 2018;91(1082):20170611.
17. Bentley K, et al. Mammography image quality: analysis of evaluation criteria using pectoral muscle presentation. Radiography. 14(3):189–94. https://doi.org/10.1016/j.radi.2007.02.002.
18. Spurr K, Poulos A. Evaluation of the pectoral muscle in mammography images: the Australian experience. EJR. p. 12–21. https://doi.org/10.1016/j.ejradi.2008.11.003.
19. Vee B, et al. Chapter 5: directions for radiographers in the quality assurance manual of the Norwegian breast cancer screening program (NBCSP), Oslo, 2011: 10. https://www.kreftregisteret.no/globalassets/mammografiprogrammet/arkiv-publikasjoner-og-brosjyrer/kval-man-radiograf_v1.0_innholdsfortegnelse.pdf
20. Miller LC. Mammography positioning basic and advanced. SBI; 2016. https://www.sbi-online.org/Portals. Accessed 2017

21. Dustler M, et al. Pattern of pressure distribution at mammography: room for improvement? ESR ECR; 2012. https://doi.org/10.1594/ecr2012/C-7251.

22. O'leary D, et al. Compression force recommendations in mammography must be linked to image quality. ECR; 2011. https://doi.org/10.1594/ecr2011/C-0427.

23. van Goethem M, et al. Influence of the radiographer on the pain felt during mammography. Eur Radiol. 2003;13:2384–9. https://doi.org/10.1007/s00330-002-1686-6.

24. Whelehan P, et al. The effect of mammography pain on repeat participation in breast cancer screening: a systematic review. Breast. 2013;22:389–94. https://doi.org/10.1016/j.breast.2013.03.003.

25. Feder K, Jens-Holger G. Is individualizing breast compression during mammography useful? Investigation of pain indications during mammography relating to compression force and surface area of the compressed breast. Fortschr Röntgenstr. 2017;189:39–48. https://doi.org/10.1055/s-0042-119450.

26. Arthur L. Effects of verbal communication experiences of discomfort in women undergoing mammography examinations. J Sci Multidiscip Res. 2013, 1;5. ISSN; 2277-0135

27. IASP. http://www.iasp-pain.org

28. Nightingale JM, et al. Breast compression-an exploration of problem solving and decision making in mammography. University of Salford. https://shura.shu.ac.uk/19045/8/Nightingale-BreastCompression%28AM%29.pdf

29. Murphy F, et al. Compression force behaviours: an exploration of the belief and values influencing the application of breast compression during screening mammography. Radiography. 2015;21:30–5. https://doi.org/10.1016/j.radi.2014.05.009.

30. Moshina N, et al. Breast compression and early performance measure in the Norwegian breast cancer screening program. ECR; 2017. https://doi.org/10.1594/ecr2017/C_0619.

31. Holland K, et al. Influence of breast compression pressure on the performance of population-based mammography screening. Breast Cancer Res. 2017;19:126. https://doi.org/10.1186/s13058-017-0917-3.

32. Mercer CE, et al. Does an increase in compression force really improve visual image quality in mammography? An initial investigation. Radiography. 2013;19:363–5. https://doi.org/10.1016/j.radi.2013.07.002.

33. Ma WK, et al. Blurred digital mammography images: an analysis of technical recall and observer detection performance, B. J Radiol. 2017;90(1071):20160271.

34. Branderhorst W. Mammographic compression: a need for mechanical standardization. Eur J Radiol. 2015;84:596–602. https://pubmed.ncbi.nlm.nih.gov/25596915/

35. Mercer CE, et al. Practitioner compression force variability in mammography: a preliminary study. Br J Radiol. 2013;86:20110596. https://pubmed.ncbi.nlm.nih.gov/23385990/

36. Waade GG, et al. Compression forces used in Norwegian breast cancer screening program. BJR. 2017;90(1071):20160770. https://doi.org/10.1259/bjr.20160770.

37. De Groot JE. Pressure-standardized breast compression in mammography, University of Amsterdam UvA-DARE (Digital Academic Repository). 2015. https://dare.uva.nl/search?identifier=ab9a2862-5bcd-410a-8bdb-e6c81793526e

38. Ng KH, et al. Large variation in mammography compression internationally. ECR; 2017. p. C-2133. https://doi.org/10.1594/ecr2017/C-2133.

# Clinical Quality Evaluation

# 12

## 12.1 Percentages of the Various Classes in PGMI and POBMI Evaluation Systems

In the **PGMI** system (P perfect, G good, M mediocre, I inadequate), the percentages of the various classes in which mammographies are sorted are listed in Table 12.1.

In the **POBMI** system in use in Italy, elaborated by Galli, V., breast radiographer, used in the Region Emilia Romagna and in other Italian regions, the Inadequate percentage is the same (<3%), in relation to PGMI, as is the sum of Perfect, Optimal, Good (Buono) and Mediocre (>97%). The percentage of the mediocre exams, on the other hand, is much lower (<12%) [1]. An example of optimum (almost perfect) exam is in Fig. 12.1.

The objective is not trivial, also as a result of the extreme variability in quality evaluation, not only between countries but also between mammographers in the same centre. This is why various automatic scoring systems based on *Artificial Intelligence (AI)* [2, 3] have been proposed and are evolving, see Chap. 24. The classes to focus the attention on to improve the radiographer's performance are the mediocre inadequate. They are also the most recognisable:

– **Mediocre exams:** (a) part of the tissue is absent, to a small extent; (b) the nipple may not be in profile, by a few degrees, but it must be in the other projection of the corresponding side [AN: to be added to the above: *in the case of breasts with upper/lower quadrants in the CC projection, and medial/lateral quadrants in the MLO projection of equal size. If they are not equal, the nipple condition in profile should not be sought*]. Specifically in MLO projection, c) the muscle may not be of the correct length, not reaching PNL by more than 1 cm (Chaps. 11 and 25) (d) artefacts and/or minimal asymmetries may be present. *Technical quality must be high, and mammogram of poor technical quality is always inadequate.*

– **Inadequate exams:** (a) a large part of the tissue is missing; (b) compression is insufficient; (c) artefacts and folds obscure the tissue and prevent it from being read [AN: to be added: *where the acquisition geometry has not been met, so in addition to the loss of tissue, the breast is deformed due to incorrect rotation and stretching*]; (d) the technical quality is poor (Chaps. 7 and 8) and does not allow for easy and sufficient reading.

© The Author(s), under exclusive license to Springer Nature Switzerland AG 2024
C. Poggi, *Breast Imaging Techniques for Radiographers*,
https://doi.org/10.1007/978-3-031-63314-0_12

**Table 12.1** PGMI system percentages

| | |
|---|---|
| P o G | =75% |
| P + G + M | >97% |
| M | <22% |
| I | <3% |

**Fig. 12.1** Almost perfect mammography examination

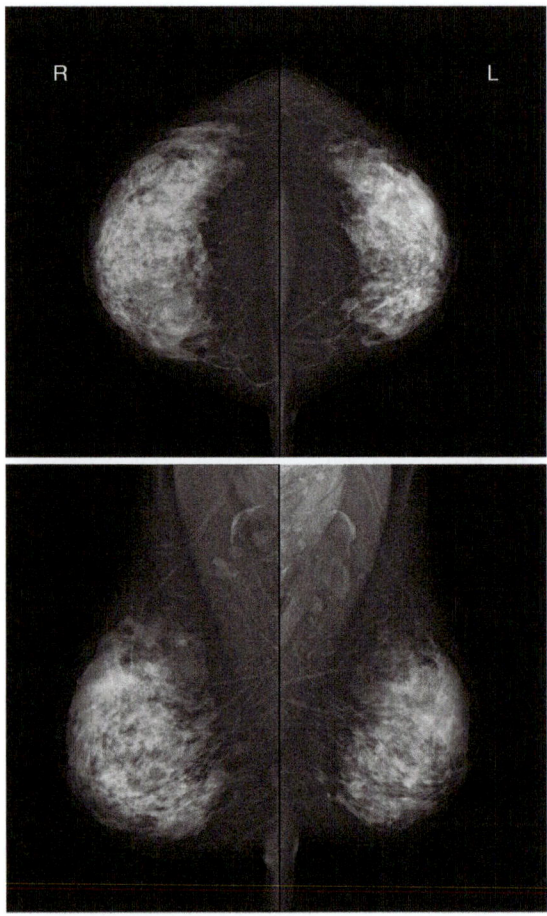

## 12.2 Common Errors in the Two Standard Projections

According to a paper presented by Reis et al. [3], at the 2014, ECR European Congress of Radiology ECR, the most common errors in CC are skin folds, hence, the presence of the other breast. Regarding MLO projections, the most common errors are the folds in the pectoralis muscle, followed closely by failure to document the IMF. The main problem observed during the work of the writer during the implementation in the VMM project, Valutazione Miglioramento e Monitoraggio, Evaluation Improvement and Monitoring of the performance of breast radiographers (Poggi C) [4], in both projections, is the incomplete documentation of tissue, in particular, of the deep tissue planes. The most difficult CC quality criteria to satisfy were the insufficient documentation of the inner quadrant and the retromammary space. Both are due to failure to meet the *acquisition geometry parameters* (Chap. 9). In MLOs, folds in the pectoralis may indeed be a problem especially in thin patients, but, according to the data collected in the VMM, the most common is the incomplete documentation of the IMF, that is either undocumented or obliterated by major folds. In some cases, also the POSTINFQ is missing (see Chap. 25). It is interesting to note that the second most difficult criterion to meet in order of importance is not the same in the different centres studied in the VMM project. This prompts reflections on the paramount importance of the initial training of radiographers who will work in Senology, the need for standardisation and frequent retraining [5].

## 12.3   When to Repeat?

An image must be re-acquired not for the sake of aesthetics, not to do the perfect examination at all costs, even when the anatomical and pathological condition of the patient does not allow it, and not to prove to someone that we have superior skills. *A mammography image is to be repeated for one reason only: The examination must be diagnostic. The PGMI system can be used as a guide to achieve a conscious review of image quality, especially in the learning phase, for the standardisation of positioning techniques.* Its validity lies primarily in identifying the areas of difficulty, i.e. those aspects of positioning that require improvement. Focused training should then be provided. It is therefore an important tool for breast radiographers to achieve a quality of mammography offered to users that is more than adequate for diagnostic purposes. In the writer's judgement, considering a training project that is wide-ranging, once all the operators in the area considered have reached a good level of quality, the assessment could be decidedly simplified. That is to say going towards the identification of systematic error, leaving aside the mere classification of examinations. This idea was supported by the project currently being implemented on the assessment of the performance of the breast radiographer, led by *ISPRO (Institute for the Study, Prevention and Oncological Network,* Florence), and proposed for the Tuscany region, the "288." The same English Guidelines for screening mammographers published in 2017 state that the PGMI system can no longer be considered sufficient [6]. In the aforementioned VMM project, implemented in 2019 in the central Tuscany area, and then interrupted by the Sars-CoV-2 pandemic, a method was proposed to assess the failure to meet the quality criteria. The system is called **POint**, was developed by the writer and takes into account "the degree of deviation" from the satisfaction of each criterion (see Chap. 27).

## 12.4   Cataloguing Errors

There are three types of errors that can be considered in mammography, **TE Technical Errors**, **TP Technical Repetitions** and **TC Technical Recalls** [7] (usually called just *inadequate* in Italy) (see Table 12.2).

The **TRs** (*repeat examinations*, or total errors), sum of TP and TC, should be analysed by *audit*, among colleagues. Very useful would be the comparison with the reporters, who may not realise the difficulties of performing this examination.

*Audit is understood as a process of quality improvement, through systematic and regular review of work. It is based on the identification of the degree of inappropriateness of processes with respect to reference guidelines, and aims to implement a plan for change, which must be constructive and plural.* Creating and participating in audits

**Table 12.2**  Type of catalogable error in mammography

| | |
|---|---|
| TE | *Technical error*: when the radiographer recognises that the projection is unacceptable from a technical quality point of view (default of the mammographic unit, non-completion of the acquisition) |
| TP | *Technical repeat*: when the radiographer makes an evaluation of the clinical quality of the newly acquired image, and realises that it is unacceptable, for (a) not correct extension or stretching of the tissue acquired, (b) due to positioning mistakes, or (c) to kinetic blurring, for example. The image is immediately repeated, *when she/he considers that conditions exist for obtaining a better image* |
| TC | *Technical Recall*: it is made by the reader who considers a projection to be inadequate and therefore insufficient for reading, and asks for it to be repeated. The radiographer had considered it to be sufficient, or that better results could not be obtained (*difficulties encountered due to the patient's lack of effective compliance, whatever the reason, must be made explicit in the notes*) |
| TR | *Total errors* = TP + TC |

is without doubts a fundamental instrument for the professional development of all health operators.

### 12.4.1 Technical Recalls

In Italy, there is a tendency to make a higher percentage of recalls in mammography screening than in other European countries, particularly compared to Northern Europe. This is mainly for patients who have the examination for the first time. However, almost all of them are recalls for suspected lesions, the so-called **second-level examinations or callbacks** (Chap. 13). Technical recalls are very few (mean data, different from a region to another). To be more precise, too few, far below the percentage recommended by the European Guidelines, set below 3% (acceptable value), and ≤1% as desirable value. This is referred to as the **"under-calling phenomenon"** [7]. Moreover, in many cases, technical recalls are not recorded, or only partially. It is certainly worth mentioning that they must be recorded, also because they add up to the dose delivered to the patient. Discarded images have to be included too. Repeated projections, whether TE, TP or TC, are actively controlled in the USA, according to MQSA rules [8].

As shown by an interesting study carried out by Vania Galli on the agreement between radiologist and radiographer on clinical quality assessment, it can be inferred that those reporting are less rigorous than those who produce mammograms [9]. Regrettably, the reader's lack of rigour has a negative impact on the radiographer's work. It must be considered the impact on the quality of the service provided, in terms of the quality of the images produced, of tissue extension and fidelity of reproduction, and consequently, in terms of the number of diagnoses [10].

### 12.5 Usefulness of a Clinical Quality Evaluation System in Mammography

The application of a clinical quality classification system, such as the PGMI, the POBMI derived from it, or the POint, is used to develop protocols to achieve high standards. Among other things, it can be shared between different centres. It allows image quality monitoring and provides the expertise that makes radiographers recognise which mammography is not optimal for diagnostic purposes [11–13]. Finally, it is useful to analyse which projections do not meet the quality criteria, in terms of type and frequency, and consequently *highlight the training needs.*

Focused training must be organised on them, as proposed in the VMM project.

The job of the breast radiographer is one of great responsibility. It is a duty to produce mammograms of a high quality, because performing mammography well, and having a closer cooperation with the reporter, means reducing the number of missed diagnoses associated with poor technique [14].

Given the complexity and subjectivity associated with the visual assessment of images produced in mammography, the use of **Deep Learning (DL)** in this field has been considered in recent years (see Chap. 24). This should be viewed as an extension and not as a restriction of the skills required for our professional role. Learning and using AI techniques is not easy to date [2, 15, 16]. Furthermore, given radiographer and reporter competence, AI implementation in breast imaging could have the potential to address, or even solve, medico-legal issues [16].

See Chaps. 25, 26, 27 and Annex 1.

### References

1. Galli V, et al. Il Protocollo di valutazione della qualità tecnica dell'esame mammografia Contributi 95. Regione Emilia Romagna; 2017.
2. Johnston L, Highnam R. White paper TruPGMI: AI for mammography quality improvement 2022. https://www.volparahealth.com/app/uploads/2022/06/AI-for-mammography-quality-improvement.pdf
3. Reis C, et al. Failure on clinical image quality criteria in digital Mammography-how can radiographers do better? PPT slide show in European Congress of Radiology. 2014. https://repositorio.ipl.pt/handle/10400.21/4781?locale=en
4. Poggi C. Valutazione Miglioramento e Monitoraggio VMM della performance del tecnico di radiologia operante in senologia nell'Area Toscana Centro, Le buone pratiche organizzative delle Aziende Sanitarie

Italiane, *Federsanità Anci*, edizione speciale Sanità 4.0. 2019.

5. Cataliotti L, et al. Guidelines on the standards for the training of specialized health professionals dealing with breast cancer. EJC. 2007;43:660–75. https://doi.org/10.1016/j.ejca.2006.12.008.

6. Borrelli C, et al. NHS breast screening programme guidance for breast screening mammographers. 3rd ed. Public Health England. Publication gateway number: 2017607; 2017.

7. FDA. https://www.accessdata.fda.gov/cdrh_docs/presentations/pghs/How_many_films_(and_what_type)_must_be_included_in_the_repeat_analysis_test_each_quarter_.htm

8. Galli V. Carcinomi di intervallo e qualità tecnica Evoluzione di un monitoraggio divenuto collaborativo, *Gisma*-Torino, 25-9-2013 PPT.

9. Blancks R, et al. NHS breast screening programme guidance on collecting, monitoring and reporting technical recall and repeat examinations. Public Health England. Publication gateway number: 2017608. 2017,

10. Boyce M, et al. Comparing the use and interpretation of PGMI scoring to assess the technical quality of screening mammograms in the UK and Norway. Radiography. 2015;21(4):342–7. https://doi.org/10.1016/j.radi.2015.05.006.

11. Reis C, et al. Quality assurance and quality control in mammography: a review of available guidance worldwide. Insight Imaging. 2013;4:539–53. https://doi.org/10.1007/s13244-013-0269-1.

12. Rouette J, et al. Evaluation of the quality of mammographic breast positioning: a quality improvement study. CMAJ Open. 2021;9:E607–12. https://doi.org/10.9778/cmajo20200211.

13. Hendersson LM, et al. The influence of mammography technologists on radiologists' ability to interpret screening mammograms in community practice. Acad Radiol. 2015;22(3):278–89. https://doi.org/10.1016/j.acra.2014.09.013.

14. Watanabe H, et al. Quality control system for mammographic breast positioning using deep learning. Sci Rep. 2023;13:7066. https://doi.org/10.1038/s41598-023-34380-9.

15. Walsh G, et al. Responsible AI practice and AI education are central to AI implementation: a rapid review for all medical imaging professional in Europe. BJR Open. 2023;5(1):20230033. https://doi.org/10.1259/bjro.20230033.

16. Sechopoulos I, et al. Artificial intelligence for breast cancer detection in mammography and digital breast tomosynthesis: state of the art. Semin Cancer Biol. 2021;72:214–25. https://doi.org/10.1016/j.semcancer.2020.06.002.

# Mammographic Findings, Recalls and Triangulation

**13**

## 13.1 Mammographic Findings

An aid to the radiographer in understanding whether the mammography produced is optimal for diagnostic purposes comes from knowing which radiological aspects the reporter looks for in the images (Fig. 13.1). They in fact may be the target of *second-level or in-depth examinations or recall, or callbacks.* **The three most important findings are microcalcifications, masses and distortions.**

The *microcalcifications are calcium deposits,* extremely small in size, ranging from a few tens to a few hundred micron (one micron is equal to $10^{-6}$ mm).

In order to be studied, they require a very low level of *blurring*, the overall technical quality must be very high, but they are characterised by *high contrast*, and, as a result, are generally well detectable (Chaps. 7 and 8).

*Masses* are lesions that occupy space in three dimensions and therefore should be seen in both projections, unless there are summation artefacts hiding them. They can, however, have a very low contrast, i.e. the same density as the healthy tissue around them. This is why *low contrast resolution* is crucial in mammography (Chaps. 7 and 8).

*Distortions* are areas of convergence associated with tissue retraction, but only in rare cases do they involve local skin retraction, the *dimpling* (Chaps. 3 and 4). Usually, they are barely noticeable.

*Asymmetry* can also be mentioned: It is defined as a dense area that is larger than the same area in the contralateral breast.

Mammography is an accurate, sensitive and specific examination (see Chap. 6). *There is an important correlation between the mammographic findings that the doctor looks for on the images, the histological characteristics of the lesion and their histological grade* (Chap. 5) [1, 2].

### 13.1.1 Microcalcifications [3, 4]

If the mammography images are of *high technical* and *clinical quality*, the reader can study the morphology, number and distribution of **microcalcifications.** If the breast has not been rigorously positioned, their location and distribution may be altered. Adequate compression is also essential for morphology. Depending on these three parameters, morphology, number and distribution, a *degree of suspicion* is assigned to the finding (Fig. 13.2); with the intermediate-low grade, a *biopsy* may anyway be recommended (Chap. 18).

### 13.1.2 Masses (Mass Lesions) [5, 6]

With regard to **masses**, the fundamental descriptor, in addition to shape, is *margin*. High spatial resolution, accuracy in positioning and adequate

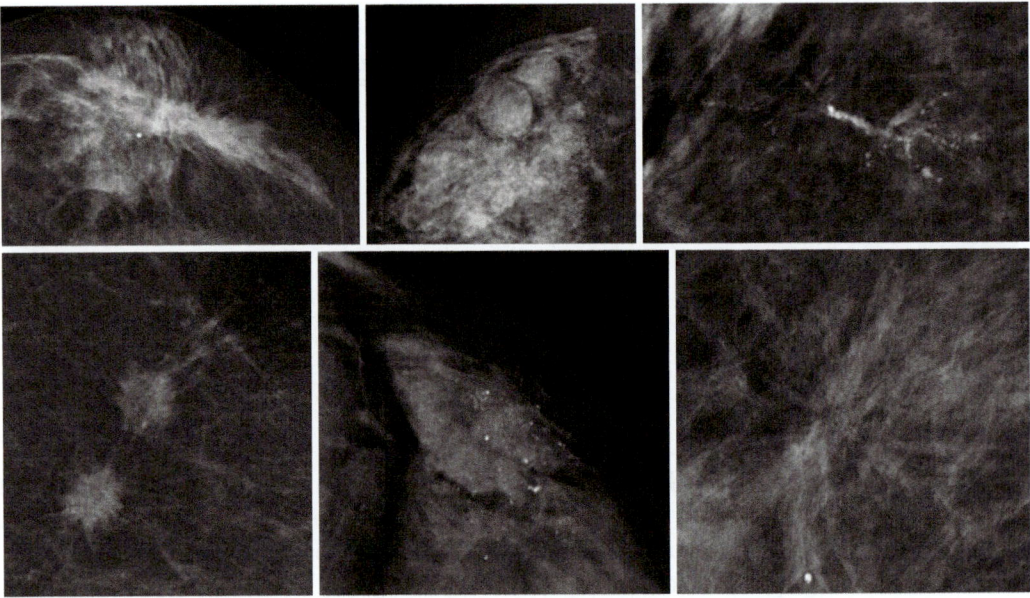

**Fig. 13.1** Mammographic findings: distortions, masses, microcalcifications

**Fig. 13.2** Classification of level of suspicion from 2 to 5 for microcalcifications, according to the BI-RADS® system

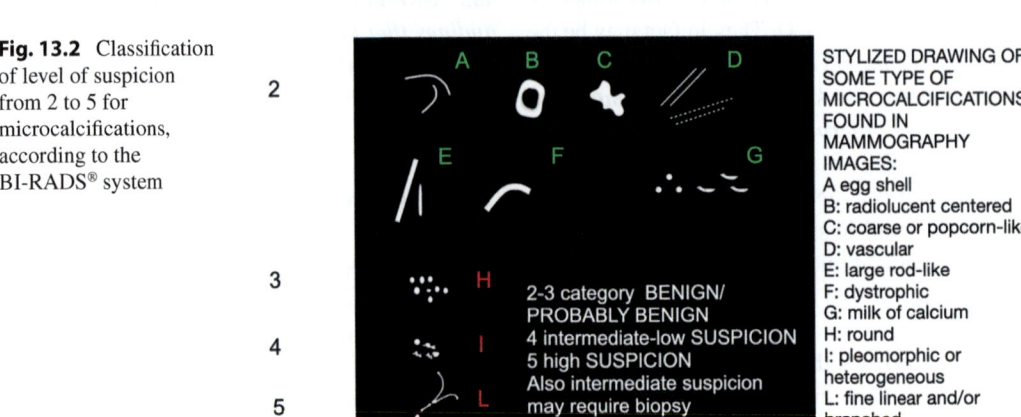

compression are again required (Fig. 13.3). Suboptimal compression introduces a blurring of the margins, i.e. it increases the *geometric penumbra* (see Annex 2). It impairs the ability to study them and be classified exactly. The most suspicious are the irregular margins, and this irregularity is due to *the invasion of the basal membrane and the surrounding tissue*, which is in turn responsible for the *desmoplastic effects* mentioned in Chaps. 3 and 4. Peritumoral features in non-spiculated and non-calcified masses are the base of *radiomics* and *deep learning (DL)* studies [7].

The increase in geometric unsharpness from inadequate compression also introduces a fictitious increase in lesion size.

### 13.1.3 (Architectural) Distortions [8, 9]

Distortions of the architecture of the Fibro-Glandular Tissue (FGT) are also an important finding, and perhaps the most difficult to diagnose, because:

**Fig. 13.3** Classification of level of suspicion, from 2 to 5 for masses, according to the BI-RADS® system

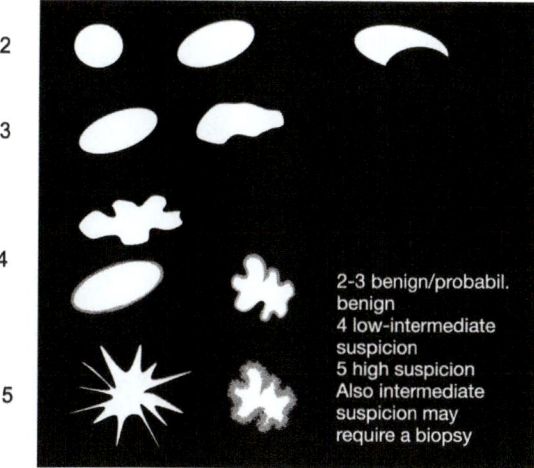

STYLIZED DRAWING OF MASSES LESIONS FOUND IN MAMMOGRAPHY IMAGES

Regular shape and well defined margins benign or low level of suspicion for malignancy

Irregular shape and ill-defined margins are more suspicious for malignancy

2-3 benign/probabil. benign
4 low-intermediate suspicion
5 high suspicion
Also intermediate suspicion may require a biopsy

1. They can be confused with benign lesions;
2. Their detection depends almost entirely on positioning and compression, and therefore on the work of the breast radiographer, which can be of varying quality. In fact, comparing examinations performed by different radiographers can be very difficult. This makes standardisation of the procedure, for positioning and compression, as repeatedly emphasised, an indispensable necessity.

### 13.1.4 Asymmetries [10]

Detecting **asymmetries** is made possible, in particular when they are very small, by the perfect symmetry of the right and left projections. Therefore, this quality criterion makes clinical sense and it is not just aesthetics. In current mammographic machines, anyway, the alignment of images on display workstations is automatic, following the *DICOM Hanging Protocols* for Mammography (see Chaps. 8 and 16).

### 13.2 Assessment or Characterisation of a Suspicious Finding: Second-Level Examinations or Recalls [11–13]

Once the suspicious finding has been verified as real and localised in both projections (but this is not always the case), in order to characterise it

("*assessment*") in itself, and with regard to its relationship with the immediately surrounding tissue, the reporter may request two different specific radiographic **examinations.** They are also called **Level 2** examinations (because after Level 1, which is the standard examination), and are:

– The *focal compression or* **spot view;**
– The *magnification view and mag spot view*.

### 13.2.1 Spot View

The same projection where the suspect finding was visualised is performed, or, if it is clearly identifiable in both, in the two projections, CC and MLO. A compression paddle smaller than in standard examination is used: It allows for greater and more effective compression, and to reach more posterior portions of tissue. Great care must be taken that the lesion under investigation is included in the FOV. The compression used in fact is such that the lesion may be pushed away from it, because is very small (the rest of the area is rendered *inactive,* see Chaps. 7, 9 and 11). The procedure involves loading the baseline examination on the image acquisition monitor, i.e. the first-level examination on which the suspected finding was found (Fig. 13.4). On it, measurements are taken, at magnification 1:1. In depth in relation to the lesion, i.e. anteroposteriorly, line 1, AB. Then, the distance from the intersection, B, between line 1 and line 2, perpendicular to each other, superolaterally in the MLO, medial-laterally in the CC, in

**Fig. 13.4** Centring procedure in spot/mag view: measurement in AP (depth), for the two projection, and laterally (CC) and superiorly (MLO) for centring the finding located in the UOQ, right breast. Line 1: lesion depth from the nipple AB; line 2, perpendicular to 1, from intersection B to lesion C. Line 3: from lesion to skin, continuation of line 2

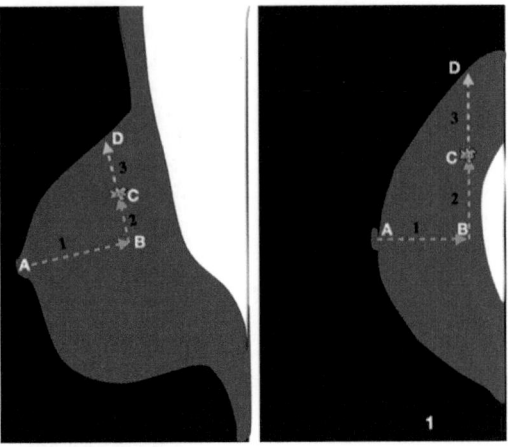

the direction of the lesion itself, C, expressed by the measurement BC. It may also be interesting to assess the distance of the lesion from the skin, line 3, CD, continuation from line 2. The measurement of the AB and BC distances is generally done using one's own fingers, as can be seen in Fig. 13.5, which is then replicated on the patient's skin to centre the acquisition.

*Positioning the patient for the acquisition of a level 2 requires that the breast is x-rayed in the same condition as in level 1 (the standard examination).* See Table 13.1 for the performing steps. Placing the breast on the detector tracing as much as possible the position of the breast in the baseline examination is not a trivial procedure, the breast being mobile and the standardisation of the positioning technique not yet achieved. This is especially true if the baseline examination has not been acquired satisfying the *acquisition geometry parameters* (Chap. 9). Generally, the radiologist indicates the position of the finding using the *quadrant* subdivision system (Chap. 3). It should also be emphasised that since the compression paddle used is much smaller, and the force is concentrated on an equally smaller area, the sensation of pressure, and discomfort, is worse than in the standard examination (with the same compression value). This must be explained to the patient, and it adds to the general discomfort of being recalled. The relational approach is therefore fundamental, understandably, which is dealt with extensively in Chap. 24.

*The spot view is generally required for the study of nodular (mass) type lesions.*

## 13.2.2 Magnification View

It is most commonly used as a level 2 examination when studying microcalcifications, or to study the margins of a lesion in detail. *Magnification* is obtained by placing a support directly on the detector that moves the breast away from the image plane. Depending on the height of the support, there will be a different magnification factor (the higher it is, the greater the magnification). **Typical values are x1.5, x1.8 or x2.** The height of the support increases the distance of the object from the image plane **Object to Image Distance (OID).** The greater the OID, the greater the magnification, but the *geometric unsharpness or penumbra* also increases. This is a parameter to be taken into account, partly compensated for by the use of an ultra-fine focus (Chap. 7). However, deep lesions, towards the chest wall, that is to say on the cathode side, will always be of a less image quality than those located anteriorly, towards the nipple. This is due to the *line focus principle* (dealt with in Chap. 7). There is in fact a greater geometric penumbra on the cathode side (see Annex 2). On the other hand, as seen in Fig. 13.6, the **Source to Object Distance (SOD)** decreases. This means that the number of intercepted photons per area increases, compared to contact mammography, and this

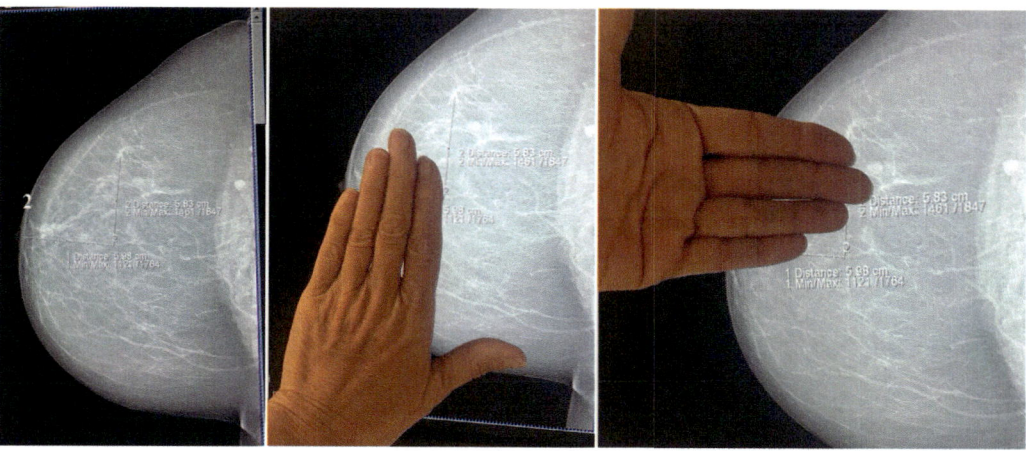

**Fig. 13.5** Fingers measurement: in the example showed, 4 fingers in depth and 4 laterally (WW and WL chosen to visualise the skin edge)

**Table 13.1** Steps in performing spot and mag view as 2 level exam

1 **Recall the first level examination**: Check that the finding indicated to be characterised is visible on the monitor of the acquisition workstation (often at a lower resolution with respect to the reporting workstation). Then, if the side corresponds with what is indicated

2 **Verify that the level 1 examination projection(s) are of high quality from the point of view of the acquisition geometry**. If not, the position of the finding will not be as indicated by the projections, and it will be necessary to repeat it/them

3 **If the first level examination has been performed well, it is possible to measure the distance of the finding antero-posteriorly from the nipple in CC, and supero-inferiorly in MLO**. The breast should be examined in the same conditions (as far as possible) in which it was X-rayed in the first level

4 **We insert the spot compression paddle (or the MAG spot paddle**, after placing the appropriate platform, see next section) **and centre the finding** possibly **in the centre of the FOV**. Measurements are taken on the first level mammography, using the two distances, to find the point of convergence between them

4 **The patient should be advised that compression may be more painful** (smaller contact area, given the smaller size of the compressor, for the same compression)

5 **The result of each projection performed by spot or mag spot paddle must be verified for clinical quality** (for sufficient diagnostic information)

leads to an improvement in SNR. Due to the ultrafine focus and low KiloVoltage, typical of mammography, there is an increased exposure time in the magnification view. This is particularly important in dense breasts and for high thicknesses of compressed tissue. There is also an increase in the risk of kinetic blurring. This is why it may be useful to ask the patient to hold her breath during acquisition.

Contrast is also improved with a magnification view, thanks to the gap (OID) between the breast and the image plane, which reduces scattered radiation. For this reason, the grid is not used in this examination; as a result, there is a reduction of the delivered dose by a factor of 2–3. However, given that the breast is closer to the source, the dose increases by approximately the same factor by the *inverse square law*. Therefore, *all else being equal, the dose in magnification is approximately similar to, or just above, that delivered in contact examinations.* As far as the centring of the lesion is concerned, the procedure used is the same as for the spot view, preceded by the placing of the appropriate platform. Even in magnification, the compression paddle is usually smaller (mag spot).

A true **lateral ML or LM** is first acquired (Chap. 10), to *triangulate* the lesion exactly (see

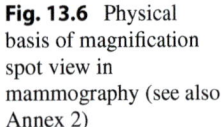 **Fig. 13.6** Physical basis of magnification spot view in mammography (see also Annex 2)

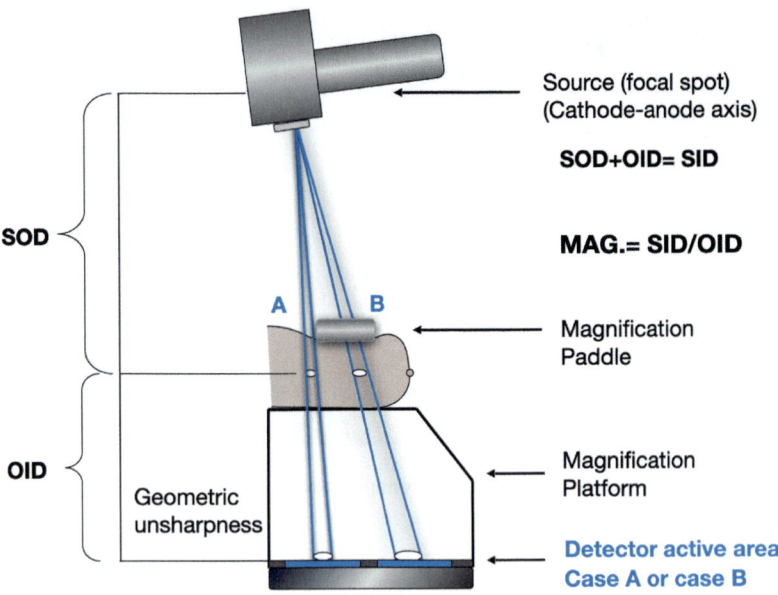

Source (focal spot)
(Cathode-anode axis)

**SOD+OID= SID**

SOD

**MAG.= SID/OID**

A     B

Magnification
Paddle

OID

Magnification
Platform

Geometric
unsharpness

Detector active area
Case A or case B

below). The positioning of the patient is the same as for the standard examination, taking care to centre the lesion in the available FOV. In addition to magnification in CC projection, the magnification in lateral projection is preferably acquired.

## 13.3    Triangulation [14–16]

*Triangulation in mammography means that a series of operations by which a lesion that can be seen in only one of the two projections can be located in the other.* The term is derived from navigation techniques, whereby a point in space is determined by the convergence of measurements from two other distinct points. It should be kept in mind that: *(1) no single projection can, under any circumstances, document all areas of the breast; (2) each quadrant is documented differently depending on the projection; (3) the nipple is the only fixed (reference) point on the image.* In other words, it must always be remembered that mammography is a two-dimensional representation of a 3D object. The purpose of triangulation is to establish whether a lesion is real or due to a summation artefact. If it is real, implement the techniques, radiological or otherwise, that offer the reporter the best possible characterisation of the lesion.

### 13.3.1    Straight-Line Triangulation Method

In the event that the lesion to be characterised is seen in the oblique projection, but not in the CC, the straight-line triangulation method can be used (Fig. 13.7). ML is performed, and the lesion location is observed. Let us assume that the lesion is seen in the CQ (central quadrant) in the MLO projection, and in the UQ in the lateral projection. A line joining the two lesions is drawn and continued to the CC projection. In the case of a right breast, as shown in Fig. 13.7, the lesion will be located in the medial quadrants (red-dotted line); if the lesion is observed in the LQ in the lateral projection, the lesion will be located in the lateral quadrant of the CC (light blue-dotted line).

It was important for the success of this technique in the analogue SF system:

- Place the three projections side by side, in this sequence ML, MLO, CC;
- That they had the same zooming;
- That the nipple was on the same level.

However, this concept can be transferred to the FFDM system (Full Field Digital Mammography, Chap. 7).

It can be observed that the actual location of the lesion in the superior inferior direction is not the same observed in the MLO projection. The lesion moves down or up, in relation to the real location, depending on where it is located in the laterolateral sense, i.e. in the CC projection. *The real location of the lesion in the superoinferior direction can only be assessed on the lateral projection.* This is why this projection (ML or LM) is required in second-level examinations.

Chapter 25 for further explanations; compare also Figs. 13.7 and 13.8.

**ITALIAN MNEMONIC HINT** *(©cpog-gimammoedu):* "si raccolgono mele nelle lande"

- **LA LESIONE MEdiale saLE ("Muffins rise")** o *MELE.*
- **LA LESIONE LAterale sceNDE ("Lead sinks")** o *LANDE.*

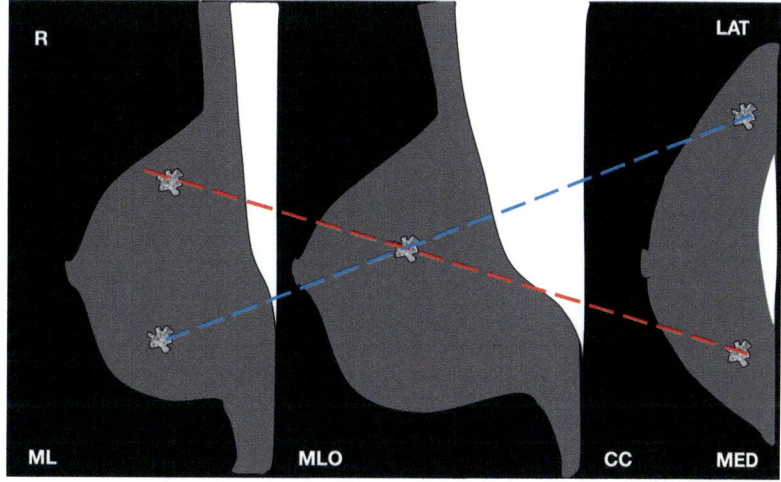

**Fig. 13.7** Straight-line triangulation method. Triangulation on the right breast, lesion "rising" on the lateral from its position on the MLO, will be in the medial portion in the CC (red-dotted line). See also Fig. 13.8 and Chap. 25

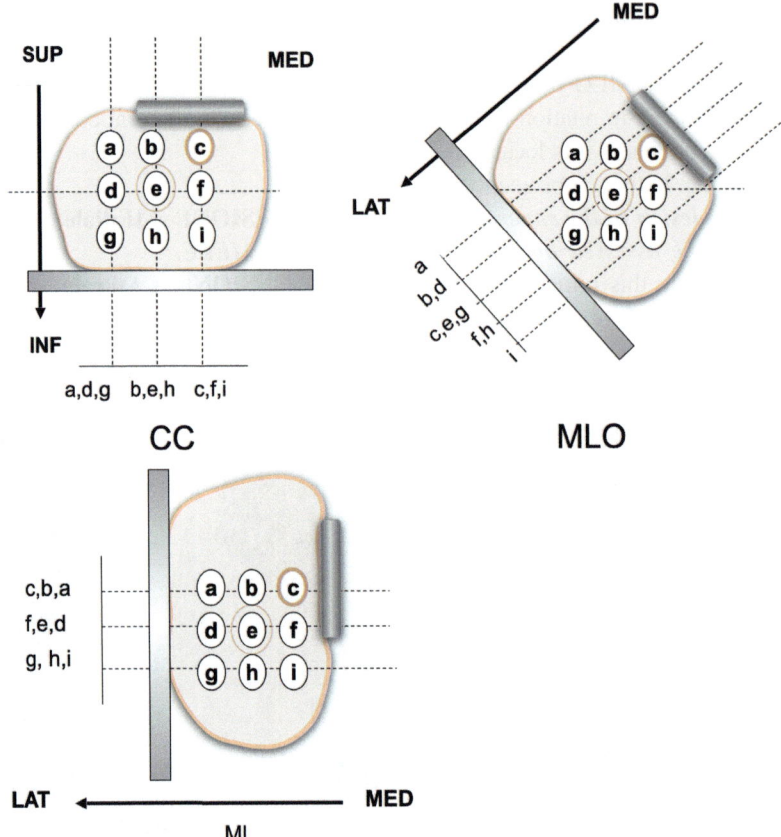

**Fig. 13.8** Subdivision of the breast with topographic points (9), for subsequent triangulation: different positions of a lesion depending on the projection: (1) the lesion in position **c** is in the medial quadrants, and the information is taken from the CC projection; (2) in the MLO, the lesion is in the central quadrants (e is the nipple): from this projection, the information taken is in the superoinferior direction. However, this is not the actual position, which is only given by the lateral projection: lesion c is actually located in the upper quadrants

## 13.4 Basic Considerations for Second-Level Examinations

As outlined earlier, the technique adopted in mammography must be such to implement a consistent and reproducible examination (Chap. 9). This is also fundamental in the case of level 2.

A breast represented in an artefactual manner (not corresponding to reality), obliges the radiographer in charge of level 2 to repeat the projections already performed in order to exactly locate the site of the lesion to be studied, thereby delivering an avoidable additional dose. The standardisation of positioning and compression must be viewed as a deontological obligation for the radiographer. The second-level basic considerations are listed in Table 13.2.

For the same subject according to the hands of the clock, see Chap. 25.

**Supplementary Material on YouTube Channel about Triangulation**

Available on Cristina Poggi YouTube channel 3 videos on the topic (2022–2023):

3. First part: https://youtu.be/fHiX8YhMBe8
4. Second part: https://youtu.be/OnNpSSu-wmV8
5. Third part: https://youtu.be/mKtqr7LXoHk

**Table 13.2** Fundamental considerations for second level examinations

| |
|---|
| 1 **Lesions in the deepest part, towards the chest, will always be less resolute than those in the front, due to the line focus principle, as well as the greater thickness of the breast** |
| 2 **The breast must be positioned in the same geometric conditions as level 1, if it is of high quality** |
| 3 **Due to the high potential for kinetic blurring,** in particular in the case of very thick breasts, and deep lesions, **it is useful to ask the patient to hold her breath during the acquisition** |

# References

1. Tamaki K, et al. Correlation between mammographic findings and corresponding histopathology: potential predictors for biological characteristics of breast diseases. Cancer Sci. 2011;102(12):2179–85. https://doi.org/10.1111/j.1349-7006.2011.02088.x.
2. De Roos MAJ, et al. Correlation between imaging and pathology in ductal carcinoma in situ of the breast. World J Surg Oncol. 2004;2:4. http://www.wjso.com/content/2/1/4
3. Naseem M, et al. Mammographic microcalcifications and breast cancer tumorigenesis: a radiologic-pathologic analysis. BMC. 2015;15:307. https://doi.org/10.1186/s12885-015-1312-z.
4. Logullo AF, et al. Breast microcalcifications: past, present and future (review). Mol Clin Oncol. 2022;16:81. https://doi.org/10.3892/mco.2022.2514.
5. Berment H, et al. Masses in mammography: what are the underlying anatomopathological lesions? Diagn Interv Imaging. 2014;95:124–33. https://doi.org/10.1016/j.diii.2013.12.010.
6. Sturesdotter L, et al. Mammographic tumor appearance is related to clinicopathological factors and surrogate molecular breast cancer subtype. Sci Rep. 2020;10:20814. https://doi.org/10.10138/s41598-020-77053-7.
7. Guo F, et al. Evaluation of the peritumoral features using radiomics and deep learning technology in non-speculated and non calcified masses of the breast on mammography. Front Oncol. 2022;12:1026552. https://doi.org/10.3389/fonc.2022.1026552.
8. Boyer B, Russ E. Anatomical-radiological correlations: architectural distorsions. Diagn Interv Imaging. 2014;95:134–40. https://doi.org/10.1016/j.diii.2014.01.003.
9. Bahl M. Architectural distortion on mammography: correlation with pathologic outcomes and predictors of malignancy. AJR. 2015;205:1339–45. https://doi.org/10.2214/AJR.15.14628.
10. Price ER, et al. The developing asymmetry: revisiting a perpetual and diagnostic challenge. Radiology. 2015;274(3):642–51. https://doi.org/10.1148/radiol.14132759.
11. Rodriguez Suarez I, et al. Diagnostic mammography: how, why and when. ECR 2018 EPOS™. https://doi.org/10.1594/ecr2018/C-1972
12. Song SE, et al. The clinical application of additional mammography for a diagnostic population: algorithm according to the lesion type, location, and patient characteristics. J Korean Soc Breast Screening. 2011;8:132–40. https://www.breast.or.kr/api/society/journal/download/40018/0802_132-140sse.pdf
13. Giess CS, et al. Interpreting one-view mammographic findings: minimizing call-backs while maximizing cancer detection. Radiographic. 2014;34:928–40. https://doi.org/10.1148/rg344130066.
14. Roberts-Klein S, et al. Avoinding pitfalls in mammography interpretation. Can Assoc Radiol J. 2011;62:50–9. https://doi.org/10.1016/j.caj.2020.07.004.
15. Mi Park J, Franken A. Triangulation of breast lesions: review and clinical application. Curr Probl Diagn Radiol. 2008;37(1):1–14. https://doi.org/10.1067/j.cpradiol.2007.09.001.
16. Atlas of breast cancer early detection. Breast imaging-mammography interpretation-Interpreting the abnormal mammogram. IARC WHO. https://screening.iarc.fr/atlasbreastdetail.php?Index=050&e=

# Mammography for Women with Breast Implants

# 14

## 14.1 Introduction

Surgical augmentation of the breast volume is an increasingly common procedure and is generally achieved by inserting **implants.** This is done in case of congenital abnormalities, for aesthetic reasons, or following mastectomy. Breast implants are composed of a polymer casing (*shell*), usually containing silicone (some are filled with saline), single chamber. They are triangular in shape, and can be placed: (1) in front of the pectoralis major muscle PM, and are called *retro-glandular* (above or below the pectoral fascia); (2) behind the PM, generally in a pocket between the pectoralis major and minor muscles (*sub-pectoral*). This second option has the advantage of a lower incidence of contracture, a complication that is in any case less frequent than it used to be, and of better visualisation of the glandular tissue on mammography images. Once in place, a fibrous capsule of scar tissue forms around the implant. It should have a density similar to soft tissue, but may present calcifications [1–4].

After mastectomy, an **expander** is placed to prepare the breast for the placement of the definitive implant. It is introduced in a collapsed form and then filled with saline solution gradually through a valve, until the volume deemed optimal is reached [5].

According to literature, breast implants can be subdivided into five generations. The latter have a high-viscosity silicone gel, with a silicone elastomer shell; the surface of the shell is generally coated with textured (rough) polyurethane. All these features inhibit the possibility of capsular contracture [6–8].

## 14.2 Positioning Breast Implant Carriers in Mammography Examination: The Eklund Technique

The gold standard for the study of breast implants is *Magnetic Resonance Imaging (MRI),* Chap. 22, which easily detects intracapsular rupture. Mammography, on the other hand, cannot fully assess the implant integrity, due to the high density of silicone that prevents the examination of the internal contents. Extravasated silicone (leakage) is easily identified, however.

The breast with an implant needs to be compressed less than a breast without it, being equal in anatomical characteristics and thickness. The aim is only to block it, to prevent patient movement. It must be said that *it is not possible to document in a mammography of a woman with implants all the tissue that is obtained in a woman without implants, other things being equal, particularly regarding the peri-implant tissue.* This is why the Eklund technique is suggested. It involves the posterior "removal" of the implants and is to be done in addition to the stan-

**Fig. 14.1** Eklund manoeuvre in CC e MLO projections, Carnesciali, E. courtesy (CRRPO-ISPRO)

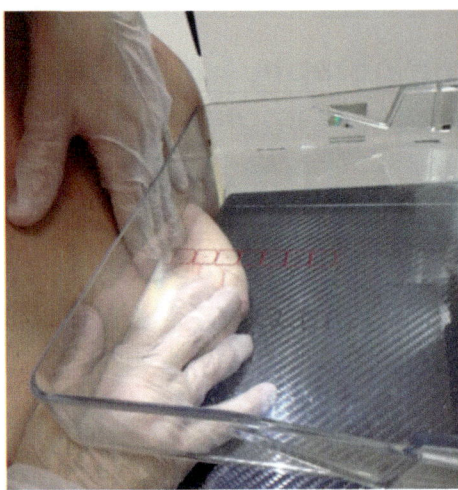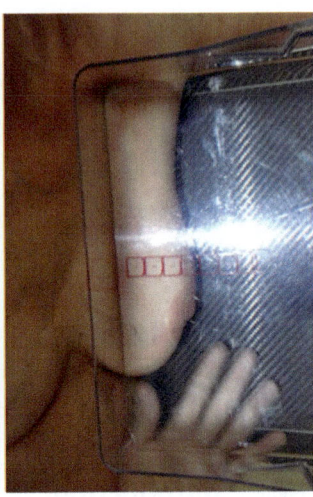

dard examination. The technique was proposed by Dr. Eklund, G.W., MD (*FACR*) [9].

**Eklund's manoeuvre, preliminary phase:** Before performing this technique, it is necessary to make sure that the patient does not have a capsular rupture. An irregular breast profile in a breast implant carrier might suggest it. Also, she has not had direct silicone injections. It cannot generally be performed in cases of major contracture. For all these reasons, it is important for the patient to sign a statement informing her of the possible need for additional mammographic projections, ultrasound (US) or MRI examinations. There is not enough evidence in the literature to indicate possible damage to the breast implant by a standard mammography exam, even with the Eklund manouevre.

**Eklund's manoeuvre, the technique**, allows patients with augmented breasts to be studied in mammography more extensively than the standard examination, primarily for the peri-implant tissue.

The positioning of the patient in the first part of the exam is the same as that described in Chap. 9; thereafter:

1. CC Eklund: The tissue in front of the implant is pulled over, with a pinch grip, while the other hand displaces the implant posteriorly and superiorly. The aim is to have the implant behind the posterior limit of the compression paddle (outside the FOV);

2. MLO Eklund: Arm and shoulder are arranged for an MLO standard projection, as explained in Chap. 9. The implant is then moved posteriorly so that an adequate compression could be applied to the tissue in front of it;

3. Since the implant is displaced, a suitable, higher compression, roughly similar to that exerted to a similar breast without implant, can be performed, for a more effective documentation of the anterior tissue.

See Fig. 14.1.

## 14.3 How Many Images to Acquire in a Breast Implant Carrier Patient [10–13]

There is no standardised protocol in Italy. In some centres, the four standard projections are performed, followed by 2 CCs Eklund. The standard projections, MLOs above all, give the reader a global idea of the implant placement and profile.

ISPRO, Toscana Centro, Sud Est e Nord Ovest areas propose a 6-image protocol, as indicated in the Tuscany regional Guide Lines (paragraph not published to date):

1. 2 CCs EKLUND (Fig. 14.2a);
2. 2 MLOs EKLUND;
3. 2 MLOs STD (Fig. 14.2b).

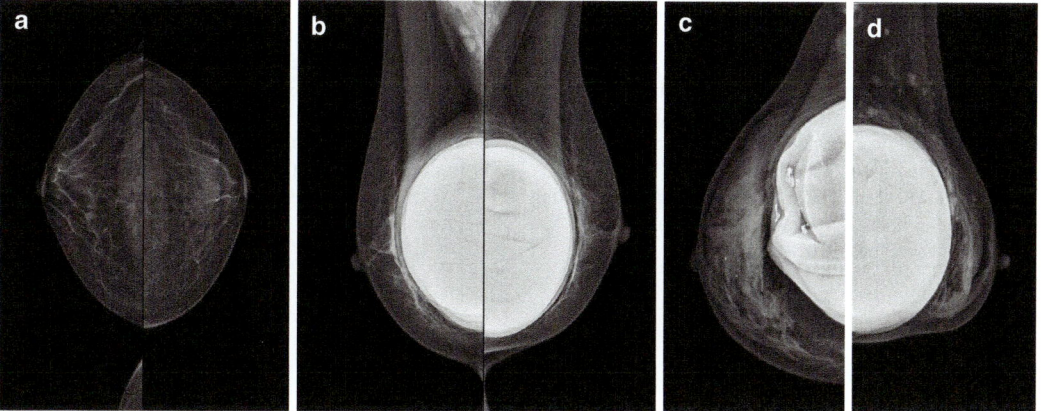

**Fig. 14.2** (**a**) CC Eklund in breast bilateral implant carrier; (**b**) MLO standard projection in the same patient; (**c**) implant deformity or distortion; (**d**) implant rupture and silicone leakage

## 14.4 The Role of Mammography in Breast Implant Imaging [14] and Latest Frontiers

The mammography examination in women with augmented breast is certainly useful in:

- The evaluation of extracapsular rupture, in some cases detectable by implant deformity or distortion (Fig. 14.2c);
- The detection of extracapsular silicone (Fig. 14.2d), even at the axillary lymph node level.

The imaging methodologies used for in-depth implant study are US and MRI, for which there is a dedicated standardised lexicon in the BI-RADS® report (see Chap. 22). In 2021, the FDA took a number of steps to improve communication of the risk that breast implant placement may entail, thus enabling patients to make informed decisions [15].

The latest frontier in breast implant surgery is 3D bio-printing technology, which uses biological units to create something that closely resembles natural tissue [16].

## References

1. Maxwell GP, Gabriel A. Breast implant design. Gland Surg. 2017;6(2):148–53. https://doi.org/10.21037/gs.2016.11.09.
2. Radiology Assistant. https://radiologyassistant.nl/breast/breast-prosthesis/breast-prosthesis-imaging
3. Seiler SF, et al. Multimodality imaging-based evaluation of single-lumen silicone breast implants for rupture. Radiographics. 2017;37:366–82. https://doi.org/10.1148/rg.2017160086.
4. Borrelli C, Vegnuti Z. NHS breast screening programme screening women with breast implants. NHS, PHE. Publications gateway number: 2017011; 2017.
5. Fairchild B, et al. Safety and efficacy of smooth surface tissue expander breast reconstruction. Aesthet Surg J. 2020;40(1):53–62. https://doi.org/10.1093/asj/sjy199.
6. Shah AT, Jankharia BB. Imaging of common breast implants and implant-related complications: a pictorial essay. Indian J Radiol Imaging. 2016;26(02):216–25. https://doi.org/10.4103/0971-3026.184409.
7. Park J, et al. Appropriate screening mammography method for patients with breast implants. Sci Rep. 2023;13:1811. https://doi.org/10.1038/s41598-023-28399-1.
8. Paap E, et al. Mammography in females with an implanted medical device: impact on image quality, pain and anxiety. Br J Radiol. 2016;89:20160142. https://doi.org/10.1259/bjr.20160142.
9. Eklund GW, et al. Improved imaging of the augmented breast. AJR Am J Roentgenol. 1988;151(3):469–73. https://doi.org/10.2214/ajr.151.3.469.
10. Soares Couto L, et al. Are all views with and without displacement maneuver necessary in augmentation mammography? Putting numbers into perspective. Asian Pac J Cancer Prev. 2022;23(1):233–9. https://doi.org/10.31557/APJCP.2022.23.1.233.
11. Deandrea S, et al. Screening of women with aesthetic prostheses in dedicated sessions of a population-based breast cancer screening programme. Radiol Med. 2021;126:946–55. https://doi.org/10.1007/s11547-021-01357-5.
12. Borrelli CD. Imaging the augmented breast. In: Hogg P, et al., editors. Digital mammogra-

phy: a holistic approach. Switzerland: Springer International Publishing; 2015. https://doi.org/10.1007/978-3-319-04831-4_27.

13. Sá Dos Reis C, et al. Study of breast implants mammography examinations for identification of suitable image quality criteria. Insight Imaging. 2020;11:3. https://doi.org/10.1186/s13244-019-0816-5.

14. Schmitt W, et al. The role of radiology in detecting prosthetic breast implant-related complications. Acta Radiol Portuguesa. 2018;30(1):23–34.

15. Le-Petross HT, et al. Assessment, complications, and surveillance of breast implants: making sense of 2022 FDA breast implant guidance. J Breast Imaging. 2023;5:360–72. https://doi.org/10.1093/jbi/wbad029.

16. Santanelli di Pompeo F, et al. History of breast implants: back to the future. JPRAS Open. 2022;32:166–77. https://doi.org/10.1016/j.jpra.2022.02.004.

# Male Breast Cancer

# 15

## 15.1 Introduction

Male breast cancer MBC is a rare disease, accounting for less than 1% of all breast cancer, and less than 1% of all male cancers (see Chap. 1). It therefore requires worldwide collaborative projects in order to be studied, so as to have statistically significant data. However, it should be noted that the incidence of male breast cancer is increasing, as it is that of female breast cancer. Often sufferers present with later-stage disease, precisely because there is no widespread awareness of this issue. BRCA2-male carriers have a much higher *lifetime risk* (Chap. 1), from 0.1% of the general population to 7%. Genetic Klinefelter syndrome carriers also have an increased risk, 20–50 times higher. Other risk factors are diseases such as liver cirrhosis and obesity. Both these conditions lead to an increase in oestrogen concentration. Also to consider testicular dysfunction and ethnicity, non-Hispanic black has a significantly higher incidence than the others, non-Hispanic white, Hispanic, Asian [1–3].

## 15.2 Breast Development in Males

In the prepubertal phase, there is a stimulation of the breast by oestrogen, leading to transient *gynecomastia*. It is defined as an increase in the amount of glandular tissue, which regresses with the physiological rise of androgens. TDLU and lobules are generally not formed. The ductal tree is atrophic and involute, and there are no Cooper's ligaments (Chap. 3). Male breast tumours are in fact almost all ductal, especially infiltrating, IDC now called NST (Chap. 5) [4–6].

Ginecomastia is the most common benign condition diagnosed [7]. The so-called "diffuse" form is typically associated with high-dose oestrogen therapies. It is therefore commonly seen in patients in transition (from assigned male at birth to female) [4].

## 15.3 The Treatment for MBC [8–13]

There are no specific treatments for this disease in men, so oncologists rely on the treatment for female BC. The psychological consequences of endocrine therapies should not be underestimated: Almost all MBC are HR+ (see Chap. 5). Sexual side effects are hardly acceptable, especially for younger patients.

## 15.4 Positioning Technique for Male Patients

The FFDM system (see Chaps. 7 and 8) has solved a good part of the problems arising from the volume of the male breast, which could be

**Fig. 15.1** Mammogram of a male breast: a different amount of gland is observable on the two sides. The breast appears radiolucent, with a prominent pectoral muscle

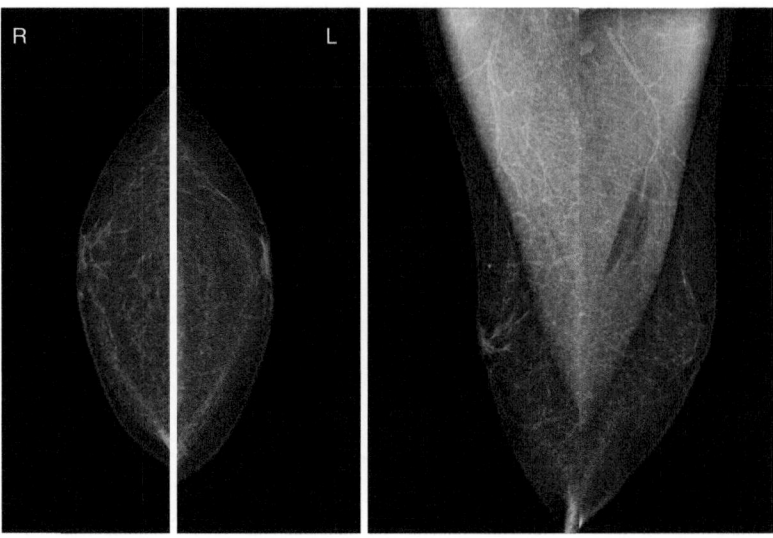

almost non-existent. Problems that can however generally arise only in CC projection. The MLO projection, given the consistency and width of the pectoralis major muscle in men, is easier. *Very important is the satisfaction of the first acquisition geometry parameter* (Chap. 9), *that is, the condition of the nipple in profile. This is because male breast pathology very often presents itself in the retroareolar site.* It should be noted that the sensitivity of mammography is very high in men, given the almost total absence of a summation artefact (see Fig. 15.1).

## 15.5    The Athlete's or Jogger's Nipple [14]

This is a pain symptom, related to dermatitis of the *nipple-areolar complex NAC* (Chap. 3), due to rubbing with clothing worn during physical activity, especially jogging, on one or both nipples. In some cases, it leads to bleeding, for which mammography may be required.

## 15.6    Screening for MBC

Individual risk assessment is particularly important for men who have a history of familial and hereditary breast cancer (see Chap. 4). In BRCA2-

gene mutation carriers, the relative risk may reach that of BC in women (about 12%). In this sense, it may be justified to include them in *selective screening* (Chap. 6). In these individuals, by the way, the peak incidence is very early, between the ages of 30 and 40. Furthermore, men diagnosed with breast cancer seem to have a rather high risk of developing a second one [1, 15].

## 15.7    The Male Breast Cancer Coalition

*The Male Breast Cancer coalition* is an association that aims to make the population aware of the existence of male breast cancer, giving the right information and a thorough understanding of the disease, thanks also to online support groups. One of the founders is a young man who has had this cancer.

## References

1. Gao Y, Heller S. Breast cancer screening in men. J Breast Imaging. 2023;5(2):104–11. https://doi.org/10.1093/jbi/wbac095.
2. Ashton J, Warren-Forward HM. Males in mammography-A narrative review of the literature. Radiography. 2019;25:392–9. https://doi.org/10.1016/j.radi.2019.05.001.

3. Zheng G, Leone JP. Male breast cancer: an updated review of epidemiology, clinicopathology, and treatment. Hindawi J Oncol. 2022;2022:1734049. https://doi.org/10.1155/2022/1734049.

4. Onder O, et al. Imaging findings and classification of the common and uncommon male breast disease. Insight Imaging. 2020;11:27. https://doi.org/10.1186/s13244-019-0834-3.

5. Charlot M, et al. Pathologies of the male breast. Diagn Interv Imaging. 2013;94:26–37. https://doi.org/10.1016/j.diii.2012.10.011.

6. ACS. 2023. https://www.cancer.org/types/breast-cancer-in-men.html

7. Blau M, et al. Anatomy of the gynecomastia tissue and its clinical significance. Plast Reconstr Surg Glob Open. 2016;4:e854. https://doi.org/10.1097/GOX:0000000000000844.

8. Chau A, et al. Male breast: clinical and imaging evaluation of benign and malignant entities with histologic correlation. Am J Med. 2016;129(8):776–91. https://pubmed.ncbi.nlm.nih.gov/26844632/

9. Korde LA, et al. Muldisciplinary meeting on male breast cancer: summary and research recommendations. J Clin Oncol. 2010;28:2114–22. https://doi.org/10.1200/JCO.2009.25.5729.

10. Johansson I, et al. Molecular profiling of male breast cancer-lost in translation? Int J Biochem Cell Biol. 2014;53:526–53. https://doi.org/10.1016/j.biocel.2014.05.007.

11. Sanguineti A, et al. Male breast cancer, clinical presentation, diagnosis and treatment: twenty years of experience in our breast unit. Int J Surg Case Rep. 2016;20S(Suppl):8–11. https://doi.org/10.1016/j.ijscr.2016.02.004.

12. Iuanow E, et al. Spectrum of disease in the male breast a pictorial essay. AJR. 2011;196(3):W247–9. https://doi.org/10.2214/AJR.09.3994.

13. Yalaza M, et al. Male breast cancer. J Breast Health. 2016;12(1):1–8. https://doi.org/10.5152/tjbh.2015.2711.

14. Sheylla Malta Purim K, Leite N. Sports-related dermatoses among road runners in Souther Brazil. An Bras Dermatol. 2014;89(4):587–92. https://doi.org/10.1590/abd1806-4841.20142792.

15. Woods RW, et al. Image-based Screening for men at high risk for breast cancer: benefits and drawbacks. Clin Imaging. 2020;60(1):84–9. https://doi.org/10.1016/j.clinimag.2019.11.005.

# Procedure Prior to Performing Mammography

# 16

## 16.1 Introduction

The phase before the mammography examination is an important step, as important as and perhaps more so than in other radiological examinations. The first thing to do, after welcoming the patient into the room, is to identify her uniquely. One must also identify oneself, as the specialist health operator, the breast radiographer, who will physically perform the examination. It must be told how many positions are required, and that it is necessary to compress the breast. This is of course especially important if it is the patient's first time. In the case of screening mammography, information must also be given on when and how the results of the test are received, and that it is possible to be called back for further tests. The mammographic exam performed by the radiographer is standard for all patients, and the reader may in some cases need to complete it with other projections, even using other imaging modalities, such as US (see Chap. 6). The anamnesis, or better, the **collection of historical data,** done by the breast radiographer, includes (1) hormonal status, that is important for radiation protection, a responsibility of our profession, but also for risk stratification; (2) whether there is a degree of familiarity (Chap. 4); (3) whether the patient has got a breast cancer diagnosis, and when, as well as a quick summary of the treatment and the surgical procedure; (4) scars, which should be carefully reported by extent and location (see below). Finally, (5) it is asked if the patient has noticed anything difference since the last mammogram, and if there are any significant symptoms, they should be reported.

## 16.2 Symptoms and Signs to Be Reported [1–3]

*Redness, swelling, local or diffuse, reduction in breast volume, discharge. Eczema or excoriations of the Nipple Areolar Complex (NAC) should also be noted.* The latter is important because it could be a sign of Paget disease, which could be associated with an underlying neoplasm (ductal in situ usually). Through the nipple, the gland has in fact a direct outlet on the skin, and it would be the neoplastic cells migrated from the gland that create these excoriations, according to an accredited theory (Fig. 16.1) [4, 5]. *Dimpling* (skin retraction, or sunken area, see Chap. 3), skin oedemas, associated with orange peel skin, should also be described. Important also to note any variation from the standard position of the nipples in relation to the median sagittal and axial plane (see Chap. 9). Congenital thoracic malformations such as *pectus excavatum* and *carinatum* (Chap. 10), and recent thoracic trauma, are also noteworthy. The breast is a very vascularised organ (Chap. 3), and even large hematomas may form, which can persist internally when the external signs have disappeared.

C. Poggi, *Breast Imaging Techniques for Radiographers*, https://doi.org/10.1007/978-3-031-63314-0_16

**Fig. 16.1** Paget disease and migration of neoplastic cells from the gland to the skin, cross-section

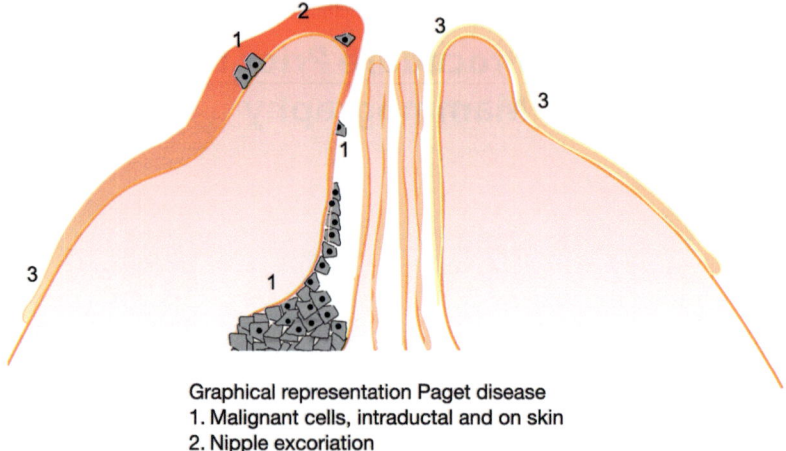

Graphical representation Paget disease
1. Malignant cells, intraductal and on skin
2. Nipple excoriation
3. Healthy epidermis

**Fig. 16.2** A warty spot of seborrheic keratosis. In MLO and CC projection, zoomed images

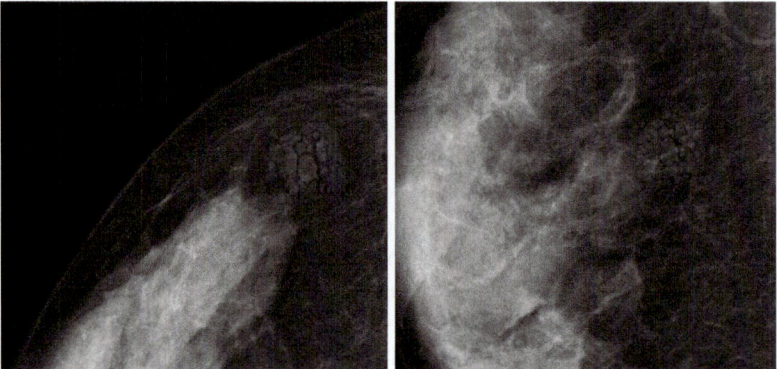

*Disfunction of the patient's joint mobility should also be noted, when these do not allow the radiographer to perform a high-quality examination. Also interesting are all those skin lesions that may appear on the reconstructed image and that can be mistaken for a lesion of the breast parenchima.* Examples are seborrheic keratosis (Fig. 16.2), skin tags (Fig. 16.3) and sebaceous cysts (Fig. 16.4). The latter may be highly radio-opaque. The four quadrants and the axillary tail, but also the axilla and two fingers below the infra-mammary fold, i.e. everything included in the image, should be checked. If the need arises, an additional projection can be acquired with a beam tangential to the skin lesion (Fig. 16.3), in order to prove its skin or dermal location.

**Fig. 16.3** Skin tag, in CC projection, tangental view, and in MLO projection

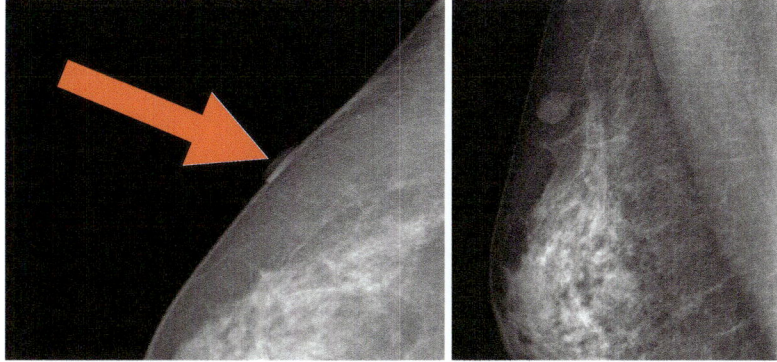

**Fig. 16.4** Sebaceous cyst, in CC and MLO projections

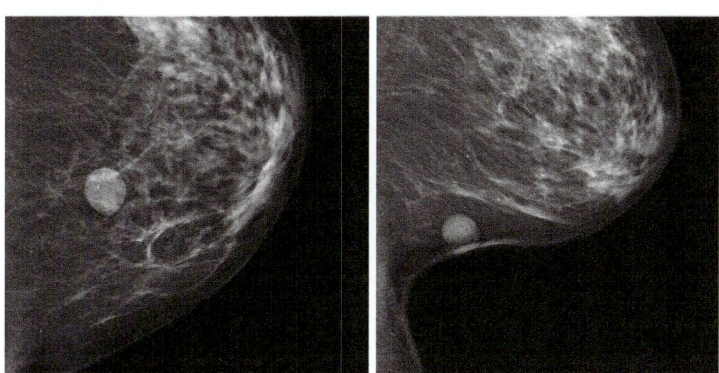

## 16.3 Skin Tears in Mammography [6]

A fact to be considered in mammography examination, brought about by compression and simple positioning technique per se, which required firm tissue stretching, is the tearing of the inframammary fold. It can be seen in patients suffering from *intertrigo.* This is a dermatological condition that includes a series of inflammatory phenomena affecting the folds, when these are subjected to rubbing, of varying severity, to which bacterial or mycological infection may be superimposed. Particularly in obese women with ptotic breasts, the IMF remains moist: This condition can become serious if associated with advancing age, in which the skin tend to become more fragile. If it is noticed, prior to the examination, that the IMF has a tear, it should be explained to the patient that having mammograms could make the situation worse, and if so, the patient should be referred to her doctor for treatment advice.

## 16.4 Historical Data Collection in Screening and Clinical Mammography

In screening programmes, data are stored in a database that can be easily consulted. However, it must be updated each time. Signs and symptoms reported by the patient are important, especially in the case of clinical mammography (Chap. 6). The form proposed in Table 16.1 is compiled example for a clinic mammography, for a synthomatic patient.

**Table 16.1** Mammography patient history collection form

Patient identification data: Name, date of birth, address, phone number, assigned identification number....

|  | | | | | | |
|---|---|---|---|---|---|---|
| Prior mammography ex. | Yes **X** | No | Date **18/2/2022** | In site | Off-site | **X** |
| Hormonal status | Fertility age | Menopause **X** | Last date of period | | Age of menopause | **52** |
| BC familial degree | 1° DEGREE (sister, mother, daughter -the same for male kinship) **MOTHER** 2° DEGREE (aunt, grandmother, granddaughter, niece, stepchildren - Same for male kinship, both maternal and paternal line) 3° DEGREE (COUSINS both maternal and paternal line) | | | | | **X** |
| Ovarian cancer | Specify only how many relatives | | | | | **1** |
| Type of surgical proc. | R **X** | Date **2014/04** | L | Date | | |
| Lumpectomy | **X** | | | | | |
| Quadrantectomy | | | | | | |
| Mastectomy | | | | | | |
| Implant placement | | | | | | |
| Mastopexy | | | | | | |
| Other | | | | | | |
| Therapies | ALND | Extended lymph nodes ex. | | | | |
| NEO adjuvant chemo | RT | Chemo | Endocrine therapy | Analogues | | |
| Signs and symptoms | R **X** | Date of occurence **1 week** | L | Date of occurence | | |
| Focal condensation/lump | **X** | | | | | |
| Pain | **X** | | | | | |
| Nipple (anat.) alteration | | | | Always **HAD** | | |
| Specify alteration: Retraction/inversion **X** | Erosion | **X** | | | | |
| Discharge | | | | | | |
| Specify colour discharge: White (milky) | Coloured | Cristal clear | Brown/red | | | |
| Note scar location (with stylized drawing of extension and shape) | | | | | | |
| And/or skin lesions (with stylized drawing of extension and shape) | | | | | | |
| Right breast | UOQ ⟲ | UIQ | Left breast | UOQ | UIQ | |
| | LOQ | LIQ | | LOQ | LIQ **SEB. KERATOSIS** ◉ | |

## 16.5   Choosing the Right Compression Paddle Dimension

In the standard examination, the compression paddles provided are basically of two dimensions, 18 × 24 and 24 × 30 cm. It should be chosen according to the size of the patient's breast; Both anteroposterior and laterolateral extensions of the breast are to be taken into account. Table 16.2 lists the main reasons why large compression paddles should not be used for small breasts. See also Chap. 26.

## 16.6   Display Layout for a Bilateral Mammography Examination [8–11]

To better assess the symmetry and inclusion of deep tissue in both projections, right and left, and also better identify any areas of kinetic blurring by comparison, it is advisable to select the two viewports layout. Right and left sides face each other back to back as mirror images (Fig. 16.5). This is the way in which the reader reports [12], and is part of the *hanging protocols* DICOM for mammography (see Chap. 8).

**Table 16.2**   Reasons why the large compression paddle should not be used for small breasts

| | |
|---|---|
| 1 | **Undue increase in dose** (even if the increase is very small in FFDM) |
| 2 | **Improper use of a large portion of the active area** (inferior abdominal tissue does not provide useful information for diagnosis |
| 3 | **Storage waste** (a large number of pixel contains air, that does not provide useful information for diagnosis) |
| 4 | **Smaller pixel effect:** Using a compression paddle of 24 × 30 cm (resulting in an active area of the same size) causes a breast reduction in the displayed image: In cases of very small breasts this effect, informally called in Italy **stamp effect,** forces the reader to use electronic zoom over the entire breast area, lengthening the reporting time [7] |
| 5 | **MLO positioning is more difficult** in cases of women with small breast and short stature |

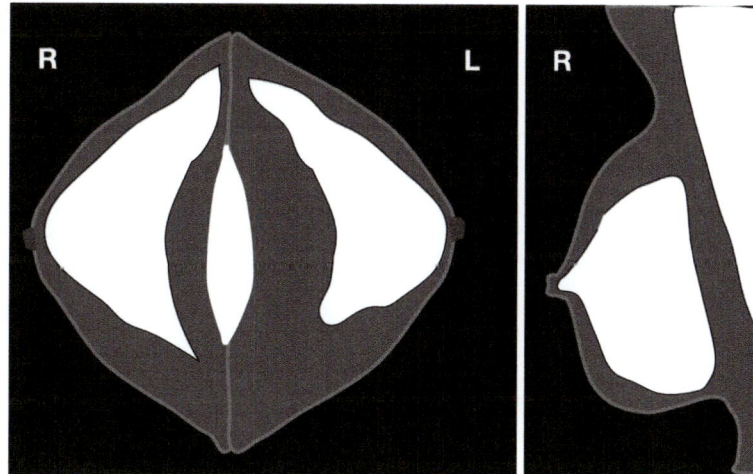
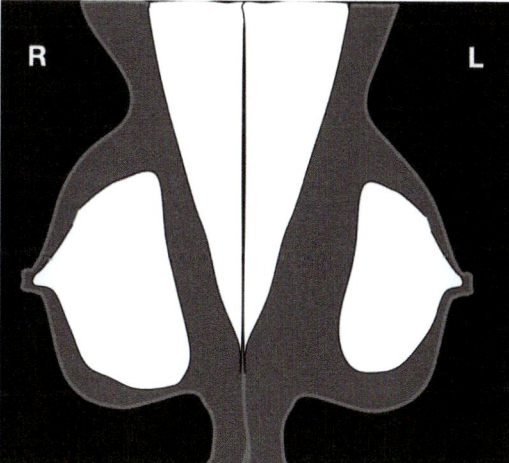

**Fig. 16.5**   1 × 2 layout (instead of full view) on the acquisition modality display, in which right and left sides face each other as mirror images, recommended for a better image evaluation in terms of technical and clinical quality, by the radiographer

# References

1. Symptoms of breast cancer Cancer Research UK. https://www.cancerresearchuk.org/about-cancer/breast-cancer/symptoms
2. Lorente Ramos RM, et al. Superficial breast lesions. A comprehensive review of skin and superficial parenchimal breast lesions with pathologic correlation, ECR 2013, EPOS™. https://doi.org/10.1594/ecr2013/C-0864.
3. Giess CS, et al. Distinguishing breast skin lesions from superficial breast Parenchimal lesion: diagnostic criteria, imaging characteristics, and pitfalls. RSNA. 2011;31(7):1959–72. https://doi.org/10.1148/rg.317115116.
4. Geoffroy D, et al. Clinical abnormalities of the nipple-areola complex: the role of imaging. Diagn Interv Imaging. 2015;96:1033–44. https://doi.org/10.1016/j.diii.2015.07.001.
5. Markarian S, Holmes DR. Mammary paget's disease: an update. Cancers (Basel). 2022;14(10):2422. https://doi.org/10.3390/cancers14102422. https://pubmed.ncbi.nlm.nih.gov/35626023/
6. Shonyo M. The impact of skin tears on patients and breast imaging centers: viewpoints from two different perspectives. https://blog.beekley.com/the-negative-fallout-of-skin-tears-in-mammography
7. Compton K, Oosterwijk H. Requirement for medical imaging monitors (part 1). https://studylib.net/doc/18570275/requirements-for-medical-imaging-monitors
8. Interpreting the Mammogram. Radiology Key, posted Jun 18, 2016. https://radiologykey.com/interpreting-the-mammogram/
9. Lamb LR, et al. Missed breast cancer: effect of subconscious bias and lesion characteristics. Radiographics. 2020;40:941–60. https://doi.org/10.1148/rg.2020190090.
10. Radiation Protection and Quality Standards in Mammography. Safety procedure for the installation, Use and control of mammographic x-ray equipment, Health Canada 2013. ISBN: 978-0-662-46361-0
11. ACR-AAPM-SIIM practice parameter for determinants of image quality in mammography Revised 2022 (resolution 46). ACR. https://www.acr.org/-/media/ACR/Files/Practice-Parameters/dig-mamo.pdf
12. Strudley CJ, et al. Mammography cancer detection: comparison of single 8MP and pair of 5MP reporting monitors. Br J Radiol. 2018;91:20170246. https://doi.org/10.1259/bjr.20170246.

# Further Reading

Hogg P, et al. Digital mammography a holistic approach. Springer; 2015. https://doi.org/10.1007/978-3-319-04831-4. ISBN 978–3–319-04830-7 ISBN 978–3–319-04831-4 (e-book)

# Main Artefacts on Full-Field Digital Mammography (FFDM)

**17**

## 17.1 Introduction

*An artefact is defined as an alteration that may be almost invisible, or very significant, of the final product of the image acquisition and reconstruction process.* This means that, due to the artefact, the reproduction of the object is not faithful to the original.

Four different sources of artefact can be considered in direct digital mammography, as presented in Table 17.1 [1–5]:

*Recognising an artefact in any branch of biomedical imaging requires a thorough knowledge of: (1) the acquisition method used; (2) the anatomy and physiology, both developmental and involutional, of the organ being studied; (3) what a high diagnostic value image can and should look like.* Internationally renowned radiologist L. W. Bassett (MD, FACR) has defined artefact as

any variation in mammographic density that is not caused by differences in actual attenuation [5]. The differences in attenuation of the incident beam between tissues, expressed by their linear attenuation coefficients, constitute the *anatomical contrast*. The breast is very low (Chap. 7), and translates precisely into different densities.

In this text, it was decided to further specify the meaning of artefact, considering in particular those related to the performance of the radiographer. In other words, the categorisation presented in the Table 17.2 was considered:

Ultimately, it is always a "deviation" of the image produced from reality, to a different degree, and in a different way, from reality, and thus, to *mammography that is not a photography of the real anatomy* (see Chap. 26).

**Table 17.1** Sources of artifacts in direct digital mammography

| | |
|---|---|
| 1 | **The radiographer** (her/his performance) |
| 2 | **The patient** (by anatomy, compliance and pathology) |
| 3 | **Hardware** |
| 4 | **Software** (including processing and archiving on PACS) |

**Table 17.2** Categorization of artifacts related to radiographer performance

| Production of images that do not reflect the actual anatomy for: | |
|---|---|
| A | **Cutaneous fold** (obliterating or otherwise disturbing the study of acquired tissue) |
| B | **Rotations inducing deformations of the acquired tissue** (non-satisfaction of the two acquisition geometry parameters) |
| C | **Inadequate stretching and/or compression, or ineffective operator/patient relationship** |

## 17.2   Artefacts Related to the Radiographer Performance, 1) A): Skin Folds [6, 7]

Skin folds are the most common radiographer performance-related artefact. The *dynamic range* of digital mammography (Chap. 8) must also be taken into account. It is much wider than analog images, allowing the visualisation of even very thin, lacking depth, radio-opaque folds. In addition to thickness and the degree of radio-opacity, it is also essential to assess the site where the folds occur.

### 17.2.1   Saturn Ring Artefact and Folds in the Axillary Extension, MLO Projection

It is located exactly at the transition between the UQ and the axillary tail, in the MLO projection (see Fig. 17.1a). It is especially common in women with a significant axillary tail thickness. It is a tissue stretching error, which cannot always be eliminated. It is generally believed that the UP&OUT manoeuvre (Chap. 9) worsens it. However, this manoeuvre cannot be avoided, otherwise the quality of the image produced will be markedly worsened, due to the loss of POSTINFQ (see Chaps. 11 and 25).

**How It Presents Itself:** Generally as a fold more or less important in density and thickness, in the shape of a semicircle with the concavity facing superiorly, approximately perpendicular to the superoinferior axis of the breast.

**Correction of Saturn's Ring and Folds in the Thick Axillary Extension:** Fundamental is the positioning of the patient's shoulder and arm, according to Poggi's positioning method, as summarised in Tables 9.2 and 9.4. Especially important is the external and upper arm rotation, the forward stretching of the arm, done with both hands, the elbow flexed and brought down. An example of incorrect positioning of the patient's arm and shoulder is presented in Fig. 17.1b. This fold may be due to an accumulation of fat, not necessarily related to high BMI. In this case, it is very difficult to eliminate, but does not generally affect the reading of the images.

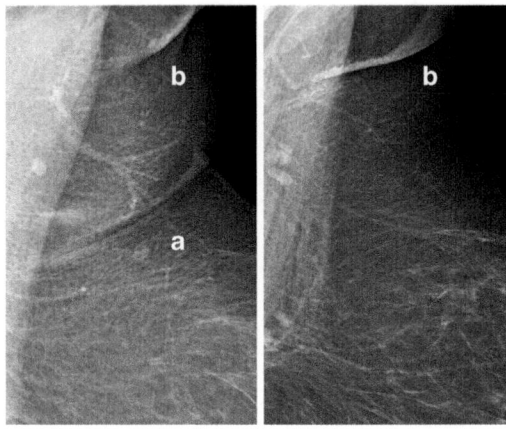

**Fig. 17.1** Saturn ring artefact in position a; in b; artefact from incorrect positioning of the patient's arm and shoulder, especially visible in the second image

### 17.2.2   Folds in the Pectoralis Major Muscle, MLO Projection

Particularly visible in women with a thin chest and small breasts, who tend to stiffen when leaning on the detector, before and during compression. This attitude leads, among other things, to a change in the shape of the pectoral muscle itself, which becomes oval-shaped, with a superior narrowing (Fig. 17.2(a)). Also indicative of the stiffening is the fold that the writer has called "trickle-like", very radio-opaque Fig. 17.2(Aa)). They are often found associated. *Folds in the pectoral muscle in the MLO projection can be subdivided according to their thickness and density, their extension and the involvement of fibroglandular tissue (FGT).*

We can speak of 3D skin folds in the case that they involve more than one tissue plane (Fig. 17.2(b and c)). They are almost always associated with women with a thin thorax, and are caused by the patient stiffening, forming a gap between the muscle and the detector. Compression therefore easily produces folds. If the fold extends into the FGT (Fig. 17.2(c), orange oval), the projection must always be repeated.

Folds in the pectoralis muscle may present themselves in various ways: for a more in-depth iconographic depiction, please refer to the videos on the subject on the YouTube channel @cristina-poggi7579. For links see below.

**Fig. 17.2** Shape and folds in the pectoralis muscle in MLO. (**a**) Oval shape of the pectoralis muscle and "trickle-like" skin fold; (**b**) 3D fold, indicated by the letter B; (**c**) 3D fold involving FGT, orange oval; (**d**) 2D fold, denoted by the letter C

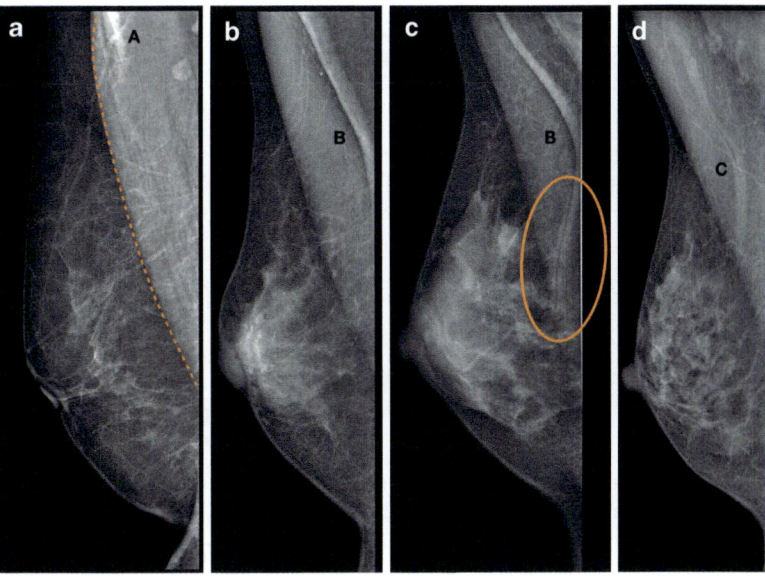

### 17.2.2.1  Correction of Thin Skin Folds in the Pectoral Muscle and Axillary Extension

The patient's arm and shoulder need to be more relaxed. One can resort to the Rosa Anna Amoruso© manoeuvre: the forearm is brought behind the detector, keeping the shoulder still. It certainly decreases the gap with the detector, but at the same time decreases the width of the pectoralis muscle (see Chap. 9, and further on). Correction from behind the thorax is also useful, smoothing out the tissues posteriorly, in order to distend the folds. It must be done very carefully not to pull away tissues that need to be documented.

**Note 1** *When the patient stiffens the arm and shoulder, a muscle bundle terminating on the humeral head can be seen, clearly visible when the arm is raised to 90°en the patient stiffens the arm and shoulder, a muscle bundle terminating on the humeral head can be seen, clearly visible when the arm is rai. 3), there is the sub-scapularis muscle, synergic with the pectoralis major. It originates in the scapular fossa and forms part of the rotator cuff. Seeing this bundle rise up over the skin is indicative of stiffening, and consequently of a high probability of* producing folds with compression. It may be helpful to apply light pressure with the fingers, drumming on this area and asking the patient to relax.

**Note 2** *The patient should always be asked beforehand if she does not suffer from joint disorders, before making shoulder-arm rotation movements. If the patient does suffer from such problems, a note should be made to indicate that it is impossible or at least difficult to obtain high-quality images.*

### 17.2.3  Folds in the Deep Lateral Tissues, MLO Projection

These folds are also often associated with women with thin chest. They are located especially in the superior and central deep tissues. The folds of the inferior lateral deep tissue, on the other hand, are more likely associated with more robust women.

### 17.2.3.1  Correction of the Folds of Superior and Central Deep Lateral Tissues

Should be done from behind the chest, with extreme care (see Fig. 17.3).

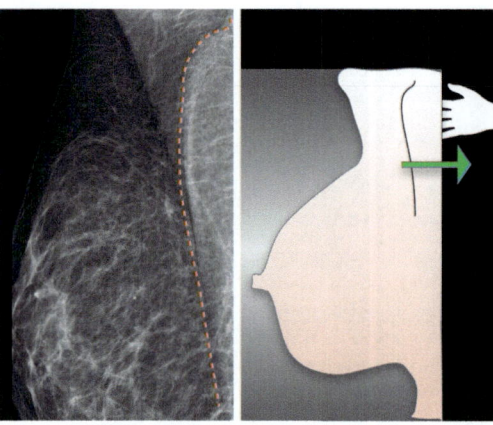

**Fig. 17.3** Deep lateral tissue fold, indicated by orange discontinuous line in front of the fold itself, superior and central (or medium) level and its correction

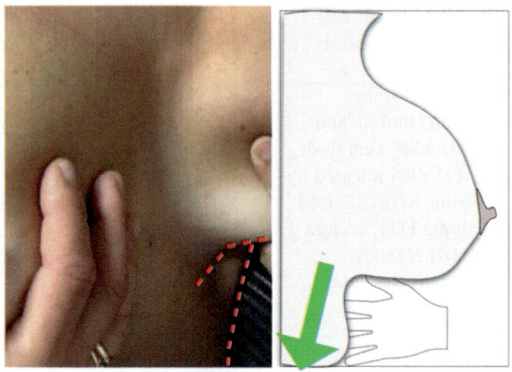

**Fig. 17.4** Folds in IMF, horizontal and vertical; making sure the breast is free behind, inferiorly. Small pinch grip not shown

### 17.2.4  Folds in IMF, MLO Projection

These folds are extremely common and fall into two types:

1. Vertical folds, which occur in deep lateral tissues, and therefore not visible to the radiographer while positioning (it is the breast part that rests on the detector).
2. Horizontal folds, which occur on the medial side, visible to the radiographer.

The former, understandably, is by far the most frequent [8].

**Correction of Vertical Folds in the IMF:** One can resort to the small pinch grip, coordinating first and second fingertips, stretching the tissues of the IMF with a vertical downward movement. Making sure first that the breast is free behind, before rotating the hips (see Chap. 9 and Fig. 17.4).

**Correction of Horizontal Folds:** The only way to avoid these folds is to perform the UP&OUT manoeuvre correctly (Chap. 9).

*If the folds also involve the POSTINFQ in addition to the IMF, they become less acceptable. This is because the portion in question can only be documented in the MLO projection.*

### 17.2.5  Folds in Fibroglandular Tissue (FGT), CC Projection

They are mostly present in women with ptotic and deflated breasts, with loose and very loose skin envelope. They occur in the inferior quadrants, those not visible because they rest on the detector. Although they are often thin and radiotransparent skin folds, if they involve the FGT they always render the projection inadequate, i.e. to be repeated.

**Correction of Folds Involving FGT in the CC Projection:** It is important to properly stretch the lower quadrants: two possible manoeuvres are recommended:

1. Mazzalupo© manoeuvre: Instead of lifting the breast with the palm of the hand, the back is used, rotating the hand clockwise and simultaneously stretching the tissues, before bringing them onto the detector. More feasible for radiographers with large hands, particularly when the breast is large and heavy.
2. Poggi© manoeuvre: *Star Hand:* Before placing the breast onto the detector, grasping it with the palm of the hand, spread the fingers apart, trying to take as much tissue as possible, and then stretching the lower quadrants with a

firm anterior movement. More practicable for radiographers with small-to-medium sized hands. It must be stressed, however, that this manoeuvre requires a fingers' divarication, in particular the hyperextension of the first finger. This may worsen the typical first finger MSD of the mammographer (see Chap. 23).

### 17.2.6  Skin Folds in the OQ, CC Projection

These folds form easily but are just as easily removed. They appear as a fan of radio-transparent and radio-opaque folds at the outermost part of the OQ (see Fig. 17.5(1)).

**Correction of Skin Folds at the OQ:** The tissue in this area is to be smoothed, vertically, upwards, while lowering the compression paddle.

### 17.2.7  Skin Folds in the InnerQ, CC Projection

Folds in the IQ are also very frequent, but are less easily eliminated than those in the OQ, being related to the anatomy of the patient's intermammary cleft, which is very variable. They can occur with varying degrees of radio-opacity and thickness. Moreover, as the deep medial portion can only be documented in the CC projection, folds in this location are negatively impacting the quality of the examination. The medial portion is one of the *forbidden zones* (Tabar, L.) [9].

**Correction of Skin Folds in the IQ:** When the patient is asked to move the contralateral breast away from the FOV, the right direction to be given to the outward movement, upwards or downwards, must be carefully chosen, depending on which direction eliminates, or at least minimises, the folds.

### 17.2.8  Folds in the IMF, CC Projection

Important in women with ptotic and deflated breasts, as they may not be detected correctly. The presence of a radio-lucent area such as that shown in Fig. 17.5(2) is indicative of this artefact: it is air trapped in the fold.

**Correction of the Folds in the IMF in CCs:** The tissues in the area are smoothed out inferiorly. It may help to ask the patient to move her pelvis slightly backwards. This movement certainly stretches the tissues, but there is a risk of their loss (deep inferior tissue). The movement must be guided carefully for this reason.

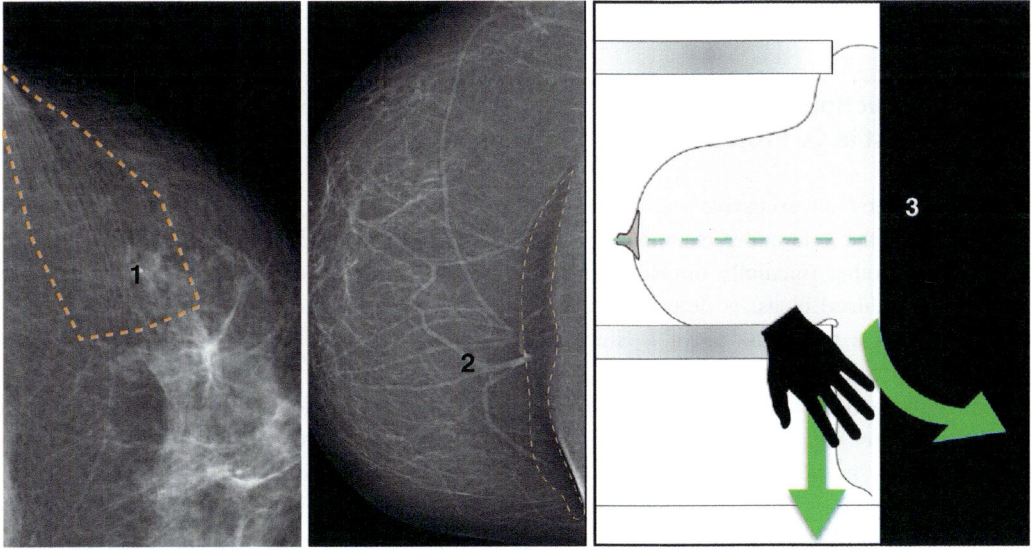

**Fig. 17.5**  (1) OQ fan artefacts; (2) IMF fold with air included; (3) correction of 2

## 17.3 Radiographer Performance-Related Artefacts 1) B): By Rotation of Tissue Acquired in Mammography, CC Projection

It must be emphasised again that the positioning technique is one of the most important factors determining the quality of the mammographic image. As reported by Taylor et al. [10], *if the whole tissue is not included in the image, or if there are artefacts that do not allow sufficient tissue documentation, all other aspects of quality totally lose their importance.* I would like to add a further aspect to be considered, which is inherent in the positioning technique, but which is very seldom described: the **acquisition geometry.** The satisfaction of the two parameters described in Chap. 9, First and Second, permits not only the documentation of the maximum extent of tissue, but what has been included will be represented as faithfully as possible to the original object. That is to say without deformations that may produce mammograms that are not well readable. It is important to remember that the retromammary space in the CC projection, also known as "no-man in the", and the area parallel to the pectoral muscle in the MLO, identified in this text with the anterior wall of the retromammary space itself (see below), known as the "milky way", are one of the *forbidden zones* already mentioned.

### 17.3.1 Production of the "Ogival" Breast in CC Projection

It is obtained by an excessive rotation of the hemithorax of the side under examination with respect to the other (medially directed). In this way, the reproduced breast is deformed, with a lateral tip (hence the term "ogive"). Since the *nipple points towards the missing tissue, the* medial tissue will be missing. It is not all: the internal structures will be displaced in an artefactual manner (especially in ptotic breasts), as shown in Fig. 17.6.

*This is an extremely impacting artefact, especially if the CC projection showed above is the*

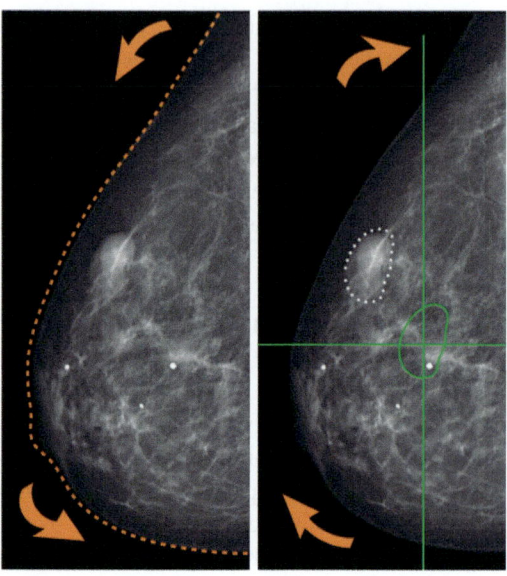

**Fig. 17.6** Ogival-shaped breast image 1: the lateromedial rotation results in a fictitious translation of the internal structures. If the projection was done correctly, cancelling the medial-directed rotation, the density shown in white (dotted line) would be deeper and more central, as shown in image 2 (green line)

*basis of a second level or callback* (Chap. 13). The finding to be studied with spot or magnification view will not actually be where it appears in the image. The baseline projection will therefore have to be repeated, with undue additional dose delivered (see also Chap. 21).

**Correction of the Ogival-Shaped Breast:** Attention must be paid to the positioning of the chest wall, which must be perpendicular to the median sagittal plane (satisfying the second acquisition geometry parameter).

### 17.3.2 Production of CCs in Which the Muscle Is Not Central and Lunette-Shaped (Semielliptical)

This artefact is induced again by an excessive rotation of the hemithorax, with failure to meet the second acquisition geometry parameter. It may be accompanied by a forceful lowering of the ipsilateral shoulder, and/or by a forceful stretching in which a direction, lateral or medial, has been impressed. It is associated with tissue loss. *The production of a pectoralis muscle that is displaced with respect to the centre, and fan-shaped or lunette-shaped, but only present laterally or medially, clearly indicates that the positioning technique has not taken into account the acquisition geometry parameters.* *Associated with translation of the nipple to an unnatural position.* Two different cases are evaluated:

1. **Outer and Inner Quadrants of the Same Size:** The nipple should be on the midline, which should coincide with the median sagittal plane. Due to the improper rotation, however, it is not (nipple incorrectly shifted to a lateral or medial position). The pectoralis muscle, if documented, is not central and lunette-shaped.
2. **Outer and Inner Quadrants of Different Sizes:** The nipple is not on the midline, it is lateral or medial to it, in a natural way. The operator incorrectly positions the nipple on the midline coincident with the mid sagittal

plane, in order to meet the quality criteria without correlating them with reality. The pectoralis muscle, if documented, is not central, and tissue from the dominant quadrant is lost (Fig. 17.7b). *The nipple is in a nonnatural position.*

### 17.3.2.1   Correction of the Not Central and Lunette-Shaped PM

1. If the quadrants are of the same size, the nipple should be on the midline/midsagittal plane. If not, it means that an incorrect rotation has taken place (Fig. 17.7a), and that tissue is missing in the direction of the rotation (including the muscle). Therefore, the rotation must be cancelled, the acquisition geometry must be restored and the second parameter be met.
2. If the quadrants are not the same size and the nipple has been forced onto the midline/midsagittal plane (Fig. 17.7b), part of the dominant quadrant is lost. In this case too, the rotation must be cancelled (see Fig. 17.7b1).

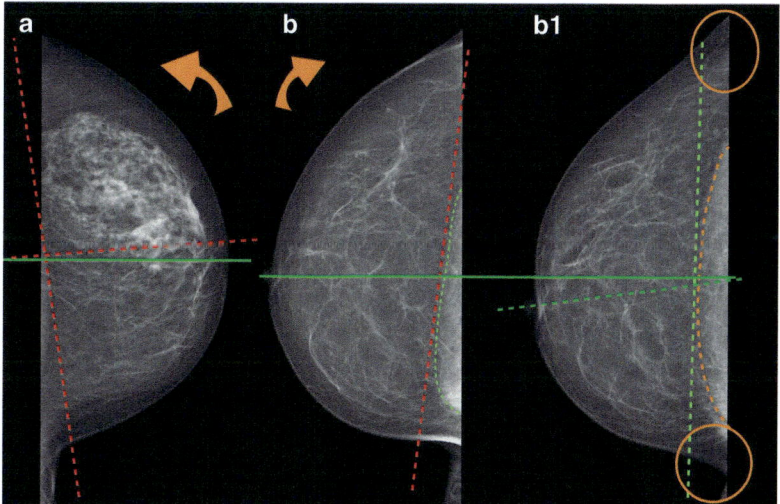

**Fig. 17.7** The muscle is not central and lunette-shaped, and the nipple is not in its natural position; (**a**) nipple shifted laterally, in a patient with outer and inner quadrants of the same size: rotation directed laterally; (**b**) nipple forced to the midline in a patient with lateral quadrant larger than medial, pectoral not central and not lunette-shaped; (**b1**) correction, wall perpendicular to median sagittal plane, pectoral muscle correctly demonstrated (with recovery of tissue lost in B, orange oval)

### 17.3.3 Radiographer Performance-Related Artefacts 1)B): By Rotation of the Tissue Acquired, MLO Projection

The correct acquisition geometry is fundamental for the production of quality mammograms. In the case of the MLO, the two acquisition geometry parameters already mentioned must be met, as for the CC. If the breast being studied has the medial and lateral parts of the same size (or about), they must be placed in parallel (First acquisition geometry parameter). When this geometrical condition is not met, the nipple will not be in profile, but more importantly, the tissue will be missing in the direction of rotation (see Chaps. 26 and 27).

### 17.4 Artefacts Related to Inadequate Compression in CCs, 1) C)

In this section, we will only refer to compression that is too low, or inadequate. In contrast to too high, a compression, which cannot be easily assessed in a physical and quantitative sense (Chap. 11), too low, a compression has a certain effect: it induces *blurring*, i.e. a degradation of the technical quality of the image [11]. This extends to the clinical quality, with possible production of *false positives* and worsening of the *summation artefact* or *anatomical noise* (Chap. 8) (see Fig. 17.8a and a1).

### 17.4.1 Artefacts Related to Inadequate Compression in MLO Projection

In some cases, inadequate compression can result in the production of mammograms that are inadequate in terms of the extent of tissue acquired, as in the case of the *droopy breast*. See Fig. 17.9a, in comparison with Fig. 17.9b: in the latter, other aspects are deficient, so it can be assumed that the positioning, as well as the compression, was incorrect.

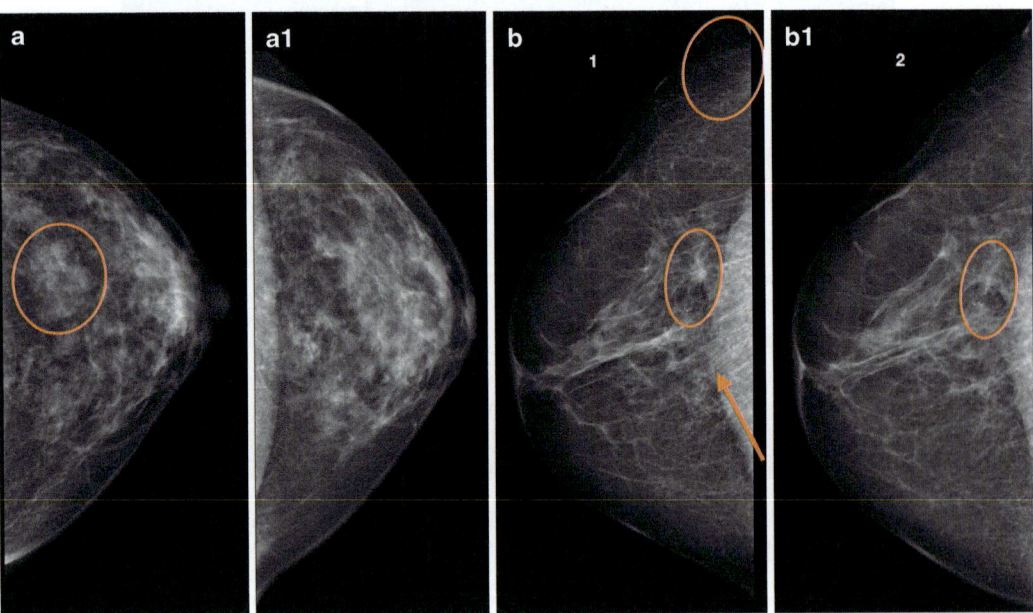

**Fig. 17.8** (**a**) Summation artefact due to inadequate compression: in the repeated projection **a1**, the central condensation disappears (the positioning technique is more correct). (**b**) Production of ogival breast with medially directed stretching, and creation of artefact (orange central oval), which disappeared in repeat **b1** (see text)

**Fig.17.9** (**a** and **b**) In **a**, droopy breast: good positioning but loss of the posteroinferior quadrant POSTINFQ (breast fall), due to inadequate compression; in **b**, another droopy breast, but with various aspects indicating an overall incorrect positioning

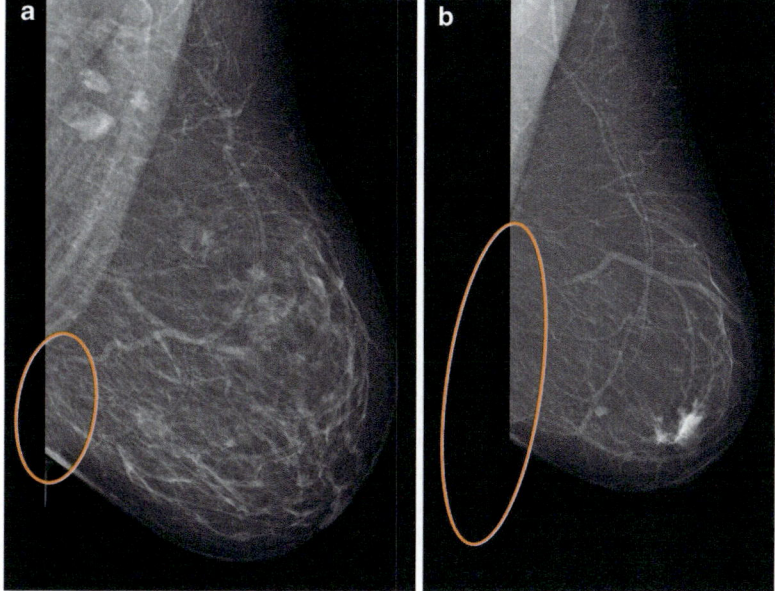

### 17.4.2 Artefacts Related to Incorrect Stretching in the CC Projection

The stretching operated by the hand of the radiographer moving anteriorly, as the compression paddle descends, must be firm. Furthermore, it must not be imparted in a lateral or medial direction, because especially in some women with too mobile breasts, with loose skin envelope, it can induce the formation of important artefacts. In Fig. 17.8b, can be seen a very common example of "enthusiastic" tissue stretching, with consequent documentation of a large part of the deep tissue, done with a not correct medial direction, leading to the formation of the external, ogival tip, and the artifactual documentation of the posterior Cooper's ligaments, medially directed (arrow, Fig. 17.8b). This led to the creation of an artefact, which disappeared in the repetition, shown in Fig. 17.8b1, proving to be a false positive.

### 17.4.3 Artefacts Related to Ineffective Stretching in MLO Projection

The stretching to be performed in both CC and MLO projections is firm and requires a fair amount of muscle strength (see for the topic MSDs, Chap. 23). It may result in poor documen-

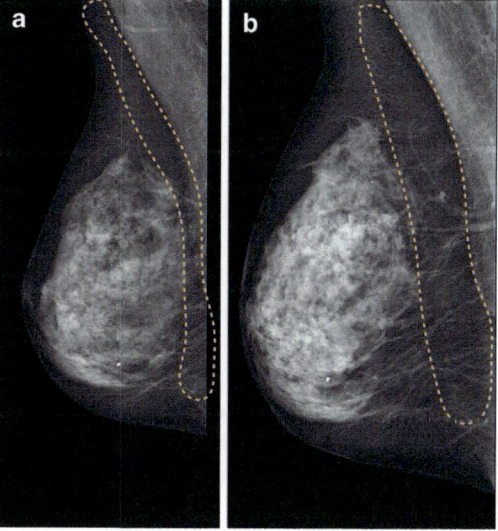

**Fig. 17.10** (**a**) Retromammary space correctly documented superoinferiorly, but not easily readable, due to ineffective stretching. (**b**) Same projection same woman (the difference in size is related to the use of the 24 × 30 cm compressor in 1, with a *smaller pixel* effect, Chap. 16). The retromammary space is open and well readable, for decisive and effective stretching

tation in particular of the deep planes if not sufficient or ineffective. Observe how the extension of the retromammary space in the superoinferior direction is correct in both images a and b (Fig. 17.10), but much less readable, as "compressed" in a. This is a case of ineffective stretching.

## 17.5 Radiographer Performance-Related Artefacts Due to Inadequate Documentation of the Pectoralis Muscle 1)C), Associated with Ineffective Operator-Patient Relationship, MLO Projection

In addition to the aforementioned oval-shaped pectoralis muscle with an upper narrowing (Fig. 17.2a), generally due to patient stiffening, various alterations in the shape of the pectoralis muscle can be observed in the MLO projection. They worsen the fidelity of reproduction, and for this reason, are considered as artefacts in this text. They are determined by various factors.

It should be remembered that the desired shape, length and width of the pectoralis muscle in the oblique projection are those shown in Fig. 17.11. They are not easily obtainable, as they are related to various physical parameters and the patient's compliance, but they should be aimed at. The zone parallel to the pectoral muscle, as shown in Fig. 17.11, represents one of the forbidden zones, to which the reporter (and the radiographer) must pay particular attention.

Extensive documentation of the pectoralis major muscle is required because it represents the posterior wall of the retromammary space; the anterior wall is indicated with the green dashed line in the figure: the space is best identified with Professor Tabar's so-called Milky Way, probable site of lesions.

### 17.5.1 Not Sufficient Pectoralis Muscle (PM) Width at Axillary Level

Often due to suboptimal performance of the radiographer, it can also be caused by the patientue to suboptimal perfoThe two-rotation manoeuvre described in Chap. 9 can only be effectively implemented if the patient does not have acute or chronic functional impotence.

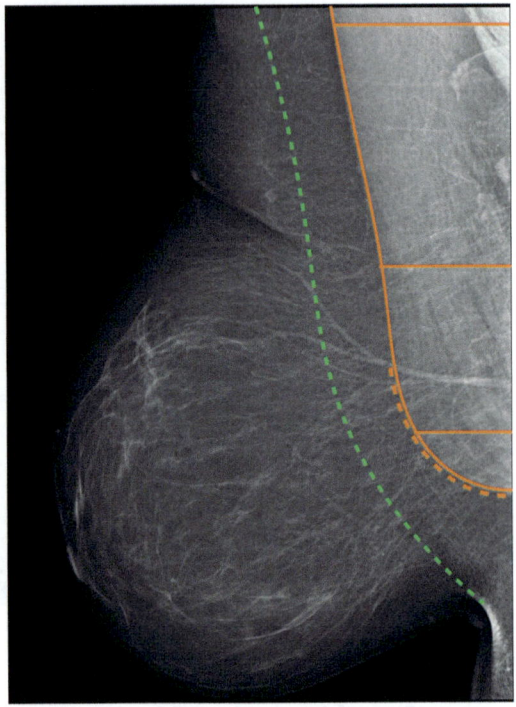

**Fig. 17.11** Pectoralis major muscle in the MLO projection: correct documentation: (1) Significant width at axillary level (with latissimus dorsi posteriorly); (2) Important width also at central level; (3) Width at a lower level, if possible with a "rounded" tail, as shown with an orange dashed line, which exactly follows the anatomy of the muscle itself; (4) Length up to PNL, and beyond (see Chaps. 12 and 25, and Annex 1); (5) Fan-shaped, convex

Sometimes, however, even simple "tension" on the part of the patient can result in inadequate documentation. The experienced breast radiographer can try "on the part with good communication. Examples in Fig. 17.12.

### 17.5.1.1 Correction in Case of PM Not Wide at Axillary Level

1. In the case of inadequate positioning: retrace the steps of positioning, as expressed in Table 9.4.
2. If determined by stiffening alone, the patient can be asked to relax her arm and shoulder, and not to squeeze the handle (see Chap. 23 for *effective and strategic relationship in healthcare*).
3. If due to a joint disorder, of course, it cannot be corrected.

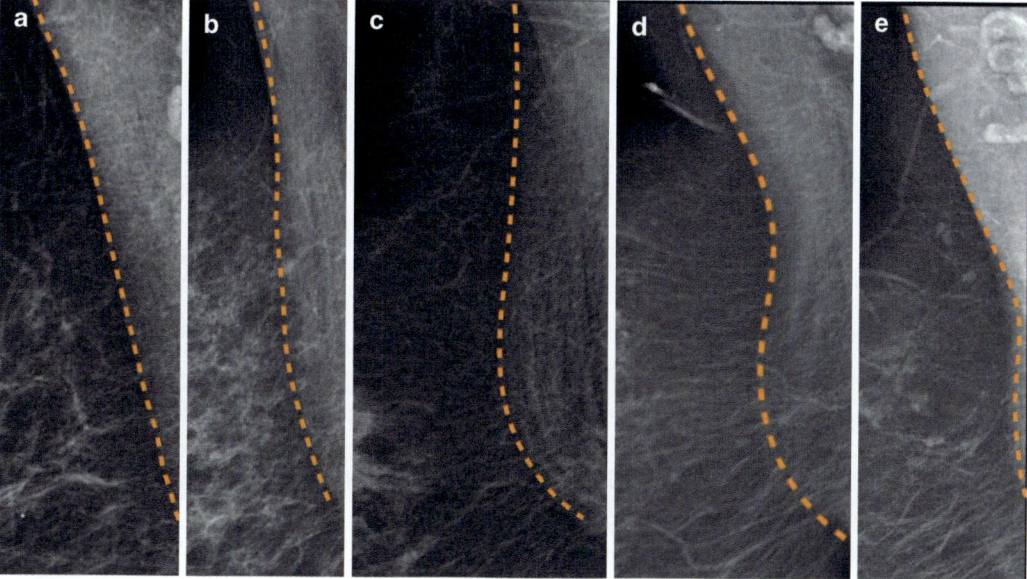

**Fig. 17.12** (**a**) Rectilinear pectoralis muscle (PM); (**b, c**) PM not wide at the axillary level that could be due to the patient's joint pathology; (**d**) PM "spool-shaped PM"; (**e**) PM concave in the middle, filiform in the lower part. See text

### 17.5.2  Concave-Shaped PM

We can distinguish, greatly simplifying, two cases:

1. The muscle is concave only in the central part, but wide superiorly and inferiorly (spool-shaped) (Fig. 17.12d).
2. The muscle is concave in the central part, and is often filiform in the lower part (Fig. 17.12e).
3. The spooled-shaped pectoral muscle may be due to the radiographer overcorrecting by moving posteriorly too much tissue (the deep lateral) away from the FOV, to smooth out the folds.
4. The muscle as depicted in Fig. 17.12e, concave centrally and then filiform, is sometimes correlated with the same error; much more often it is associated with a patient with pectus excavatum or in general with malformations of the rib cage.

#### 17.5.2.1   Corrections for Concave PM

1. Great attention must be paid to the positioning of the patient, when she is guided towards the detector, so that no folds are formed. This is difficult to achieve, especially if the patient is very thin. It is usually necessary to stretch the tissues from behind, and therefore the possibility of losing something grows.
2. For mammography in women with pectus excavatum, it may be useful to increase the degree of obliquity of the C-arm, from 50°–55°. The correction must be noted.

### 17.5.3  PM Not Extending to PNL

This is perhaps the most important parameter, as the pectoralis muscle partially represents the posterior wall of the retromammary space. If the muscle is not fully represented in length, a portion of tissue in which a lesion may be present could be lost (Fig. 17.13 and Chap. 27). The area shown in the figure corresponds approximately to Professor Tabar's Milky Way. In the case of shoulder functional impotence, or otherwise difficulty on the part of the patient to follow the steps indicated, documentation of the pectoralis muscle in length becomes more complicated. Skill and experience of the dedicated radiographer are tested.

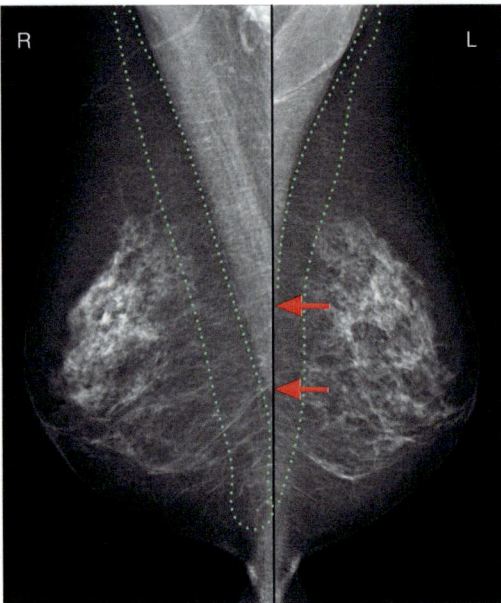

**Fig. 17.13** PM non-extending to PNL (Appendix 1): part of the retromammary space is missing, indicated by the red arrows. The left shoulder shows stiffening with the presence of the fold in the axillary region

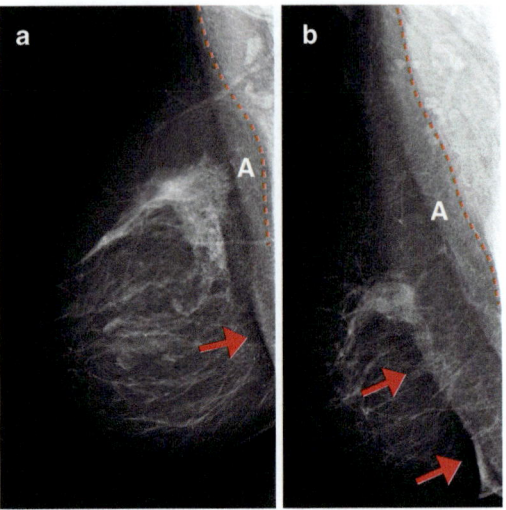

**Fig. 17.14** (**a**) Misrepresentation of the latissimus dorsi muscle in length (orange dotted lines), accompanied by folds and significant artefacts (red arrows). In **b**, the extensive inclusion of the latissimus is related to the patient's incorrect posture, torso forwards and hips backwards

**Correction for Muscle Not Extending to the PNL:** Deep medial tissues (on the sternum side) are missing. The patient must therefore be rotated effectively (laterally, towards the detector) to reach the lost tissues, as far as possible. The documentation of the pectoralis major muscle does indeed depend on many factors, including the patient's compliance. *Obviously, there are no corrections to be done if the shape of the pectoral muscle, or its unusual density, is related to anatomical or pathological reasons.*

### 17.5.4 Latissimus Dorsi Represented Too Extensively in Length 1)C)

Latissimus dorsi is not mentioned in the quality criteria list. It is however recommended in this text: this is because it represents the posterior part of the axillary fossa, the only part visible in mammography. Being the pectoralis muscle, the anterior part, having both means to have documented all the axillary fossa. It is difficult to

include this artefact in one of the three mentioned categories: sometimes, however, it may be related to an "enthusiastic" collaboration on the part of the patient, which results in a non-effective one. It is seen as a more radio-opaque triangle of the pectoralis major, in the *top right corner* of the MLO image (Fig. 27.5). A more extensive documentation, especially in length (which can happen especially in women with a very thin thorax), can be accompanied by the formation of important folds. From Fig. 17.14a and b, not only the breast tends to fall (even more if the patient's posture is not correct, Chap. 26).

**Correction of the Over-Extended Latissimus Representation:** The steps in Table 9.4 are to be followed. More precisely, the first rotation of the arm, which aims to bring the upper and deep tissues onto the detector. It is important to make the patient relax as much as possible, with a good strategic relationship (Chap. 23), paying particular attention to: (1) the leaning of the deep lateral side against the detector, which is perceived as very uncomfortable by patients with a slender chest, and (2) her posture: torso and hips must be on the same line (Chaps. 9 and 26).

## 17.6 Patient-Related Artefacts 2) [5, 12]

They are of various kinds. Those due to ineffective operator-patient collaboration were extrapolated and placed in category 1)C).

### 17.6.1 Artefact Due to Patient Movement During Acquisition [11]

It is the most common artefact associated with kinetic blurring. It may affect the whole breast, but also only a part of it (especially the area of the axillary extension, or the POSTINFQ).

**Correction of Patient Motion Artefact:** Kinetic blurring, even if it affects a circumscribed area of the breast, always makes the mammogram inadequate, i.e. to be repeated. It is recommended to:

1. Arrange the arm and shoulder appropriately, so as not to have a large axillary tissue thickness that can induce the breast to fall during acquisition. Having a large axillary extension thickness also requires going up a lot with the compression value, in order to obtain an effective fixation of the breast itself, and this increases the patient's discomfort and the probability for her to move.
2. Ask the patient not to move arm and shoulder, using words of motivation.
3. Ask not to squeeze the handle with her hand, or in any case not to stiffen the muscle. This would increase its thickness and decrease its compressibility, at the same time increasing the patient's discomfort and thus her likelihood of moving.
4. Ask the patient, in the case of very thick and/or very dense breasts, for which a significant compression value is necessary (and a long exposure time), not to breathe during the acquisition.

### 17.6.2 Artefacts Due to Body Creams, Anti-Perspirants, Healing Ointments or Talcum Powder

Before having a mammogram, especially in the summertime, it may be good advice to ask the patient if she uses creams, ointments, or talcum powder. Or, for instance in the case of patients with very large and ptotic breasts, if they use *intertrigo* healing ointments (Fig. 17.15). See Chap. 16 for the approach in case of significant intertrigo, and material on YouTube and Facebook, links below.

**Correction of Artefacts Due to Creams, Ointments, Talcum Powder:** The patient is asked to wash the IMF and the axilla with detergent. We are to explain to her that the products she has used may create artefacts that may produce diagnostic doubts (Fig. 17.15(1)).

### 17.6.3 Occlusive Artefacts

The various sources of this artefact are: (1) hair, earrings and in recent times, the protective mask worn upside down (Fig. 17.15(2)); (2) the chin, the other breast and the shoulder (Fig. 17.15(3)); (3) the opposite hemithorax (Fig. 17.15(4)), especially in cases of congenital thoracic malformations. Each of those can project itself onto the studied breast, partially hiding it.

**Correction of Occlusive Artefacts:** Pay particular attention, with the light field on, that nothing is projected onto the FOV.

#### 17.6.3.1 Pseudo-Artefacts
1. From the sternalis muscle
2. Polka-Dotted breast

1. It is a particular artefact, which is actually a *pseudo-artefact*, determined by the **sternalis muscle.** It is an accessory muscle, which is generally only seen in CCs, in the deep medial portion (Fig. 17.16).

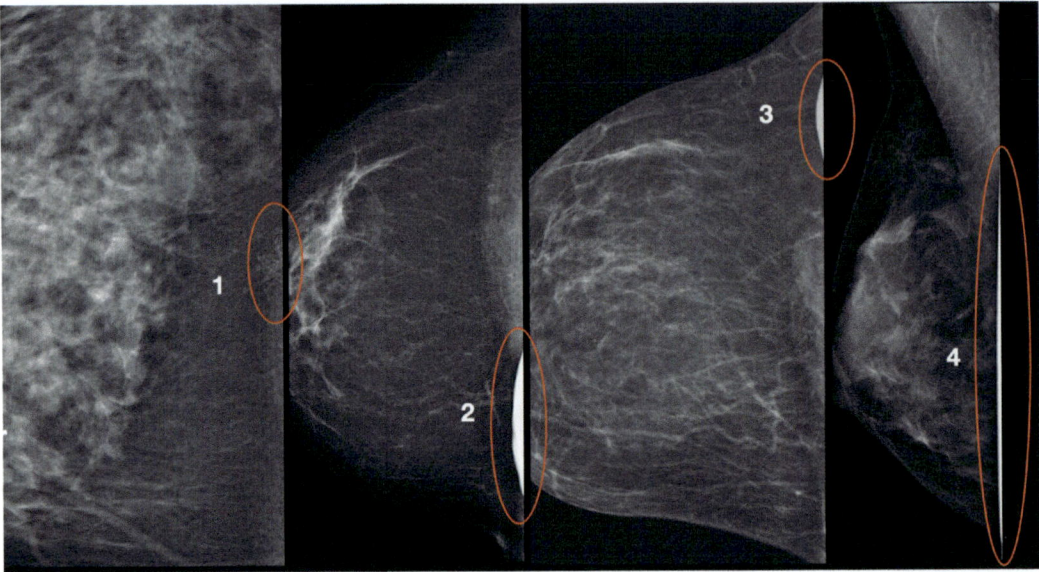

**Fig. 17.15** 1. Artefact from intertrigo healing ointment (Chap. 16), magnification view; in the following, occlusive artefacts, 2. from facial mask, 3. from shoulder and 4. from opposite hemithorax

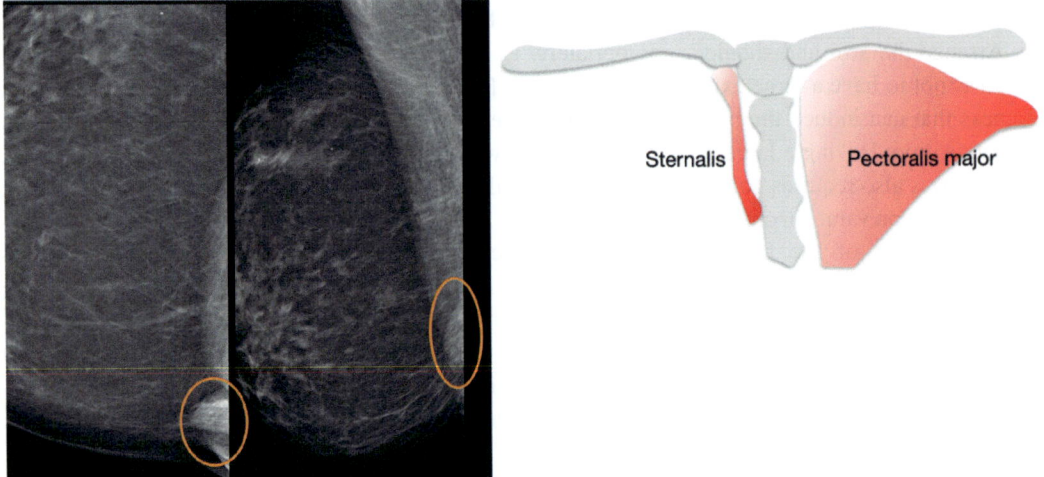

**Fig. 17.16** Visualisation of sternal muscle, in CC and MLO (much rarer), and drawing of the muscle itself. Pseudo-artefact

2. It is another interesting pseudo-artefact that makes the **"polka-dotted breast"** appear (not shown). It is presumably due to skin cavities in which columns of hypodermis fat are inserted. They appear round as axial sections of a cylinder, and radio-lucent as they are made of fat.

### 17.6.4 Artefacts Due to the Presence of Major Skin Lesions

Skin lesions that may project into the breast, in the fibroglandular tissue, must be carefully reported by the radiographer for size and location (see Chap. 16).

### 17.6.4.1   Cristina Poggi YouTube and Facebook Supplementary Material

Please refer to the four lectures published on YouTube, and on the Facebook profile (see the back of the book), for a more extensive iconographic treatment of the topic of artefacts (2021):

1. Basic radiographic anatomy, patient-related artefacts, Chap. 1. https://youtu.be/ojaxqorf_6l
2. Radiographer-related artefacts: skin folds from incorrect distension, Chap. 2. https://youtu.be/G_fAmZDt7ms
3. Extension and rotation mistakes in mammography positioning, CC projection: the quality criteria, Chap. 3. https://youtu.be/RVhPZUqp-rs
4. Extension and rotation mistakes in mammography positioning, MLO projection: the quality criteria, Chap. 4. https://youtu.be/3HCivhdMEfQ

In addition to the two chapters on the pectoral muscle, in four videos (2022):

1. In the CC: first part https://youtu.be/TvYITfNNPKU
2. In the CC: part two https://youtu.be/9kDcWmalQhY
3. In the MLO: part one https://youtu.be/lREhJKwooTE
4. In the MLO: part two https://youtu.be/fN-hRRJcCNE

---

## 17.7   Main Hardware-Related Artefacts in FFDM 3) [13–15]

Detector-related artefacts, the most significant ones are mentioned:

– Dead pixels (and misread pixels).
– Vertical lines (vibration artefact).
– Ghosting.
– Blooming.
– Collimator misalignment (Chap. 7).
– Correlated to AEC (Chap. 7): salt and pepper artefact.

– Sensitive area activation error (Chaps. 7, 8, and 11).

**Dead pixels,** or **bad pixels,** are generally well visualised (they are actually clusters of pixels). They appear as white or black dots, and always remain in the same position in different projections. They can often be corrected by *flat-field calibration QC* (Chap. 8). Amorphous selenium systems are characterised by intrinsic non-uniformities: they can be detected in the images produced. If the problem is not resolved, it may indicate the need to replace the detector.

Also related to the detector are the electrical interferences that can occur when reading digital data. They can manifest themselves as vertical black lines, or as alternating black and white, horizontal lines, which are also called *vibration artefact.*

*Ghosting* refers to the persistence of a previously acquired image on a newly acquired one. Again, calibration can remove the memory of the old image. Ghosting was more common in the past, due to the high sensitivity to changes in the operating temperature of the amorphous selenium detector (see also Chaps. 7 and 23).

**Blooming:** This is an artefact that can be seen in many biomedical imaging modalities, including MRI. It is related to high-density (or high-signal in MRI) objects, where the object itself appears larger than it actually is.

**Misalignment of the Collimator** (with respect to the light field, itself coinciding with the active area): It is a fairly common phenomenon. It presents itself as a radio-opaque line (representing the limit of the collimator itself projecting onto the FOV, see Chap. 7), at one edge of the image, due to misalignment. It usually requires the intervention of the equipment manufacturers technical support.

In some cases, the image may not be reconstructed, or may be displayed with a high level of noise (**salt and pepper artefact**, Fig. 17.17a). This can be due to: (1) an **imperfect calibration of the AEC**, (2) very dense breast, (3) post-radiotherapy effects, (4) the dose delivered which was higher than the maximum set limit, (5) exposure that has been mistakenly aborted. It may happen that the area delimited by the chosen

**Fig. 17.17** (**a**)
Unreconstructed image,
salt and pepper artefact
(high noise level). (**b**)
Activation error of the
sensitive area, which
should have been
18 × 24 cm

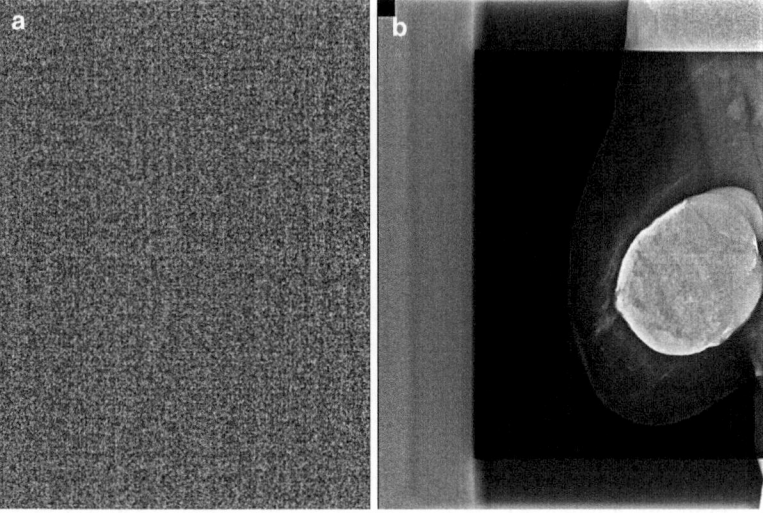

compression paddle dimension is not exactly activated (Fig. 17.17b), usually for the reason (4) listed above.

## 17.8   Main Software-Related Artefacts (Processing and Archiving) 4)

– Horizontal lines.
– Loss of edge.
– Breast within a breast sign.
– Vertical processing bars artefact.
– Related to archiving.

A software-related artefact may appear as a **white horizontal line or lines**. It is due to the failure of the detector to read the data lines (Chap. 7). It is possible that this artefact is self-corrected by the software.

In the presence of patients with PORT, or Pace Maker (PM) or other high-density, strongly radio-opaque devices, an image-processing artefact may occur. It is caused by the *gradient* (high-density difference) between neighbouring tissues, at the periphery of the object itself, and it presents itself with a black signal (*dark Halo*). Even breasts that have undergone radiotherapy, which results in varying degrees of increased fibrosis, and thickening of the skin, may show a correlated processing artefact. For the same reason, i.e. if

very high densities are present, a *loss of the skin edge* itself due to beam saturation can be observed.

*Breast within a breast* is an artefact that can occur in the case of a thickness or density gradient between the central and peripheral regions, due to a failure of the software algorithm. It creates a clearly delineated transition between the two areas, which is not real.

The *vertical bar* artefact presents itself as a series of low-exposure areas. This is an error in the pre-amplification of the signal (see Chap. 7).

*Processing artefacts* are caused by the failure of dedicated algorithms, and occur when the software system fails to compensate for differences in exposure perceived by the entire detector.

There are also *artefacts caused by the archiving system PACS,* which does not reconstruct the images properly so that they are not (properly) displayed. This happens when the information contained in the **DICOM Header** (Chap. 8) of the image, which contains the display parameters, is not interpreted correctly.

Failure to identify lesions on the mammography examination may be due to the above-mentioned artefacts, of each of the four categories already indicated (Table 17.1). In the case of high technical and clinical quality, and high competence of the reporter, it may depend: (1) on the type of lesion itself [16]; (2) on the anatomical-radiographic characteristics of the patient; (3) on certain biases related to the diagnostic decision-making process [17]; (4) on the fatigue from high number of working hours.

Interestingly, an article published in Lancet Oncology, and mentioned by AuntMinnie on 3 August 2023 [18], points out that the use of AI as a second reader in the screening programme, in low- and medium-risk cases, results in a reduction of working hours, and a consequent improvement of the reader's performance.

For tomosynthesis and CESM artefacts, see Chap. 20.

## References

1. Milosevic ZC, Nadrljanski M. Classification system of artifacts in direct digital mammography, ECR 2012, EPOS™. https://doi.org/10.1594/ecr2012/C-0922.
2. CHOI JJ, et al. Mammographic artifacts on full-field digital mammography. J Digit Imaging. 2014;27(2):231–6. https://doi.org/10.1007/s10278-013-9641-4.
3. Geiser WR, et al. Challenges in mammography: part 1, artifacts in digital mammography. AJR. 2011;197:W1023–30. https://doi.org/10.2214/AJR.10.7246.
4. Bassett LW, et al. Digital mammography: clinical image evaluation. Radiol Clin North Am. 2010;48:903–15. https://doi.org/10.1016/j.rcl.2010.06.00616.
5. https://ec.europa.eu/programmes/erasmus-plus/project-result-content/cbb7e7ba-a519-4368-9d3e-168f43188f77/IO3_Mammographic%20artefacts.pdf
6. Boyce M, et al. Comparing the use and interpretation of PGMI scoring to assess the technical quality of screening mammograms in the UK and Norway. Radiography. 2015;21(4).342–7. https://doi.org/10.1016/j.radi.2015.05.006.
7. Guertin M-H, et al. Clinical image quality in daily practice of breast cancer mammography screening. Can Assoc Radiol J. 2014;65:199–206. https://doi.org/10.1016/j.carj.2014.02.001.
8. Miller LC. Mammography positioning basic and advanced. SBI. https://courseware.cutm.ac.in/wp-content/uploads/2020/06/Mammo-for-Techs-Positioning-pdf.pdf
9. Theberge I, et al. Screening sensitivity according to breast cancer location. Can Assoc Radiol J. 2019;70:186–92. https://doi.org/10.1016/j.carj.2018.10.007.
10. Taylor K, et al. Mammographic image quality in relation to positioning of the breast: a multicentre international evaluation of the assessment systems currently used, to provide an evidence base for establishing a standardized method of assessment. Radiography. 2017;23:343–9. https://doi.org/10.1016/j.radi.2017.03.004.
11. Abdullah A, et al. The impact of simulated motion blur on lesion detection performance in full-field digital mammography. Br J Radiol. 2017;90:20160871.
12. Schueler B. The art of the image in mammography artifacts in 2D and 3D breast imaging: their origin, presentation, and remediation. Mayo Clinic Rochester, AAPM Spring Clinical Meeting 2018, PPT.
13. DE Visschere P. Artifacts in digital mammography. Universiteit Gent, PPT. 2018. http://www.semicomedia.be/Kingconventions/Imaging/Presentations2018/presentation8.pdf
14. Geiser WR, et al. Artifacts in digital mammography PPT. https://www.aapm.org/meetings/amos2/pdf/41-10046-70873-266.pdf
15. Fayadevan R, et al. Optimizing digital mammographic image quality for full-field digital detectors: artifacts encounters during the QC process. Radiographics. 2015;35:2080–9. https://doi.org/10.1148/rg.2015150036.
16. Mario J, et al. Benign breast lesions that mimic cancer: determining radiologic-pathologic concordance. Appl Radiol. 2015;44(9):24. https://appliedradiology.com/Articles/benign-breast-lesions-that-mimic-cancer-determining-radiologic-pathologic-concordance
17. Lamb LR, et al. Missed breast cancer: effects of subconscious bias and lesion characteristics. Radiographics. 2020;40:941–60. https://doi.org/10.1148/rg.2020190090.
18. Allegretto A. Swedish team advocated AI risk assessment for breast screening. AuntMinnie, 3 August 2023. https://www.auntminnieeurope.com/index.aspx?sec=sup&sub=wom&pag=dis&ItemID=624222

# Part IV

# On the Report, Other Breast Imaging Modalities; Radiation Protection in Senology

# Mammography Report: Cytological and Microhistological Sampling: Stereotactic Biopsy

# 18

## 18.1 The Mammography Report, R-Labelling; BI-RADS® Classification

In the screening programme, radiologists sort mammograms into two groups: **negative** and **suspicious** (i.e. with doubtful lesion positivity). In the latter case, *further investigation, 2° level or recalls* are performed (Chap. 13). The mammograms are then labelled with a standardised code, presented in Table 18.1 [1]:

The system is simple but not perfectly reproducible. The classification system **Breast Imaging Report and Data System BI-RADS®**, *American College of Radiology (ACR)* [2], is spreading also in Italy. It is a structured mammography reporting system, designed to standardise the interpretation of breast imaging, encompassing all modalities, even MRI (Chap. 22). It is also used to classify density in mammography (in 4

categories, from almost entirely fatty breast to extremely dense breast, see Chap. 3). Australia uses the RANZCR synoptic scale, which is similar to the BI-RADS fourth edition [3].

Despite the use of standardised report, however, subjective differences persist, and studies confirm that reader experience and training are crucial in increasing diagnostic efficacy [4].

## 18.2 Percutaneous Breast (Micro) Biopsy

The implementation of nationwide screening programmes in Europe and the United States [5] has led to an increase in the detection of small or otherwise non-palpable, radiologically indeterminate lesions. This in turn has led to an increase in the number of *percutaneous biopsy procedures that* can rapidly ascertain benignity or malignancy [6]. Prognosis is in fact directly related to the stage of development of the disease at diagnosis (Chap. 6). In the case of lesions classified as BI-RADS 4 or 5 (Table 18.2), biopsy is considered mandatory.

*The term biopsy refers to the taking of a sample of tissue or cells by percutaneous procedure, using a hollow needle of different diameters, and then its evaluation (under the microscope).* A cytohistopathological diagnosis is obtained, to establish whether a lesion is benign or malignant and other useful information, for therapeutic purposes.

**Table 18.1** "R"-Labelling in mammography report

| | |
|---|---|
| R1 | Negative or normal test result: no further investigation necessary |
| R2 | Lesion with benign characteristics; no further investigations necessary |
| R3 | Probably benign, but with abnormalities of undetermined significance: Further investigation or close monitoring required |
| R4 | Lesion with suspicious features: Cytological or histological finding required |
| R5 | Positive for malignant changes with cytological/ histological confirmation |

**Table 18.2** Mammography examination classification according to BI-RADS®

| Mammography exam classification results (suspicion) | Recommendations | Probability of Ca |
|---|---|---|
| **Category 0:** Incomplete Previous exams assessment | Recall | Not assessable |
| **Category 1:** Negative | Routine screening invitation | 0% |
| **Category 2:** Benign | Routine screening invitation | 0% |
| **Category 3:** Probably benign | Early follow-up invitation | Between 0 and 2% |
| **Category 4:** Suspect Subcategories A, B, C, D low to very high | Biopsy | > 2% up to <95% |
| **Category 5:** Very suggestive of malignancy | Biopsy | ≥ 95% |
| **Category 6:** Malignancy proven with biopsy | Possible surgical exeresis | Already evaluated |

**Table 18.3** C labelling for cytology report

| C1 | Negative or inadequate cytology report |
|---|---|
| C2 | Benign |
| C3 | Atypical cytology in benignity (doubtful) |
| C4 | Suspicion for malignancy (inconclusive) |
| C5 | Positive for malignancy |

Most biopsies are performed in the outpatient setting under ultrasound (US) guidance by the radiologist. Micro breast biopsy can be divided into two groups: **needle aspiration (FNAC),** and **Core Needle Biopsy (CNB)**, or *thick needle biopsy.* Also to be considered are stereotactic and surgical biopsy.

### 18.2.1 Needle Aspiration, FNAC or FNAB

*Needle aspiration refers to cytological sampling,* i.e. *the aspiration of individual cells, with an extremely fine hollow needle.* It is also referred to by the acronyms **FNAC Fine Needle Aspiration Cytology** or **FNAB Fine Needle Aspiration Biopsy.**

#### 18.2.1.1   FNAC [7–10].

FNAC is used if the image and clinical investigations document the presence of a breast lump suspicious enough to require biopsy (definitely BI-RADS 4 and 5, in some cases even 3), that may or may not be palpable. FNAC is usually done under US guidance. Currently, the preferred system for masses, however, is CNB. FNAC remains the best procedure in case of cystic lesions, or suspicious axillary lymph nodes. FNAC is quick and simple, if performed by an experienced radiologist (the procedure is in fact highly operator-dependent), and rarely causes complications. However, cytological analysis requires a high degree of specialisation of the cytopathologist/laboratory technician (see Chap. 6), higher than that required for histological analysis. The physician may choose to apply a mild local anaesthetic; however, its injection may be more disturbing than the sampling itself. The needle used is extremely thin, usually 23–21 G (gauge). The *gauge* is a system for measuring the diameter of hypodermic needles: the higher the number, the smaller the diameter. It is less than a millimetre from 20 G upwards. Several samples are usually taken by suction and moving the needle tip back and forth (*plunger system*). The collected material is transferred to a slide, on which it is swiped and fixed for sending to the laboratory. The sample is labelled and enclosed with a case report. A major disadvantage is that the lesion may not be exactly centred, resulting in a false negative, or the material taken may not be sufficient (*inadequate*). No information on the invasive nature of the lesion is obtained. The classification given in the European Guidelines for FNAC reporting is in Table 18.3:

### 18.2.2 Core Needle Biopsy CNB or Microhistological Biopsy [9–11]

The sensitivity of sampling by means of **CNB Core Needle Biopsy** under ultrasound guidance is definitely high. It shows a concordance with the results of surgical biopsy estimated on average at around 96%. Many authors point out that the high sensitivity of CNB is based on various factors, such as (1) the number of samples taken (4–5 usually); (2) the depth reached by the instrument used for sampling, which increases the volume of material collected; (3) the immediate placement of the material in formaldehyde solution.

It is a safe procedure in which serious complications are rare. Among the complications can be mentioned the pneumothorax, the risk of which becomes higher in the case of very small breast, and when the lesion is medial or in the axilla. However, it is always a low risk. Milder complications such as pain, oedema, minor haemorrhages and vasovagal reactions may be observed more frequently. Bleeding is more common in women suffering from hypertension and in those who have undergone radiotheraphic treatments.

In the case of women of childbearing age, it would be advisable to avoid biopsies in the perimenstrual phase, and in the early luteal phase, when the breasts are particularly sensitive. It is also important to stop taking certain drugs, such as anticoagulants (when possible), and nonsteroidal anti-inflammatory drugs. Patients have to be informed about all these aspects, given an information sheet, and asked to sign a consent form. The doctor should explain the procedure, the risks, the benefits and the existence of possible alternatives.

Micro-histological sampling may be required in case of (1) inadequate C1; (2) doubtful C3 cytology; (3) lesions that can only be appreciated by mammography (such as microcalcifications); (4) discordance between the clinical-instrumental picture and cytology; (5) the need to define the *histotype of the lesion* with a view to surgery (Chap. 5). The instrument to perform CNB is a device in which a needle of around 22 mm in length and 14 gauge is inserted. The procedure is also called **TRU CUT** or **shearing needle**; It is performed under US guidance, with a high-quality probe. The instrument has a spring-loaded, two-step needle-loading mechanism. It has an inner needle which contains a sampling notch that is "fired" first, and carried deep into the tissue. The second action requires the "firing" of a hollow cannula, which wraps around the first needle and cuts the tissue. The needle must be removed each time to collect the tissue sample. The doctor studies the mammography images, including any recall to precisely *locate* the lesion, using the *o'clock position system* (Fig. 18.1 and Chap. 25). A small incision can be made in the skin beforehand, but many doctors do not consider this necessary. Three to six passes are required, more in the case of microcalcifications, to reduce sampling error. The method of choice for micro, however, is *stereotaxis* (see below).

The doctor makes sure that the tip of the needle is on the lesion, before starting the sampling, with two US images perpendicular to each other. Since air often enters the needle, it is its presence, appearing as a hyper-echogenic (white) line that perfectly delineates the trajectory. Once the procedure is complete, the area of the breast involved is compressed, to avoid the risk of haematoma formation.

**Fig. 18.1**  o'clock positions, right breast; TRU CUT phases

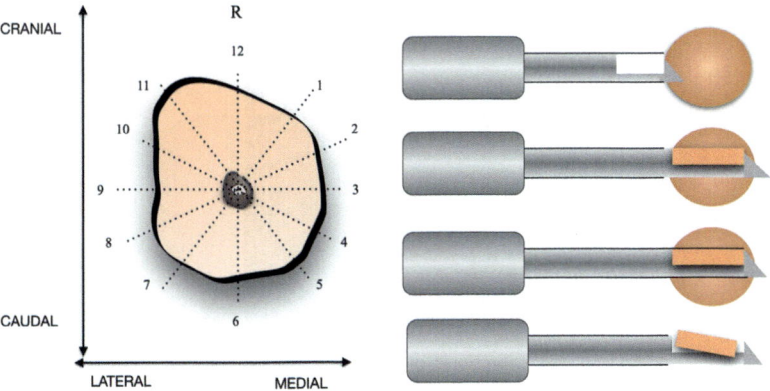

A final report has to be filled in, e.g. using the BI-RADS system® for lesion classification, location and number of samples collected. The patient will then be called back by the centre where she took the biopsy once the results have arrived from the pathology laboratory. The safety, accuracy and convenience of CNB, including the possible sequelae to the patient, have led to its use instead of surgical biopsy for most lesions requiring tissue sampling.

*ImmunoHistoChemistry (IHC)* analyses are conducted on the material to assess prognostic and predictive biomarkers (Chap. 5). The results correlate effectively with those performed on the surgical specimen, also comparing them with those obtained with VAB [12], see below.

## 18.3  Stereotactic Biopsy VAB [13–19]

Stereotactic **Vacuum Assisted Biopsy (VAB)** or **Vacuum Assisted Breast Biopsy (VABB)** is a procedure in which histological biopsies of non-palpable breast lesions are performed, usually BI-RADS 4 or 5, seen exclusively, or at best, on mammographic images. They are mainly micro-calcifications, but also asymmetries or areas of architectural distortion (Chap. 13) not identified by the US. Accurate visualisation of the finding is required, through the acquisition modality monitor. It is a *secondary monitor,* i.e. one with characteristics that are generally not as high in terms of spatial resolution and *luminance,* as those of *first-level or reporting monitors* (see Chap. 23). The stereotactic procedure requires high-quality mammographic monitors.

Stereotaxis is a system that allows for the sampling of more tissue than CNB, and it is also referred to as *large core biopsy*, or minimally invasive surgery. There is the single insertion of a needle, of a large diameter (12 to 7 gauge), preceded sometimes by a scalpel incision for the insertion of a guide, through which a rotating blade operates. Serial contiguous samples over 360° are collected. The samples are then transported out of the collection chamber by a *vacuum back-aspiration mechanism* (hence the name of the method). The suction is maintained at constant values by a control module. The whole system is connected to the mammography machine which uses the calculations made during the procedure to adjust the positioning of the needle in the x-y plane and in depth (z), according to the principles of *stereotaxis. Stereotaxis refers to the use of two simultaneous 2D images at different angles, which create the illusion of a 3D image, to locate and exactly centre a non-palpable lesion.* The data obtained are then used by the computer to guide the needle over the lesion for the removal of the tissue to be studied.

The technique involves first of all choosing the patient's position, which must be the one that allows the best approach to reach the lesion (usually the shortest distance from the skin). The breast must then be positioned to obtain a CC projection or a lateral projection (in the case of a stereotactic sitting position system, see below). The breast is then compressed so that the lesion is in the centre of the **biopsy window.** The compression paddle has a window for needle access, Fig. 18.2, outlined in red. *Stereotactic localisation of a lesion requires a fixed coordinate sys-*

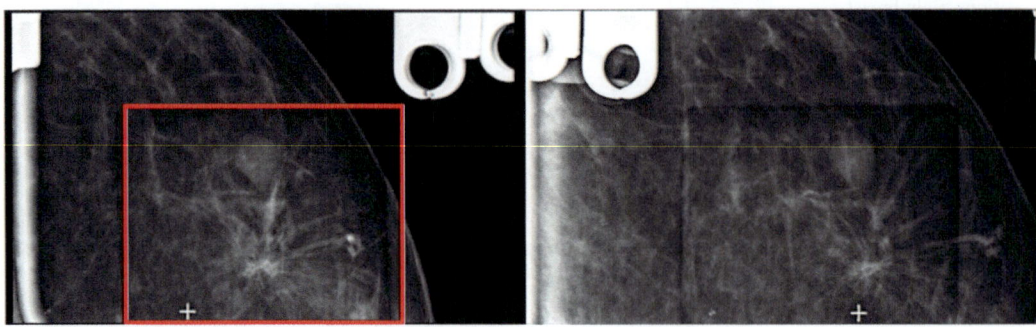

**Fig. 18.2** Stereo pair; biopsy window shown in red. Siemens Healthineers™, Mammomat Inspiration

*tem.* The breast is locked in position and compressed, so that its location is not lost in any way. This can be described by the x, y and z coordinates, relative to a reference point (0,0,0). The total Z-dimension is given by the total thickness of the compressed breast. To locate the *x, y* coordinates, i.e. the horizontal (laterolateral) and vertical (anteroposterior) positions of the lesion, in the centre of the window, one proceeds as follows:

1. The baseline examination is studied and **the patient is positioned congruously**, as if centring the lesion for a second-level study;
2. **A 0°, reference image** is acquired, in which the centring of the lesion with respect to the centre of the biopsy window is verified. Multiple acquisitions may be required for exact localisation;
3. **Two images** are then acquired, **at −15° and +15°, called stereo pair of projections,** with a left and right tube swing, relative to the 0° position of the lesion. They are also called *pre-fire* acquisitions because they precede the movement of the needle over the lesion, and its launch or "firing" for sampling (Fig. 18.3). The two images are displayed on the monitor: The radiographer positions the cursor over the target (the lesion) on both images. The shift of the reference point on the two images with respect to the 0° image is called **parallax** and is proportional to the depth of the lesion. Knowing then the tube angles at which the images were acquired, the software performs a *triangulation* to determine the last coordinate, the z of the lesion, which expresses its depth.

All **coordinates are transmitted to the needle, which is guided by the computer to the indicated position**. The tip of the biopsy system will then point to the lesion. The area where the needle will be inserted is disinfected and anaesthetised. In some cases, a small incision is made in the skin to facilitate the passage of the biopsy needle, which is advanced deep into the lesion. Tissue samples are drawn. The biopsy needle has a cavity or receptacle that allows samples to be

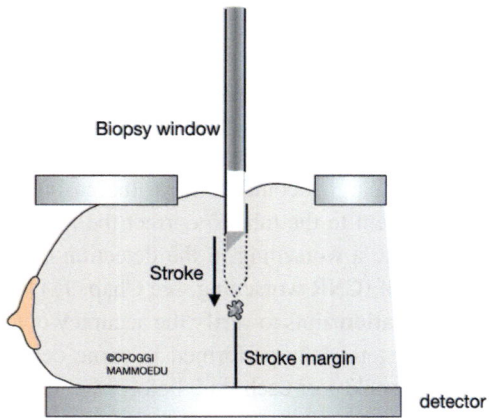

**Fig. 18.3** Stroke and stroke margin in stereotactic biopsy; superoinferior approach, seated patient, central lesion

collected continuously without removing it from the target. A total of 12 samples are the standard with a 10–11 gauge needle, collected by rotating the needle through 360° (about 1–2 centimetres in diameter). **A metal clip is inserted into the site** to indicate the position of the lesion for follow-up studies. Episodes of clip migration are reported, after loosening of the compression (*accordion effect*), or due to haematoma formation and resolution [16]. A pair of *post-fire images* is acquired to verify the sampling success, and then **a radiographic image of the specimen**, especially in the case of microcalcifications.

**Stroke Margin and VAB Limits:** The most advanced biopsy systems have a system to control the so-called *stroke margin*, defined as the distance between the tip of the "fired" needle and the surface of the detector. There is a tolerance range, beyond which using the biopsy manoeuvre involving the firing of the needle leads to damage to the detector, as well as causing an injury to the breast with tearing of the skin. It is necessary to know exactly where the tip of the needle will be once it has been fired. This depends on:

1. The length of the needle;
2. The *stroke*, i.e., the power of the shot, which can be very variable from one system to another, and must be controlled (Fig. 18.3).

*Very small breasts are therefore at risk, and the minimum compressed breast thickness considered to be safe is at least equal to 3 cm* [17]. Very large and thick breasts may require multiple 0° images for centring, and significant blurring of the lesion margins could be seen. Increasing the kV or current to the tube to correct the problem may lead to a worsening in the detection of the lesion itself (CNR worsening, see Chap. 7) [18].

**Calibration** aims to verify the accuracy of the biopsy system. It is performed in some centres daily, or weekly, or each time before use. It consists of assessing how accurate the positioning of the needle tip is in relation to a given point in space (phantoms are used), with an acceptable tolerance of less than 1 mm in all directions.

**Pre- and postbiopsy procedure:** The biopsy site must be pressed for 4–5 min, for haemostasis, and then, a special medication is applied. The patient can go home with an instruction form, which must also be offered orally. The biopsy site must not be wet for 2 days; if the patient feels pain, she can use a painkiller, but not aspirin. Exertion on the day of the biopsy should be avoided. Applying ice before the procedure may also be helpful to limit bleeding afterwards. The entire step-by-step procedure is shown in Table 18.4.

## 18.3.1 Stereotactic Systems with Sitting or Prone Position: A Comparison

The imaging equipment used for biopsy guidance is always the mammographic machine. However, there are two systems for stereotactic biopsy, with a dedicated table, or with a chair [18–20]. In the dedicated table system, the patient is placed prone, with the breast under study descending into an opening. The imaging and biopsy equipment is under the table. The position of the patient and the visual barrier to the biopsy system result in less movement of the patient, and a low incidence of vasovagal reactions. However, these systems take up a lot of space and are more expensive than the chair-based system. It must be considered that many patients have difficulty maintaining the

**Table 18.4** Procedure In Stereotactic Biopsy Exam (with chair system)

| | |
|---|---|
| 1 | Prior to biopsy, if required by the system, **calibration** is performed **on the phantom** to verify the correct functioning of the stereotactic system |
| 2 | The standard and second level mammography images in which the lesion to be biopsied has been identified are viewed. This allows the **best position to be chosen for the patient, depending on the position of the lesion in her breast:** |
| | 1. If the lesion is central, the needle approach may be either with the patient seated, superoinferiorly (example Fig. 18.3) or with the patient in lateral decubitus; |
| | 2. If the lesion is in OQ, lateral decubitus may be chosen, with a LATEROMEDIAL approach; |
| | 3. If the lesion is in IQ, lateral decubitus may be chosen, with a MEDIOLATERAL approach |
| | **That is, care will be taken to choose the position through which the needle's trajectory towards the lesion is the least possible, or in any case the easiest to reach, considering (a) the patient's comfort, (b) the need to avoid vessels, and therefore bleeding and trauma, as far as possible.** The competence of the radiographer to reassure, prepare, and accurately position the patient is fundamental |
| 3 | **Reference image** acquisition **at 0°** |
| 4 | **Stereo image pair** acquisition |
| 5 | On the acquisition monitor: Place the **REFERENCE POINT** or cursor on the lesion, zooming the image in order to Centre it as precisely as possible (according to x and y coordinates) |
| 6 | **The coordinates are transmitted to the system,** which will have identified, by calculation of the parallax shift of the lesion, the coordinate $z$ |
| 7 | Anaesthesia, needle insertion |
| 8 | (It may be necessary to check that the anaesthetic has not in any way 'displaced' the lesion relative to the biopsy window by taking a pair of images). The **PRE-FIRE image pair is acquired** (before sampling) in any case |
| 9 | The material is aspirated, which is then collected from the chamber and placed in a tray for radiographic inspection; the clip is inserted |
| 10 | The **POST-FIRE image pair is acquired**, to check the positioning of the clip and successful aspiration of the target lesion |
| 11 | Images of specimen are taken if appropriate (depending on the nature of the lesion) |

prone position, and there are weight limitations. In addition, the chair system is added to the standard mammography equipment, without the need for a dedicated room and equipment for biopsy only. In the chair system, the patient can sit upright or in a lateral decubitus position, the chair can be placed at 180°, which often allows better access to the posterior tissues. However, vasovagal reactions are generally more likely. For biopsy with tomosynthesis, see Chap. 20.

## 18.4 Pre-operative Localisation of Non-palpable Lesions [21–24]

Mammographic lesions detected in the screening programme are often small, non-palpable, and clinically occult. That is lesions that can be excised by conservative methods, aiming at complete removal, with adequate resection margins (Chaps. 5 and 19), preserving healthy tissue as far as possible.

There are various planning techniques to guide the surgeon in the surgery procedure:

- **Metallic wire:** The standard used to be the insertion of a *wire*, the distal tip of which was placed adjacent to the lesion, and the proximal tip protruding externally on the skin. Although this technique is still used, it has some contraindications, mainly concerning its possible dislocation. For this reason, the distal part generally has a hook. It should preferably be positioned on the day of surgery;
- **Tissue marker (clip):** The clip is generally placed after biopsy, as explained above. It is often made of titanium.
- **Sterile carbon powder diluted with saline solution: Carbon Nanoparticle Suspension (CNS):** This is a safe system and is also used for thyroid or gastrointestinal tract surgeries. It is stable and generally does not tend to spread. It can therefore be inoculated days before surgery. It is injected near the lesion via US guidance, with a continuous release until a small amount is left on the skin, creating a trail to guide the surgeon. Difficulties have been reported in CNS injections in very dense and in very large breasts, and in very deep lesions, near the chest wall, or for multi-focal lesions; CC and ML of the side under examination should be taken, to check the position of the clip;

**Table 18.5** General procedure for pre-operative localisation of non-palpable lesions

| | |
|---|---|
| 1 | The localisation device is placed at the site of the lesion, preferably using US or rarely, MRI guide; sometimes using stereotaxis, in DBT or FFDM mode |
| 2 | If the guidance is US, a mammogram of the side under examination is taken, post-procedure, in CC and ML(LM) projections. It is to assess the exact position of the device, and its possible migration |
| 3 | The phenomenon of *marker migration* must be carefully considered, especially in the case of small breast and superficial lesions. There are no internationally accepted standardised solutions. To mitigate this phenomenon, it is certainly useful to: (1) do the post-insertion marker decompression manually and slowly; (2) re-acquire CC and ML projections before surgery, to be compared with those at the end of the procedure |
| 4 | Charcoal can be released using VAB or DBT-VAB: When possibile the approach to be chosen is the superoinferior (CC projection). While releasing the carbon solution the breast is to be slowly decompressed. CC and ML are acquired before the injection to verify the clip position |

- Other solutions have been proposed, involving the use of different types of **markers, magnetic, radioactive**.

However, the general procedure remains the same, as shown in Table 18.5.

## References

1. Protocollo diagnostico terapeutico dello screening per la diagnosi precoce dei tumori della mammella della regione Emilia Romagna, 4 edizione-Anno. 2012. https://salute.regione.emilia-romagna.it/normativa-e-documentazione/rapporti/contributi/contributi_69_PDT_mammella.pdf
2. ACR BI-RADS Atlas. Mammography 2013 reporting system. 5th ed. ACR; 2013.
3. Hadadi I, et al. Breast cancer detection across dense and non-dense breasts: markers of diagnostic confidence and efficacy. Acta Radiologica Open. 2022;11(1):1–9. https://doi.org/10.1177/20584601211072279.
4. Trieu PD, et al. Reader characteristics and mammogram features associated with breast imaging reporting scores. Br J Radiol. 2020;93:20200363.
5. Funaro K, et al. Screening mammography utilization in the United States. J Breast Imaging. 2023;5(4):384–92. https://doi.org/10.1093/jbi/wbad042.

6. Bick U, et al. Image-guided breast biopsy and localization: recommendations for information to women and referring physicians by the European Society of Breast Imaging. Insight Imaging. 2020;11:12. https://doi.org/10.1186/s13244-019-0803-x.

7. Nakano S, et al. Significance of fine needle aspiration cytology and vacuum assisted core needle biopsy for small breast lesions. Clin Breast Cancer. 2015;15(1):e23. https://doi.org/10.1016/j.clbc.2014.07.001.

8. Mahmoud OM, et al. Fine-needle aspiration cytology versus core needle lymph node biopsy in axillary staging of breast cancer. Egypt J Radiol Nucl Med. 2022;54:219. https://doi.org/10.1186/s43055-022-00895-w.

9. Bhatta UM, et al. Comparison of fine needle aspiration cytology and core needle biopsy findings with excision biopsy in breast malignancy. J Pathol Nepal. 2019;9:1564–70. https://doi.org/10.3126/jpn.v9i2.25031.

10. Shashirekha CA, et al. Fine needle aspiration cytology versus trucut biopsy in the diagnostic of breast cancer: a comparative study. Int Surg J. 2017;4(11):3718–21. https://doi.org/10.18203/2349-2902.isj20174893.

11. Cadavid-Fernàndez N, et al. The role of core needle biopsy in diagnostic breast pathology. Curr Topics Breast Pathol. 2022;35(S2):S3–S12. https://doi.org/10.1016/j.senol.2022.04.006.

12. Elsharkawy M, et al. A ten-year, single-center experience: concordance between breast core needle biopsy/vacuum-assisted biopsy and postoperative histopathology in B3 and B5a cases. PLoS One. 2020;15(5):e0233574. https://doi.org/10.1371/journal.pone.0233574.

13. Jonna AR, et al. Stereotactic breast biopsy: an update in the era of digital tomosynthesis. Appl Radiol. 2018;47(9):17–20.

14. Reiser I. Physics of stereo vs. tomosynthesis-guided breast biopsy PPT Department of Radiology. The University of Chicago; 2020. http://amos3.aapm.org/abstracts/pdf/155-53849-1531640-157537.pdf

15. Tsai HY, et al. Accuracy and outcomes of stereotactic vacuum-assisted breast biopsy for diagnosis and management of non palpable breast lesions. Kaohsiung J Med Sci. 2019;35(10):640–5. https://doi.org/10.1002/kjm2.12100. Epub 2019 Jul 4

16. Hadley R, Jacobs S. Breast biopsy marker migration: significance and potential solutions, Winter-2023-SBI-Newletter.pdf. https://assets-002.noviams.com/novi-file-uploads/sbi/1_25_23_digital.pdf

17. Yeow Y-J, et al. A cohort study of mammography-guided vacuum-assisted breast biopsy in patients with compressed thin breasts (≤3cm). Asian J Surg. 2023;46:4296–301. Science Direct https://www.sciencedirect.com/science/article/pii/S1015958423005869?via%3Dihub

18. Shin K, et al. Tomosynthesis-guided core biopsy of the breast: why and how to use it. J Coin Imaging Sci. 2018;8:28. https://doi.org/10.4103/jcis.JCIS_10_18. https://www.ncbi.nlm.nih.gov/pmc/articles/PMC6085842/

19. Wunderbaldinger P, et al. Comparison of sitting versus prone position for stereotactic large-core breast biopsy in surgically proven lesions. AJR Am J Roentgenol. 2002;178(5):1221–5. https://doi.org/10.2214/ajr.178.5.1781221.

20. Vijapura CA, et al. Upright tomosynthesis-guided breast biopsy: tips, tricks, and troubleshooting. RadioGraphics. 2021;41(5):1265–82. https://doi.org/10.1148/rg.2021210017.

21. Franceschini G, et al. Image-guided localisation techniques for surgical excision of non-palpable breast lesions: an overview of current literature and our experience with preoperative skin tattoo. J Pers Med. 2021;11:99. https://doi.org/10.3390/jpm11020099.

22. Kapoor MM, et al. The wire and beyond: recent advances in breast imaging preoperative needle localization. RSNA. 2019;39:1886–906. https://doi.org/10.1148/rg.2019190041.

23. Zhou Y, et al. Evaluation of carbon nanoparticle suspension and methylene blu localization for preoperative localization of nonpalpable breast lesions: a comparative study. Front Surg. 2021;8:757694. https://doi.org/10.3389/fsurg.2021.757694.

24. ACR Practice parameter for the performance of preoperative image-guided localization in the breast (Resolution 28). 2021. https://www.acr.org/-/media/ACR/Files/Practice-Parameters/Preop-Image-Guided-Breast.pdf

# On the Management of the Surgical Specimen

19

## 19.1 Introduction

Radiography of the surgical specimen allows a quick assessment of the resection margins status and direct a possible margin enlargement in case of tumour involvement (positive margins) [1–5]. See also Chap. 5.

## 19.2 New Approaches

Documenting the surgical specimen with an X-ray used to mean implementing the same acquisition geometry for a standard mammography, i.e. in two projections. The appropriate rotation of the surgical specimen to obtain the CC and MLO standard projections was allowed by the surgeon's insertion of metal landmarks indicating the three directions in space. Only in the case that the specimen contained microcalcifications, the X-ray had to be taken with magnification. For many years now, there has been widespread use of devices that allow radiography of the surgical specimen directly in the operating room, during surgery, thus cutting down the time needed for the patient's anaesthesia. The margins of the lesion are assessed in real time, for the eventual enlargement of the resection. A single projection is generally requested, although the approach is unfortunately not standardised.

*In the case of mammography, the X-ray of the surgical specimen is acquired always with magnification, even in the absence of microcalcifications.* The exposure data must be entered manually and changed according to the size of the surgical specimen.

Considering the subsequent anatomopathological evaluation by sagittal sections, according to the orientation code chosen by the surgical unit, which must be *anatomically relevant*, i.e. useful for the evaluation of the margins of the piece, and standardisable [6], a marking with

1. stitch for the superior margin;
2. stitches for the medial margin;
3. stitches for the inferior margin

could be done. See Figs. 19.1 and 19.2. It is necessary to arrange the different length wires terminating with the metal stitches so as to move them away from the surgical specimen itself, allowing a clear view of it. The stitches have to be counted (the number identifies the side); all have to be included in the FOV so as to be correctly visualised in the reconstructed image. It should be possible to observe also the clip inserted during biopsy, within the lesion.

The image is acquired with compression, although some studies would indicate the need to acquire one without compression as well [7].

*Radiography of the surgical piece is considered mandatory in cases of non-palpable lesions requiring localisation and is recommended for procedures involving extensive local excisions.*

C. Poggi, *Breast Imaging Techniques for Radiographers*,
https://doi.org/10.1007/978-3-031-63314-0_19

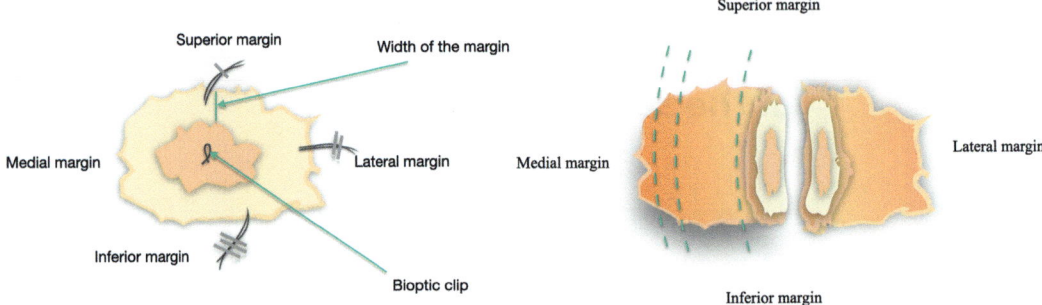

**Fig. 19.1** Positioning of the surgical specimen and landmarks identifying the superior lateral and inferior margins, and sagittal sections, perpendicular to the medial-lateral plane

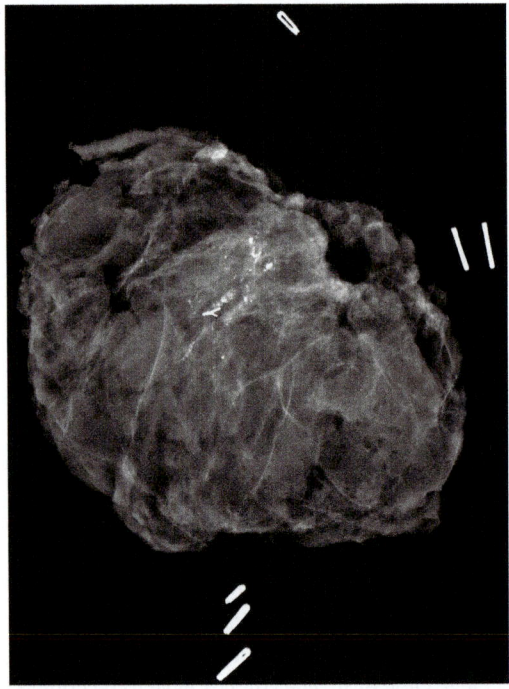

**Fig. 19.2** X-ray of the surgical specimen with dedicated HOLOGIC® Biovision device™ System. Presence of the lesion in the centre of the piece is identified by the clip. New Prato S. Stefano Hospital, Dr. Battaglia, A., courtesy

**Table 19.1** Radiographer's surgical specimen management

| 1 | Patient identification data (assigned id number) |
| 2 | Viewing mammography examination, done before the surgery |
| 3 | Correct identification of the side of the surgical specimen |
| 4 | Double-checking the documentation about surgical specimen labelling (exact locating of the radio-opache stitches, for correct specimen orientation) |

## 19.3   Radiographer's Role

The basic steps of the procedure are listed in Table 19.1:

Radiography and report, if the radiography is performed in the senology department, take precedence over standard examinations so that immediate feedback is sent to the waiting surgeon.

The gap between in vivo histology and radiological imaging in terms of margins and extent of the lesion remains wide [8, 9]. There are many studies fielded in recent years with the aim of narrowing it, relying on artificial intelligence (AI), and different diagnostic imaging methodologies [10–13]. In the histopathological field, Deep Learning (DL) techniques (see Chap. 24) in particular have been successfully used, especially for assessing the presence of lymph node micro-metastases from breast cancer [14].

## References

1. Funk A, et al. Efficacy of intraoperative specimen radiography as margin assessment tool in breast conserving surgery. Breast Cancer Res Treat. 2020;179(2):425–33. https://doi.org/10.1007/s10549-019-05476-6. Epub 2019 Oct 25
2. Rua C, et al. Evaluation of lumpectomy surgical specimen radiographs in subclinical, in situ and invasive breast cancer, and factors predicting positive margins. Diagn Interv Imaging. 2012;93:871–7. https://doi.org/10.1016/j.diii.2012.07.010.
3. Corsi F, et al. Preoperative localization and surgical margins in conservative breast surgery. Int J Surg Oncol. 2013;2013:793819. https://doi.org/10.1155/2013/793819.

4. Kim JY, et al. Indications and methods of intraoperative specimen radiography in breast-conserving surgery. Breast Cancer Res Treat. 2020;179:425–33. https://doi.org/10.21037/tcr-20-2859.

5. Teo KAT, Mallon EA. Breast pathology update. 2021. https://doi.org/10.1016/j.mpsur.2021.11.013

6. Bundred JR, et al. Margin status and survival outcomes after breast cancer conservation surgery: prospectively registered systematic review and meta-analysis. BMJ. 2022;378:e070346. https://doi.org/10.1136/bmj-2022-070346.

7. Kim JY, et al. Indications and methods of intraoperative specimen radiography in breast-conserving surgery. Breast Cancer Res Treat. 2020;9(11):6625–8. https://doi.org/10.21037/tcr-20-2859.

8. Tot T, et al. The pressing need for better histologic-mammographic correlation of the many variations in normal breast anatomy. Virchow Arch. 2000;437(4):338–44. https://doi.org/10.1007/s004280000301.

9. van Doremalen RFM, et al. Novel breast specimen orientation approach through 3D visualizations for relocating inadequate margins based on the surgical clips: feasibility study. ResearchSquare Preprint. https://doi.org/10.21203/rs.3.rs-819800/v1.

10. Mertzanidou T, et al. 3D volume reconstruction from serial breast specimen radiographs for mapping between histology and 3D whole specimen imaging. Med Phys. 2017;44(3):935–48. https://doi.org/10.1002/mp.12077.

11. van Riet YE, et al. Is specimen radiography still necessary in patients with non-palpable breast cancer undergoing breast conserving surgery using radioactive I-125 seed localization? Clin Imaging. 2021;69:311–7. https://pubmed.ncbi.nlm.nih.gov/33045475/

12. Abe H, et al. Comparing post-operative human breast specimen radiograph and MRI in lesion margin and volume assessment. J Appl Clin Med Phys. 2012;13(6):3802. https://doi.org/10.1120/jacmp.v13i6.3802.

13. Wienbeck S, et al. Breast lesion size assessment in mastectomy specimens. Medicine. 2019;98(37):e17082. https://doi.org/10.1097/MD.0000000000017082.

14. Ektefaie Y, et al. Integrative multiomics-histopathology analysis for breast cancer classification. NPJ Breast Cancer. 2021;7:147. https://doi.org/10.1038/s41523-021-00357-y.

## Further Reading

Tabar L, Dean PB. Teaching atlas of mammography. 4th ed. Thieme; 2012. ISBN 978-3-13-640804-9

# On Digital Breast Tomosynthesis and Mammography with Contrast Medium: Notes on Molecular Breast Imaging

**20**

## 20.1 Introduction

Mammography is still considered the gold standard for early detection of breast cancer and is the only screening tool recommended by the European Union for that purpose. Difficulty of assessing dense and very dense breasts still remains, due to *anatomical noise or summation or masking artefact* induced by the two-dimensional nature of the method (Chaps. 3, 7 and 8).

In 2011, the *Food and Drug Administration (FDA)* approved the clinical use of **Digital Breast Tomosynthesis (DBT)** [1]; in recent years, it has emerged as an additional or even alternative technology to *FFDM* (Chap. 7), with the creation of *2D Synthetic Mammography SM* [2]. It is a method that can minimise the masking artefact, enabling an improvement in lesion detection, characterisation and localisation. In addition, the *quasi-three-dimensional information* should make the imaging work-up more efficient than with classical digital mammography, with a reduction of recalls (Chap. 13). The FDA approves the use of DBT in combination with FFDM or SM.

Another important emerging method that will be addressed is the **contrast-enhanced spectral mammography (CESM).**

**Molecular Breast Imaging (MBI)** examinations are also mentioned in this chapter. It stands as an alternative to traditional methods, in the face of the remarkable evolution of NM Nuclear Medicine imaging in the last twenty years.

## 20.2 Digital Breast Tomosynthesis (DBT) [3–7]

*Tomosynthesis* involves the acquisition of a series of projections views of the breast. They are made at different angles, at low dose, while the tube moves over a set arc, from 15 to 50°, depending on the manufacturer. The single views are then reconstructed by an algorithm into thin slices, usually 0.5–1 mm each. Generally, the greater the angular range of the tube's swing, also known as **scan angle**, the more tomographic information is obtained, and thus a better separation between slices, or vertical resolution (on the **z-axis**, or out of plane, see Fig. 20.1). At the same time, increasing the angle of movement of the tube requires an increase in the number of projection views in order to have sufficient sampling. In these reconstructed images, all the structures of the specific slice are in focus, everything shallower or deeper is out of focus. The reader then switches from one reconstructed slice to the next, and the whole dataset represents the overall breast parenchyma (pseudo-3D-reconstruction). However, ***the range of motion is not 360°, and the dataset is highly under-sampled,*** which is why many artefacts occur, especially in the z-direction. The image series produced, or *stack*, is acquired in the two

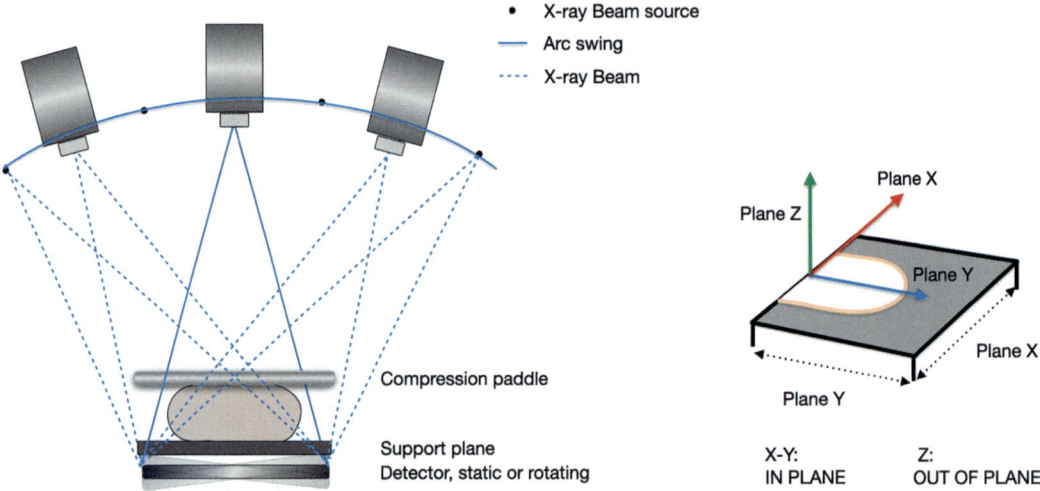

**Fig. 20.1** Image acquisition geometry in DBT: $x$, $y$ and $z$ planes (in plane; out of plane)

standard projections CC and MLO, parallel to the median axial and median sagittal planes, respectively.

DBT images are associated with an increase in acquisition and reading time (the amount of data produced is significant), as well as an increase, albeit small, in the dose delivered. For this reason, the **synthetic mammography (SM),** which uses all the data acquired, was developed as a possible replacement for classic 2D acquisition.

### 20.2.1 Image Acquisition Geometry in DBT

The acquisition geometry is very similar to that of standard digital mammography. The difference is that the tube rotates in a plane around the compressed breast, acquiring a series of images, one for each position of the tube. The detector can be static or rotate, in order to maintain the characteristic of perpendicularity with the X-ray beam; generally, however, it is static (Fig. 20.1).

The series of projections is processed and reconstructed with an algorithm based on the position of the internal structures at each location. The comparison makes it possible to identify their exact location in the vertical direction ($z$-coordinate), and to deduce their 3D spatial distribution. However, due to the fact that the swing

angle of the tube is not 360°, **the spatial resolution is strongly anisotropic**, very high in the plane parallel to the detector ($x$-$y$ plane, or in plane), similar to the FFDM system, and much lower in the plane perpendicular to it ($z$ plane, out of plane). Nevertheless, the problem of anatomical noise is substantially reduced. To optimise the tomographic system, some mammographic machine manufacturers have developed a variety of solutions that make it highly specialised. So much so, however, that it can no longer acquire standard mammography images, which is generally not appreciated by users.

The factors to be considered are as follows:

- The reading of the data, which is desired to be as fast as possible, in order to minimise the total acquisition time;
- The *ghosting* artefacts (Chap. 17 and later), which you want to contain;
- The reduction in *DQE* (Chap. 7) resulting from the low exposure per single acquisition, which must be kept above a given limit for the image to be readable.

**The movement of the X-ray source can be continuous or performed in a *step-and-shoot* manner.** In the first case, the scanning time is shortened, but a blur is produced in the direction of movement. In the second case, the acquisition time inevitably becomes higher, as the tube has to stop at each projection, stabilise itself to avoid vibrations, before acquiring. The likelihood of movement on the part of the patient also increases.

*The scan angle is defined as the maximum angle described by the movement of the tube from the first to the last image. Conversely, the number of projections acquired in a single scan determines the angular sampling* (between two consecutive projections).

In-plane (*x-y*) resolution improves for small scan angles, while larger scan angles improve resolution along z, out of plane. However, it is not possible to increase the scanning angle beyond a given limit, due to the fact that in most cases, the detector is static, and therefore, as the angle increases, the visible FOV decreases (out-of-FOV or truncation). In addition, increasing the number of views would require decreasing the dose (which is fixed, and must be distributed for radiation protection reasons among the various projection views). *Quantum noise* and *electronic noise* increase, as a result (Chap. 8). Increasing the number of projection views does not actually increase the lesion detectability, even if it certainly reduces some artefacts. The degradation of spatial resolution caused by the higher obliquities of the incident beam must also be considered. Another thing to note is that *a wide scan angle improves the ability to detect low-contrast lesions, the masses, which are described by low spatial frequencies* (unless they are very small, Chaps. 8 and 22), *best sampled with wide scan angles.*

Given the acquisition geometry, of non-alignment between source and detector, the use of grids is generally not possible. Therefore, the contribution of scattered radiation, both for contrast and dose, must be considered. Higher energy beams are used, compared to 2D digital mammography (Chap. 7), and this leads to a deterioration of contrast between tissues. In DBT, the stack is reconstructed to compensate for this problem as much as possible. Moreover, in order to speed up data readout time and reduce the detector noise, some manufacturers make use of so-called **pixel binning**. With this system, a group of pixels, e.g. 4 ($2 \times 2$), are assimilated as

if they were a single super-pixel. In addition to the actual reduction in readout time and noise, and the increase in SNR, there is, however, a decrease in spatial resolution.

## 20.2.2 Image Reconstruction in DBT [8, 9]

The data obtained in the DBT are not truly 3D, due to the scanning angle and number of views, making the reconstruction of the image not an easy task. The anisotropic geometry degrades resolution along the *z*-axis, which is reconstructed and not acquired directly. A number of different types of reconstructive algorithms have been proposed and implemented. However, they can be roughly divided into two categories: those based on **Filtered Back Projection (FBT)**, and those on **iterative methods**. The first category, FBT, is the same as that used in CT; it is an efficient system, but has a tendency to produce very noisy images in DBT. The second category consists of comparing the data collected in successive steps, assessing the differences found, and generating continuously updated estimates of the images produced. There is significantly less noise and, among other things, it is also possible to incorporate special algorithms into the system for an overall improvement in image quality.

## 20.2.3 Artefacts in DBT [4, 10, 11]

In contrast to CT, which is a real 3D method, in DBT, there is only a partial cancellation of out-of-plane structures. This is less or more important depending on the scanning angle. It leads to the creation of a series of artefacts inherent in the insufficient sampling along the *z*-axis.

Some of the most significant are mentioned here.

**Artefact due to patient movement:** Given the longer acquisition time compared to FFDM, this is the most common. It may not be so obvious due to method-related blurring. In order to ascertain its presence, 2D mammography must be carefully reviewed.

**Blurring artefact** is determined by the acquisition process in DBT, which does not allow the anatomical noise from planes outside the reconstructed one to be completely eliminated. It presents itself perpendicular to the swing arc.

**Truncation artefact** is due to the finite size of the detector and determined by the reduced scan angle. Breast tissues at the lateral ends can be "eliminated" from the reconstruction in the more oblique projections. As a result, some anatomical structures that "enter and exit" the FOV are only present in some of the projections. They appear as streaks perpendicular to the direction of the tube swing, at the boundaries of the reconstructed image. This is a **stepped artefact**, which gradually decreases as one approaches acquisition at $0°$. In the SM, the individual steps add up to form a single white band.

It is also called truncation artefact that one induced by some dense and/or thick peripheral anatomical structures (e.g. the axilla), which attenuate the beam at the periphery of the image, creating a **bright edge artefact**. Sometimes, this artefact can be eliminated merely by repositioning the patient. Obviously, however, an additional dose is delivered.

**"Halo" artefact:** A high-density object that is represented along the x-y plane may appear with a dark halo around it. This artefact is caused by the attenuation of the X-ray beam due to the presence of the object itself, which inhibits the arrival of photons at the detector around it.

**Zipper or ripple artefact:** Along the scan angle path, the beam may be attenuated if it encounters high-density objects (clips, or macrocalcifications for example). In the reconstruction process, the pixel values corresponding to the attenuation may present an erroneous attenuation estimate along the entire scan angle. This error then can propagate over the entire stack. High-density objects exhibit blurred edges and distorted, elongated shapes, to the point of producing copies of themselves, as many as there are the projection views acquired. This artefact grows proportionally as the distance from the object that caused it increases.

**Shadowing or slinky artefact** occurs in the form of dark lines, which are associated with dense objects. The shadowing artefact in the SM, if adjacent to a lesion, presents itself in such a manner to hinder the study of the lesion.

**Skin edge artefacts:** The skin in DBT appears brighter and thicker than in FFDM. This may be due to an overcompensation of the edge equalisation algorithm (Chap. 8), which allows the visualisation of both the skin and the denser internal structures in 2D images. In SM, the artefact may also include the entire subcutaneous layer. In the case of very thick breasts, the opposite artefact can occur, i.e. the skin edge disappears. The dose required for a thick breast is higher, and peripheral X-rays passing through the skin and subcutaneous tissue can saturate the detector.

**Relocation of skin lesions:** Due to DBT image acquisition and reconstruction system, skin lesions located on the anterior surface of the breast- especially around the areola- can be reconstructed as if they were deeper.

**Ghosting (see also Chap. 17):** It is related to the response of the detector, which changes over time. Ghosts of previous images may appear on new acquisitions. This artefact can be seen particularly when switching from FFDM to DBT acquisition.

**Calcifications in DBT:** Lesions with calcifications as a dominant feature may not be seen in DBT, or appear less suspicious than they would have been in FFDM. In doubtful cases, a magnification view should be performed. In this case, the localisation of the lesion does not necessarily require the acquisition of the *true lateral* projection (see Chaps. 10 and 13).

**Pseudo calcifications in SM:** During the reconstruction of synthetic mammography, a *high-pass filter* is sometimes used (Chap. 8), to improve the spatial resolution of the image. Any microcalcifications that are present may appear more important for this reason, or, they may appear totally artificial (meaning that they are not really present). The reason lies in the quantum and structured noise (Chap. 8) emphasised by the reconstruction process.

A comparison then with FFDM is important.

When in doubt, a magnification view is necessary.

## 20.2.4 Use of DBT in the Biopsy Procedure: DBT-VAB [12, 13]

Tomosynthesis can be performed in the biopsy procedure, not only for lesions seen exclusively with DBT but also for those detected with mammography (Chap. 18). The great advantage of DBT lies in the $z$-axis information: Triangulation obtained with stereo images is not required. The subsequent procedure is the same. This means that the entire available FOV could theoretically be used for initial localisation with $0°$ reference image. The fact that the lesion does not need to be triangulated can reduce the total procedure time by up to 50%. However, lesions with microcalcifications are, as already mentioned, difficult to visualise. An increase in the number of biopsies required has been reported, at least in the first round of screening with tomosynthesis. DBT-VAB is looked as an interesting asset to locate suspicious findings detected by MRI and CESM [14]. See also Chap. 22.

## 20.2.5 Dose Delivered in DBT and DBT-VAB [2, 15]

Tomosynthesis has been suggested as a replacement technique for FFDM, although it is generally still thought as an additional technique. The use of SM is not yet widespread in Italy. In DBT, the estimation of the *average glandular dose (AGD)*, Chap. 21, must take into account another conversion factor in addition to those in use for FFDM, which is the number of projection views acquired.

*Currently, the dose delivered in DBT is similar to/superior to that of FFDM, depending on the equipment, including tube output and beam spectrum, imaging protocol and breast thickness.* It is estimated to be around 30% higher for a bilateral DBT examination than for FFDM.

An increase in mammographic density leads to an increase in dose in both FFDM and DBT, but affects the former more.

As far as DBT-VAB dose is concerned, it is worth noting that the entire glandular tissue is exposed, since the compression paddle is X-ray permeable. In FFDM-VAB, the irradiated tissue is within the active area of the biopsy window only, usually $5 \times 5$ cm.

## 20.2.6 Clinical Pros and Cons of DBT [3–18]

The impact of tomosynthesis in screening and clinical breast studies varies widely, depending on multiple factors. Generally, the increase in diagnostic accuracy is emphasised by the reduction of masking artefact in dense breasts, with a general improvement in *detection rate* (Chap. 6), especially in dense breasts, and for invasive low-grade cancers. This may lead to an increase in *overdiagnosis*. See Chap. 6. The decrease in recalls is mainly associated with asymmetries, thanks to the multiple-section study. At the same time, the possible increase in recalls concerns *masses* and *distortions*, which can be both malignant and benign (Chap. 13). With regard to *architectural distortions*, DBT shows greater accuracy in their detection, and these are lesions that are commonly poorly visualised in FFDM, and sometimes associated with *Interval Cancers IC* (Chap. 6).

Main pros and cons are listed in Table 20.1.

Many studies on DBT suggest that cancers are more conspicuous, i.e. more detectable, on CC than on MLO projection. This should be due to the fact that in CCs more direct force is exerted on the parenchyma than in MLO. Namely, part of the compression value is "absorbed" by high-density and thicker portions, such as the pectoral muscle and juxtasternal tissues. It must be emphasised, however, that these studies do not take the quality of the performance of the breast radiographer into account, both for positioning and compression, which have a considerable weight in the distribution of the compression, in particular precisely in the MLO projection (Chaps. 9 and 17).

**Table 20.1** Advantages, equivalences and disadvantages of DBT versus FFDM

| DBT/ FFDM Advantages | Equivalence | Disadvantages |
|---|---|---|
| Higher diagnostic accuracy for benign calcifications | · | Decreased accuracy for malignant calcifications |
| Higher diagnostic accuracy in dense breasts | Similar accuracy for non-dense breasts | |
| | Dose that can be similar to FFDM, using SM (depends on the characteristics of the mammographic unit) | Definitely higher dose, if in addition to FFDM |
| Higher diagnostic accuracy for architectural distortions, small spiculated masses | | – Lower SR, due to the type of acquisition, that may determine a reduction in the conspicuity of a lesion (Chap. 8) <br> – Increased false positives (see Chap. 13) |
| Reduced second-level us recalls (in addition to FFDM) | Recalls for second level similar with SM | |
| | Similar overall specificity in the two systems | |
| Increased detection of smaller and lower grade invasive cancer (see Chap. 5) | | Possible consequent increase in overdiagnosis |
| Biopsy does not require the use of stereotactic projection for the triangulation of the lesion (information z already present, see also Chap. 18) | | Biopsy rate increase for architectural distortions and radial scars |

## 20.2.7  The Future of DBT

The time for the radiologist to read DBT data is expected to gradually decrease, also due to the advent of new image display methods, such as *slabbing* [19]. In this method, several sections are grouped together to form thicker slices. Machine Learning (ML) detection algorithms have also been developed for DBT, and recently approved by the FDA. In addition, studies are underway on DBT with contrast medium, which, from initial results, seems to have a similar performance to *CESM* (see following paragraphs). According to the latest *European Commission Initiative on Breast Cancer (ECIBC)* recommendations for women with dense breasts, considering the ionising radiation sensitivity of the fibro-glandular tissue (Chaps. 3 and 21), it is preferable not to do both FFDM and DBT, but possibly to choose only the latter [20].

## 20.3  CESM or Dual Energy Mammography

**Contrast-enhanced spectral mammography (CESM)** is an emerging technique, which requires the administration of an iodine-based contrast medium to visualise the *process of neo-angiogenesis* (see Chap. 22) and a dedicated mammographic machine as acquisition modality [21–25].

CESM is also referred to as contrast-enhanced mammography (CEM) or contrast-enhanced digital mammography (CEDM), also as dual energy, spectral or contrast medium mammography. Both 2D FFDM digital mammography and DBT are based on anatomical changes induced by the presence of a lesion: CESM offers *functional information* (see more below). Although studies on CESM are still in their infancy, they suggest that it can improve the sensitivity and specificity of anatomical-based methods. It is also a more accessible and less expensive system than MRI, but comparable in performance to it.

### 20.3.1 Acquisition Protocol in CESM

The parameters are not yet standardised, and this mainly concerns the concentration of the contrast medium, the rate of administration, and the time interval between the administration of the agent and the acquisition of the images. Comparing the results therefore becomes difficult. However, there are general guidelines on which a certain degree of international agreement has been reached. The contrast medium is iodinated, with low osmolarity, with a concentration ranging between 300 and 370 mg/mL. The bolus volume is approximately 1.5 mL/kg of patient weight, preferably administered via an automatic injector, intravenously, at 3 mL/s. It must be followed by a bolus of saline. This keeps the media bolus compact, as experienced in both CT and MRI examinations. The acquisition of images, in the two standard projections CC and MLO, takes place approximately 2 min after injection. It is essential that there is no contamination of the detector with the agent. The radiographer has the task of preparing the patient for the examination, providing her with all useful information and establishing a good relationship (Chap. 24).

A low-energy image is acquired first, followed immediately by a high-energy image, for each projection, during which, as in mammography, the breast under investigation remains compressed.

Total time: about 10–15 min.

**Low energy image LE (Low Energy):** Between 26 and 33 kV, i.e. below the peak of iodine absorption, with an anode/filter combination similar to standard mammography. See Fig. 20.2.

**HE (High Energy) image:** Between 44 and 50 kV voltage, i.e. above the iodine absorption peak, with an anode of the same material as FFDM (Chap. 7), but with combined filters of copper or titanium. The result is a non-diagnostic image: It is used in post-processing to generate the **recombined image.** This is obtained by co-registering LE and HE images, to cut down the background signal, leaving visible only possible areas of enhancement. It is similar to the "subtraction" of MRI, Chap. 22: in CESM, however, this is not a temporal subtraction, before and after contrast, but between images of different energy both after contrast media injection (Fig. 20.2).

Some studies would suggest the possibility of acquiring more images in the late phase (after 7–10 min after injection). The persistence of enhancement, also visible in LE images of the post-biopsy specimen, would indicate the feasibility of performing stereotaxis with CESM, even on several lesions [26, 27].

The total breast compression time per single exposure depends on the thickness of the breast, and its composition: from a few seconds as in standard mammography, to about twenty.

No kinetic curves are created for the temporal study of lesion enhancement, as is the case in MRI (Chap. 22), since only one time point is studied.

ACR-BI-RADS® supplement for standardised CESM reporting is available from 2022 [28].

### 20.3.2 Physics of CESM

The probability of the photoelectric effect occurring in the X-ray biological matter interaction depends on the energy of the photon itself (see Chap. 7). It is highest if the photon has an energy equal to, or better just above, the electron binding energy. This is the process that leads to the production of *characteristic radiation.* If the incident photon has an energy large enough for ionisation, it can succeed in removing an electron from the innermost orbital, the k. The vacuum created makes the atom unstable, so an electron from the outermost orbital will drop to occupy it, creating a photon of energy equal to the difference in the binding energies of the two orbitals involved. The photon is completely absorbed, and maximum contrast is achieved.

This is what we want to happen with the high-energy image in CESM: hitting the k orbital of the iodine, and increasing the absorption probability of the x-photon by the photoelectric effect.

This is referred to as the *absorption peak* or *edge* of the iodine, which is 33.2 kV.

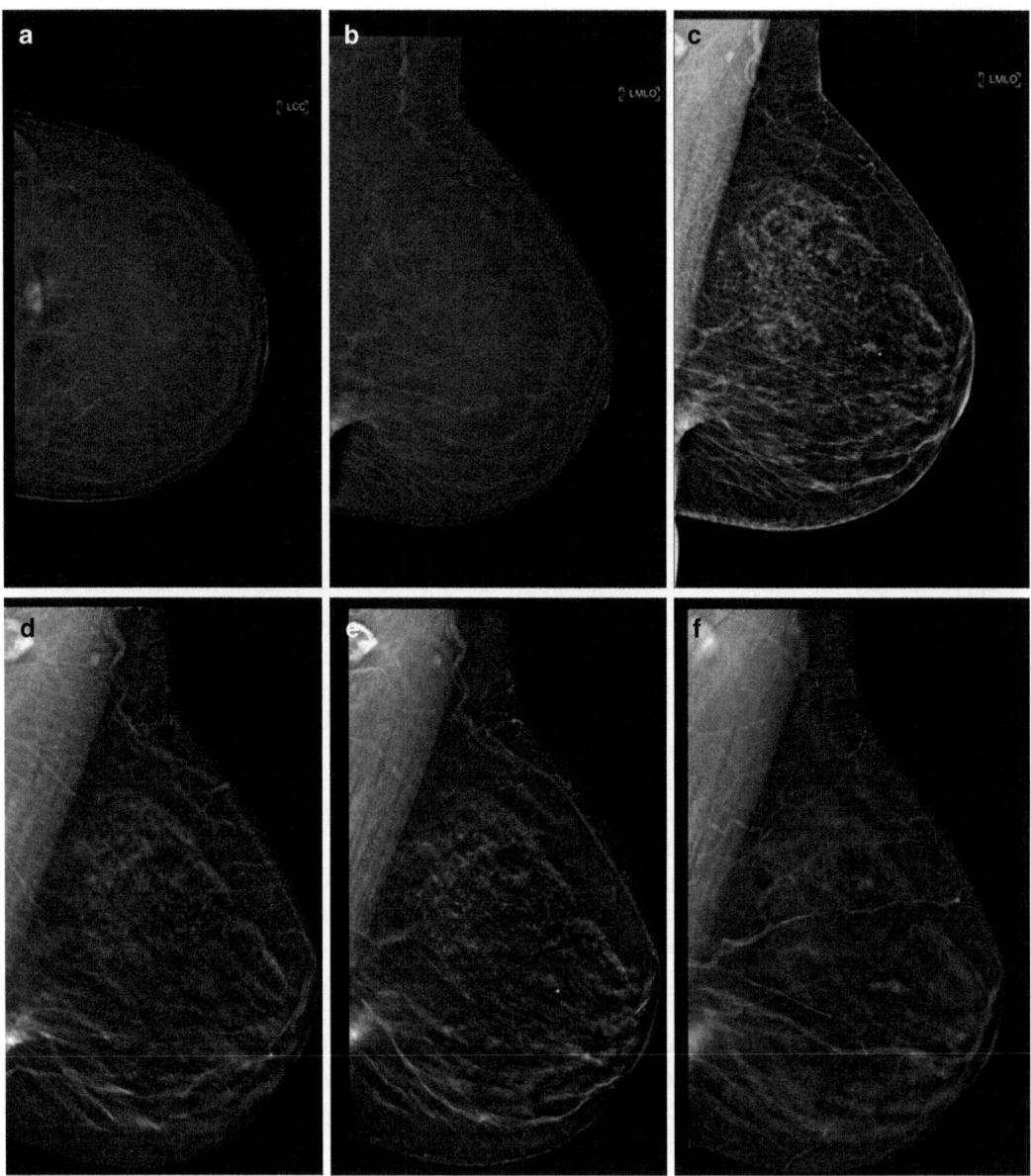

**Fig. 20.2** (**a**, **b**) CESM in two projections, recombined images; (**c**): CESM LE, low energy image; (**d–f**): tomosynthesis on MLO, after contrast, on a deep finding. Note the major skin fold in both projections (due to tissue retraction in important lesion and/or sub-optimal positioning and stretching by the radiographer), which tends to resolve in the over- and under-slices

### 20.3.3 Indications, Limitations (Vs. MRI), and Dose Delivered in CESM

Although the use of CESM appears to improve the sensitivity of FFDM, several considerations must be made in this regard:

1. Even benign lesions can take contrast agents;
2. Globally, to date, it appears that there are no clear advantages of CESM over FFDM for the study of microcalcifications, for example;
3. Preoperative assessment with CESM could actually be one of the most important indications.

It is in fact suggested that CESM could replace MRI, about which there is controversy due to cost, limited access, and low specificity. However, unlike MRI, this method does not allow an extensive study of the axillary cavity. Further studies are also awaited on the correlation between the menstrual phase and enhancement of glandular parenchyma, and on any correlated fluctuations in lesion enhancement, as seen in MRI. MRI is recommended for screening women at high risk of developing breast cancer. It remains the most sensitive method in this respect, also relying on its ability to detect *neoangiogenesis*. CESM is proposed for screening medium-risk women, especially those with dense breasts, for whom there are no established guidelines, and where there is also insufficient evidence to recommend MRI screening. CESM can be regarded as an alternative examination, based on vascularity, for patients who cannot undergo MRI [29]. ECIBC recommendations indicate that CESM is preferable to MRI, due to its more favourable cost, logistics and access in preoperative planning in patients with invasive cancer [30].

The most important limitation of this examination is the possibility of reactions to contrast media, which however appear to be rare. Patients with a history of specific allergy should not undergo this test. A renal function test (glomerular filtrate) is required in any case.

*The lesion site is also important: If it is in the deep inner quadrant, or just close to the chest wall, it could be lost with CESM.*

Artefacts are similar to those of FFDM (Fig. 20.2), apart from the ones related to contrast media administration, due to detector contamination. They are visible and disturbing in the recombined image. Also to be considered is the artefact caused by the patient's movement between the first and second acquisition: Immobility should be recommended.

Another aspect to consider is the *dose delivered* (Chap. 21). For a bilateral examination, *the dose in CESM is around 30% higher than with FFDM* [24–31], similar to that provided by bilateral DBT. Other studies indicate an increase in *AGD* (Chap. 21) in CESM compared to FFDM by 70%, and by 30% compared to DBT. The increase in AGD in CESM is closely related to the features implemented by the mammography machine manufacturer, which makes a generalised comparison difficult. However, the functional information obtained would appear to be particularly interesting, for patients at increased risk, with dense breasts, carefully weighing the cost/benefit ratio.

## 20.4   Molecular Breast Imaging (MBI) or Breast-Specific Gamma Imaging (BSGI) [32–34]

The remarkable evolution of Nuclear Medicine (NM) over the last twenty years has seen an improvement in the typical low spatial resolution, and a reduction of the high dose delivered. This has made it possible and desirable to use this set of methods, referred to as **Molecular Breast Imaging (MBI)**, or **Breast Specific Gamma Imaging (BSGI),** for studying the breast. These examinations require the use of a *radiopharmaceutical* which is administered to the patient in very small quantities. It is composed of a biologically relevant molecule, labelled with a radioactive isotope, which does not alter its behaviour. The radiation emitted is captured by a detector sensitive to gamma photons or positrons. This radiopharmaceutical accumulates in a specific organ or cells, delineating a specific function at the biochemical level. The images show how the tracer itself is distributed in the patient, in a spatio-temporal sense, creating a map of disease sites. It is also expressing the intensity of the process in which the radiopharmaceuticals are involved (*degree of uptake*). This is referred to as **functional imaging.** The detectable concentrations of radiopharmaceuticals are in the order of picomoles, i.e. these methods are extremely sensitive. They are in fact detecting cellular changes in some cases prodromal to structural or anatomical changes, targets of conventional examinations that make up the **morphological imaging.**

### 20.4.1 Physics of MBI

MBI physics is based on an interaction between photons and biological matter, called *pair production.*

**Pair production:** This interaction can only occur if the incident photon has an energy greater than 1.02 MeV, greater than the upper limit of the energy used in conventional and cross-sectional radiology. The photon interacts with the atomic nucleus, creating an electron-positron pair, which loses energy through successive excitations and ionisations. When the positron- a form of anti-matter- arrives at a state of rest, it interacts with an electron, annihilating itself and producing two photons heading in opposite directions, each of 511 keV. When added together, those photons give precisely the minimum energy required for this interaction to occur.

It is actually a process of transforming mass into energy, according to Albert Einstein's famous equation:

$$E = mc^2$$

Annihilation photons are detected by specific, ring-shaped detectors, for the structure and characteristics of which please refer to dedicated texts. However, it can be said that it is a suboptimal system from a physical point of view, since the capacity to capture the emitted radiation is around 1%. It is a percentage that is nevertheless comparable to that of the x-photons produced in the tube in radiology.

The most important characteristics to be taken into consideration with regard to the detection of the annihilation photon pair are four:

1. Both photons produced must leave the patient's body (i.e. not be attenuated or scattered);
2. Both photons produced must reach the detector;
3. Both photons must interact with the detector (detection efficiency);
4. Both signals must be such that they pass the selection criteria to compete for the production of images.

The dose delivered is measured in *radionuclide activity*, the unit of which is the *Bequerel (Bq).*

### 20.4.2 Whole Body Positron Emission Tomography (WBPET) [35–37]

Today's scanners combine advances in acquisition technology with advances in iterative 3D reconstruction and increased computational power. These characteristics have finally enabled a true total-body study, thanks also to the implementation of *time of flight* reconstruction. The improvement in spatial resolution must, however, be coupled with a high photon capture capacity. This is in order to reduce the data-related noise that tends to propagate on the final reconstructed image. PET uses radioactive tracers with a short *half-life*, obtained by marking molecules normally present in biological tissues, such as sugar. One of the most widely used tracers in breast imaging is in fact **FDG (fluoro-deoxy-glucose), labelled with Fluorine 18.** The metabolic energy status of the breast cancer (BC) is an important indicator. BC exhibits a metabolic reprogramming, with a **high/very high rate of glycolysis.** This is the breakdown of sugar for energy production, growth and proliferation of the lesion [37], and it can happen even under anaerobic conditions. It is also called the *Warburg effect*, which appears to occur in 80% of cancers, not just breast cancer. FDG uptake is also influenced by breast tissue density, although to a lesser extent than in cancer. The intensity and pattern of uptake are also directly related to the biological characteristics of the lesion, its aggressiveness and molecular type (see Chap. 5).

[18]F-FDG imaging is used for staging BC determining tumour subtype, and monitoring therapy (Chap. 5). However, it is not recommended for the diagnosis of a primary cancer, at least not routinely.

*PET is very sensitive to neoplastic breast lesions, but is limited by their size.* The sensitivity drops from around 95% to 60% if the lesion is less than 1 cm. In addition, there are subtypes that demonstrate low uptake.

WBPET is an essential complementary exam to morphological image modalities, especially for staging, for directing possible changes in the treatment plan, which happens in a significant number of patients, also useful for detecting hidden metastases on conventional imaging. Scans are acquired about 1 h after administration of the tracer, when its uptake is high enough to be detected, and its distribution has reached a plateau phase.

As far as the maximum administered activity of FDG-F18 is concerned, considering the Dose Reference Levels (DRL), it should stay below 530 MBq (the patient's weight must anyway be considered). See Chap. 21.

PET is currently offered clinically mainly as **PET/CT** and in some cases, as **PET/MRI**. Morphological and functional images are co-registered. Breast PET/MRI has been gaining ground lately, and some scholars are proposing it to decrease the false positives of MRI. It must be said that MRI is an examination that can obtain both morphological and functional information and is still considered the most sensitive image modality (Chap. 22). Furthermore, its diagnostic value will grow further with the advent of techniques employing artificial intelligence (AI), see Chap. 24. The dose in hybrid imaging, considering PET/CT, includes a double exposure, for the radiopharmaceutical activity and for the CT dose: In hybrid equipment, the device is in fact *low-dose* [38].

For the lymph nodes study, we rely on conventional imaging and *lymphoscintigraphy* (see below).

### 20.4.3 Positron Emission Mammography (PEM); The Dose Delivered

The whole body system is not suitable for the study of breast lesions, not only because of the supine position. A dedicated system has therefore been developed: It is called PEM. It comprises two planar or curved detectors, opposite each other, moving in a linear fashion and at a small angle, which scan the breast with slight compression. The patient is seated. The spatial resolution is certainly better than in PET, but the acquisition geometry has major limitations at the end of the chamber field (at the chest wall) and, in addition, has problems with overlapping structures as in standard mammography. After injection of the tracer, 18F-FDG, the two CCs and the two MLOs, right and left, are acquired, as in the mammographic examination. The time required for a PEM is between 5 and 10 min per projection [39, 40].

*The images are displayed as a tomographic stack of 12 slices, the thickness of which is equal to the thickness of the compressed breast divided by 12.*

Interestingly, it is possible to perform a biopsy procedure during the examination itself, with a specific device connected to the imaging system.

*Currently, the dose delivered in PEM is around 370 MBq, which results in an estimated effective dose of around 6.2–7 mSv, much higher than that delivered in the FFDM system.* Consideration must be given to the fact that **exposure in MBI affects the whole body**, due to the systemic injection of the radiopharmaceutical. The overall dose is therefore the sum of the doses to individual organs, weighted according to specific factors.

However, by reducing the radiopharmaceutical dose, and making every possible effort according to the *ALARP principle* (Chap. 21), according to some authors, it should be possible to achieve an effective dose in PEM more comparable to the one delivered in FFDM.

### 20.4.4 MBI with Other Tracers; Dose Delivered in SLNB; and Lymphoscintigraphy

One of the most widely used tracers, besides FDG, is **technetium-99 m sestamibi, 99mTC**. Developed in the 1980s for the cardiological study in nuclear medicine, it was inadvertently discovered that it behaves like a tumour tracer. It is probably based on neoangiogenesis and on the increased concentration of mitochondria in tumour cells.

**Lymphoscintigraphy** is an examination used to map the lymphatic system. This is closely connected to the vascular system and consists of a vast network of vessels, organs and tissues. The propulsive thrust of the *lymph* in the lymphatic system is due to various factors. It derives from the interstitial fluid, through which exchanges between blood and cells take place. The presence of a tumour induces over time an increase in lymphatic pressure in its surroundings, but not in its interior. By pressure gradient then, tumour cells pass into the lymphatic flow. Besides this, the lymph nodes reached by the cancer present a resistance to lymphatic flow, which will be diverted to other sites, with an ever-widening distribution of metastases.

*Lymphoscintigraphy* is used for staging and preoperative planning, but most importantly, for the identification of the **Sentinel Lymph Node SLN** (Chap. 5). This is the first lymph node station to receive drainage from the tumour site. The procedure makes it possible to decide whether to proceed with the biopsy **SLNB**, which can also involve more than one lymph node, and possibly with a more or less extensive exeresis in the event of positivity [41–43].

Lymphoscintigraphy is not always totally reliable for determining the extent of lymph node metastases. In some cases, the sentinel lymph node cannot be visualised. In fact, the lymph node and lymphatic study in general are undergoing major changes, including, for example, the use of *lymphangioMRI* [42], and *Single-Photon Emission SPECT-CT* [43]. The latter method can be used in cases where lymphoscintigraphy did not visualise the SLN. The significance of non-visualisation is not yet well understood [44, 45].

**SLNB:** The radiopharmaceutical generally used is *technetium 99-albumin*, $^{99m}$*T-albumin*, in nanocolloid form. It is injected peri-areolar, intradermal or superficial subcutaneous, or in the peritumour site. Less widely used is the intratumour administration.

The dose administered depends on the time interval between injection and surgery (for lymph node exeresis), with the *activity of approximately 30 MBq at injection, one day before surgery* [45].

Two phases are therefore considered: (1) the first involves imaging, with injection of the radiopharmaceutical and the photon measured by PET, and subsequent *dermographic marking*; (2) the second is detection in the operating room with a collimated probe. Image acquisition should start immediately after injection, up to 30–60 min later.

### 20.4.5  Purpose of MBI

Breast cancer is an extremely heterogeneous disease (Chap. 5), and the different subtypes have different biological characteristics. This has an impact on prognosis, response to therapy, and recurrence rates.

Molecular imaging of the breast emerges as a method to obtain broader biological information on the tumour by developing specific biomarkers to visualise physiopathological processes in vivo.

Recent studies on the use of MBI in breast screening would seem to indicate it as an effective tool, especially in view of the development of MBI-guided biopsy and the gradual reduction of the dose delivered.

Another interesting development in NM, in general, concerns the *theranostic approach*. The term **theranostics** [46] refers to the combination of therapy and diagnostics, in which MBI techniques are used to identify the target, to be hit for instance with ionising radiation, in the field of precision oncology.

## References

1. Lee CI, et al. The effect of digital breast tomosynthesis adoption on facility-level breast cancer screening volume. AJR Am J Roentgenol. 2018;211(5):957–63. https://doi.org/10.2214/AJR.17.19350.
2. Durand MA. Synthesized mammography: clinical evidence, appearance, and implementation. Diagnostics. 2018;8:22. https://doi.org/10.3390/diagnostics8020022.
3. Caumo F, et al. Digital breast tomosynthesis two-dimensional images versus full-field digital mammography for population screening: outcomes from the verona screening program. Radiology.

2018;287(1):37–46. https://doi.org/10.1148/radiol.2017170745.

4. Tirada N, et al. Digital breast tomosynthesis: physics, artifacts, and quality control considerations. Radiographics. 2019;39:413–26. https://doi.org/10.1148/rg.2019180046.

5. Sechopoulos I, et al. A review of breast tomosynthesis. Part I. The image acquisition process. Med Phys. 2013;40(1):014301. https://doi.org/10.1118/1.4770279.

6. Bagnalasta M. Digital breast tomosynthesis Principi di funzionamento e applicazioni cliniche. Tesi: Università degli Studi di Padova, Dipartimento di fisica e astronomia Galileo Galilei, anno accademico; 2017–2018. https://thesis.unipd.it/handle/20.500.12608/25400

7. Chong A, et al. Digital breast tomosynthesis: concepts and clinical practice. Radiology. 2019;292:1–4. https://doi.org/10.1148/radiol.2019180760.

8. Krammer J, et al. Evaluation of a new image reconstruction method for digital breast tomosynthesis: effects on the visibility of breast lesions and breast density. Br J Radiol. 2019;92(1103):20190345. https://doi.org/10.1259/bjr.20190345.

9. Sechopoulos I, et al. A review of breast tomosynthesis. Part II. The image reconstruction, processing and analysis and advanced applications. Med Phys. 2013;40(1):014302. https://doi.org/10.1118/1.4770281.

10. Lay Y-C, et al. Digital breast tomosynthesis: technique and common artifacts. J Breast Imaging. 2020;2(6):615–28. https://doi.org/10.1093/jbi/wbaa086.

11. Geiser WR, et al. Artifacts in digital breast tomosynthesis. AJR. 2018;211:926–32. https://doi.org/10.2214/AJR.17.19271.

12. Rochat CJ, et al. Digital mammography stereotactic biopsy versus digital breast tomosynthesis-guided biopsy: differences in biopsy targets, pathologic results, and discordance rates. Radiology. 2020;294:518–27. https://doi.org/10.1148/radiol.2019191525.

13. Ambinder EB, et al. Tomosynthesis-guided vaccum-assisted breast biopsy of architectural distortion without a sonographic correlate: a retrospective review. AJR. 2021;217:845–54. https://doi.org/10.2214/AJR.20.24740.

14. Ward P. Clinical support builds for DBT-guided breast biopsies. December 20, 2023. https://www.auntminnieeurope.com/clinical-news/womens-imaging/article/15660580/clinical-support-builds-for-dbtguided-breast-biopsies

15. Feng SSJ, Sechopoulos I. Clinical digital breast tomosynthesis system: dosimetric characterization. Radiology. 2012 Apr;263(1):35–42. https://doi.org/10.1148/radiol.11111789.

16. Johnson K, et al. Tumor characteristics and molecular subtypes in breast cancer screening with digital breast tomosynthesis: the Malmö breast tomosynthesis screening trial. Radiology. 2019;293(2):273–81. https://doi.org/10.1148/radiol.2019190132.

17. Horvart JV, et al. Calcifications at digital breast tomosynthesis: imaging features and biopsy techniques. Radiographics. 2019;39:307–18. https://doi.org/10.1148/rg.2019180124.

18. Li J, et al. Diagnostic performance of digital breast tomosynthesis for breast suspicious calcifications from various populations: a comparison with full-field digital mammography. Computat Struct Biotechnol Technol J. 2019;17:82–9. https://www.ncbi.nlm.nih.gov/pmc/articles/PMC6317146/

19. Pujara AC, et al. Digital breast tomosynthesis slab thickness: impact on reader performance and interpretation time. Radiology. 2020;297:534–42. https://doi.org/10.1148/radiol.2020192805.

20. Digital breast tomosynthesis (DBT). https://healthcare-quality.jrc.ec.europa.eu/sites/default/files/Guidelines/EtDs/Updated/2020/ECIBC_GLs_EtD_DBT_vs_DM.pdf

21. Jochelson MS, Lobbes MBI. Contrast-enhanced mammography: state of the art. Radiology. 2021;299:36–48. https://doi.org/10.1148/radiol.2021201948.

22. Sung JS, et al. Performance of dual-energy contrast-enhanced digital mammography for screening women at increased risk of breast cancer. Radiology. 2019;293:81–8. https://doi.org/10.1148/radiol.2019182660.

23. Kornecki A. Current status of contrast enhanced mammography: a comprehensive review. Can Assoc Radiol J. 2022;73(1):141–56. https://doi.org/10.1177/08465371211029047.

24. Sensakovic WF, et al. Contrast-enhanced mammography: how does it work? Radiographics. 2021;41:829–39. https://doi.org/10.1148/rg.2021200167.

25. Avramova-Cholakova S, et al. Performance comparison of systems with full-field digital mammography, digital breast tomosynthesis and contrast-enhanced spectral mammography. Radiat Prot Dosim. 2022;197(3–4):212–29. https://doi.org/10.1093/rpd/ncab172.

26. Kowalski A, et al. Contrast enhanced mammography-guided biopsy: initial trial and experience. J Breast Imaging. 2023;5:148–58. https://doi.org/10.1093/jbi/wbac096.

27. Alcantara R, et al. Contrast-enhanced mammography-guided biopsy: technical feasibility and first outcomes. Eur Radiol. 2023;33:417–28. https://doi.org/10.1007/s00330-022-09021-w.

28. Lee CH, et al. Contrast enhanced mammography (CEM) (A supplement to *ACR BI-RADS®* Mammography 2013) 2022. https://www.acr.org/-/media/ACR/Files/RADS/BI-RADS/BIRADS_CEM_2022.pdf

29. Li L, et al. Contrast-enhanced spectral mammography (CESM) versus breast magnetic resonance imaging (MRI): a retrospective comparison in 66 breast lesions. Diagn Interv Imaging. 2017;98:113–23. https://doi.org/10.1016/j.diii.2016.08.013.

30. Planning surgical treatment: Contrast-enhanced mammography in European guidelines on breast cancer

screening and diagnosis. https://healthcare-quality.jrc.ec.europa.eu

31. Gennaro G, et al. Radiation dose of contrast-enhanced mammography: a two-center prospective comparison. Cancers. 2022;14:1774. https://pubmed.ncbi.nlm.nih.gov/35406546/

32. Smith KA, et al. Molecular breast imaging in the screening setting. JBI. 2023;5(3):240–7. https://doi.org/10.1093/jbi/wbad011.

33. Li H, et al. Radionuclide-based imaging of breast cancer: state of the art. Cancers. 2021;13:5459. https://pubmed.ncbi.nlm.nih.gov/34771622/

34. Dibble EH, et al. Molecular breast imaging in clinical practise. AJR. 2020;215:277–84. ISS-L0361-802X/20/2152-277

35. Vanderberghe S, et al. State of the art in total body PET. EJNMMI Phys. 2020;7:35. https://doi.org/10.1186/s40658-020-00290-2.

36. Whal RL. Quo Vadis: PET and single-photon molecular imaging, vol. 57. Society of Nuclear Medicine and Molecular Imaging, Inc. p. 3S. https://doi.org/10.2967/jnumed.115.159202.

37. Zheng X, et al. Energy metabolism pathways in breast cancer progression: the reprogramming, crosstalk, and potential therapeutic targets. Transl Oncolol. 2022;26:101534. https://doi.org/10.1016/j.tranon.2022.101534.

38. Ming Y, et al. Progress and future trends in PET/CT and PET/MRI molecular imaging approaches for breast cancer. Front Oncol. 2020;10:1301. https://doi.org/10.3389/fonc.2020.01301. eCollection 2020

39. Narayanan D, Berg WA. Use of breast-specific PET scanner and comparison to MRI. Mag Reson Imaging Clin N Am. 2018;26(2):265–72. https://doi.org/10.1016/j.mric.2017.12.006.

40. Yanai A, et al. Newly-developed positron emission mammography (PEM) device for the detection of small breast cancer, Tohoku. J Exp Med. 2018;245:13–9. https://www.jstage.jst.go.jp/article/tjem/245/1/245_13/_pdf/-char/en

41. Ranzenberger LR, Roshan BP. Lymphoscintigraphy, January 2022. https://www.ncbi.nlm.nih.gov/books/NBK563213/

42. Lu Q, et al. Imaging lymphatic system in breast cancer patients with magnetic resonance lymphangiography. PLoS One. 2013;8(7):e69701. https://doi.org/10.1371/journal.pone.0069701.

43. Marino MA, et al. Lymph node imaging in patients with primary breast cancer: concurrent diagnostic tools. Oncologist. 2020;25:e231–42. https://doi.org/10.1634/theoncologist.2019-0427.

44. Chahid Y, et al. Risk factors for nonvisualization of the sentinel lymph node on lymphoscintigraphy in breast cancer patients. EJNMMI Res. 2021;11:54. https://doi.org/10.1186/s13550-021-00793-8.

45. Giammarile F, et al. The EANM and SNMMI practice guideline for lymphoscintigraphy and sentinel node localization in breast cancer. Eur J Nucl Med Mol Imaging. 2013;40:1932–47. https://doi.org/10.1007/s00259-013-2544-2.

46. Gomez Marin JF, et al. Theranostics in nuclear medicine: emerging and re-emerging integrated imaging and therapies in the era of precision oncology. Radiographics. 2020;40:1715–40.

# Radiation Protection in Mammography

21

## 21.1 Introduction

Radiation protection is an interdisciplinary science that aims to preserve the health and well-being of workers and individuals, their offspring and the population as a whole. It aims to reduce the health risks arising from the use of ionising radiation, in activities that must be justified by the benefits derived from them [1].

## 21.2 Ionising Radiation and Interactions with Biological Matter

**Ionising radiation** is defined as the *radiation* or propagation of energy, which has sufficient energy to eject electrons from electrically neutral atoms, and therefore transform themselves into charged atoms, or *ions*. The X-rays used to produce images in mammography are among them. In particular, **X-rays are indirectly ionising radiation,** i.e. by interacting with matter, they set particles in motion, and it is these that ionise. Because of their ability to ionise the atoms of matter they pass through, X-rays have a damaging action on it. There is a transfer of energy that is responsible for biological damage. *X-rays transfer energy to matter through a series of complex interactions with atomic nuclei and electrons, mainly through the Compton and photoelectric effects.* See also Chap. 7.

In the *Compton effect,* an electron is moved away from its orbital, with a certain kinetic energy that it loses through successive ionisations, and it is a contribution to absorbed dose (see Sect. 21.3). The rest of the energy is collected by a secondary photon, deflected from the original trajectory of the primary. The deflected *photon,* also *backscattered,* can subsequently be absorbed by the photoelectric effect. ***The photoelectric effect is a threshold effect.*** The incident photon must have higher energy than the binding energy of the electron, usually of the innermost orbitals (where the electron density is higher, and thus, the probability of interaction increases). The photon gives up all its energy and disappears. The vanished electron creates a "gap" or electron absence, which induces a rearrangement. An electron passes from the outermost orbitals, and there is the emission of the *characteristic X-ray beam*, or Auger electrons. The latter process is more likely for elements with a low atomic number Z: it has therefore relevance in radiobiology for calculating the absorbed dose. Since the photon is totally absorbed, without scattering, the photoelectric effect allows for maximum contrast in radiology. However, it has a negative side-effect: the patient receives more doses than all other mechanisms of X-ray interaction with matter. ***All imaging techniques must be based on the best achievable compromise between image quality and the delivered dose, which is desired to be as low as possible.*** It should also be emphasised that X-rays are high-penetration radiation, which means that the risk is present even at a distance from the source.

## 21.3  General Dosimetric Quantities and Health Detriment

X-rays are characterised by a low **Linear Energy Transfer (LET)**, defined as the average energy transferred from a charged particle to a medium, per unit length. This means that they have a low probability of interaction, i.e. a low ionisation density in the traversed medium.

**Absorbed dose D** is defined as the quantity that evaluates the average energy released by ionising radiation per unit mass. The unit of measurement is the **Gray (Gy)**, corresponding to 1 Joule per 1 kg (J/Kg).

The effects of ionising radiation on health are classified into two types, *stochastic* and *non-stochastic or deterministic*.

**Stochastic effects:** The probability of their occurrence is without a threshold dose, and their severity does not depend on the dose itself. They can also arise many years after irradiation. *The fact that a threshold dose cannot be determined means that there is no dose below which the effect does not occur, and that the severity of the effect is independent of the dose.*

**Non-stochastic or deterministic effects**: Their severity varies as a function of dose, above a given threshold. The latency period is short (acute effects).

Stochastic effects induced by ionising radiation for clinical use include cancer and other heritable effects (see also Chap. 4).

*Health detriment is defined as the reduction in the duration and quality of life that occurs in a population as a result of exposure. Individual health detriment as the sum of clinically observable harmful effects manifested in individuals and their descendants, the onset of which is immediate or delayed.*

*Health detriment* is the concept used to quantify the stochastic effects of low-energy radiation exposure (of radiology examinations). The absorbed dose is not sufficient to predict both the severity and probability of the effects: this is why the **equivalent dose H** was introduced. It is the absorbed dose in the tissue or organ, with a weighting factor that takes into account the type and quality of radiation. In other words, a quantity such as to assess the *different degrees of biological effect of the radiation for the same dose absorbed by a given organ or tissue*. The unit of measurement is the **Sievert (Sv)**, 1 Sv = 1 J/kg [2–5]. The difference between Gray and Sievert is that, although they are expressed by the same unit of measurement, for the same dose, Sievert produces different biological effects, depending on the type of radiation considered. In the case of X-rays, the weighting factor is 1 so that the equivalent dose coincides with the absorbed dose. The weighting factor of the equivalent dose expresses the **Relative Biological Effectiveness (RBE)** of different types of radiation.

The **effective dose E** developed by the *International Commission on Radiological Protection (ICRP)* is the dosimetric quantity that takes into account the different radio-sensitivity of tissues. It can therefore be used to protect against stochastic effects, especially cancer. It is expressed as the sum of the equivalent doses in all tissues and organs of the body after exposure, with the weighting for the radiation and the tissue or organ. *Equivalent and effective doses are used in radiation protection to define exposure limits for workers and the population, as well as to assess the risk/benefit ratio of diagnostic radiographic activities.*

## 21.4  Mammography Dose Descriptor Parameters and Diagnostic Reference Levels (DRLs) [6, 7]

Over the past two decades, increasing importance has been given to various factors that help differentiate the sensitivity of different population groups with regard to exposure to ionising radiation, depending on gender and age at exposure. *It is very important to assess the exposure of the supposedly healthy population, for exam-*

ple in screening programmes. There are still debates about the percentage of reduction in breast cancer mortality and morbidity achieved by screening. However, many international studies have shown it to be overwhelmingly favourable. *In mammography, the only part of the body that receives a significant dose during the examination is the breast* [8–12]. The increase in thyroid cancer correlated to the participation in the breast screening, as erroneously and dangerously claimed (due to the resulting decline in adherence to the screening programme), has been refuted several times by large and important studies. See also Sect. 21.6. The main factors on which the dose delivered to the breast in mammography depends are presented in Table 21.1.

The x-beam in mammography (Chap. 7) is calibrated to produce a specific and known dose, relative to a standard breast under given exposure conditions. Among the most important factors in determining the dose are (a) the sensitivity of the detector; (b) the setting of the AEC system; (c) the anode-filter combination and the kilovoltage, i.e. the energy of the beam. Chapters 7 and 8. For example, if it is necessary to decrease the kilovoltage, in order to obtain the exposure required to produce a high-quality image, the mAs must be increased, which results in a higher dose.

*The reference parameter for estimating absorbed dose in mammography is the Average or Mean Glandular Dose (AGD or MGD), expressed in mGy.* The AGD is an accurate estimation of the *effective dose* to the patient. It could be correlated with *Dose Area Product (DAP)* or *Kerma Area Product (KAP)* for projective radiol-

ogy in general; with *Dose Lenght Product (DLP),* in mGy × cm for CT; *radiopharmaceutical activity* in nuclear medicine. AGD was chosen because it is based on the assumption that it is the glandular tissue, and not the adipose one, to be sensitive to radiation-induced effects. It is therefore a quantity that can be reasonably related to the risk posed by the different mammographic procedures. *AGD cannot be measured directly.* It can be deduced from the output of the X-ray tube, which can be measured directly, and from the exposure parameters. *The dose in soft tissue is approximately proportional to the exposure, defined as the capacity of X-rays to produce ionisation in air (C/kg).* The exact composition of the breast, on the other hand, is not known, and it has an important influence on the average glandular dose. An estimate of this is calculated using conversion factors, according to the model of Dance et al., with a PMMA phantom (see Table 21.2):

$$AGD = k.g.c.s$$

where $k$ is the **incident air kerma (IAK),** measured at the upper skin surface of the breast. *Kerma is* defined as the kinetic energy released in a material. In diagnostic radiology, kerma is equal to the absorbed dose D. Air kerma is measured from the source to the skin, along the cen-

**Table 21.1** Factors on which the dose delivered to the breast depends

| 1 | The intrinsic characteristics of the mammographic unit, and the modality of examination (contact or magnification) |
| 2 | Selected exposure parameters (mainly in automatic mode with AEC) |
| 3 | The size (especially thickness) and density of the breast (the *distribution of* glandular tissue also counts) |
| 4 | The quality of the positioning technique, including adequate compression |

**Table 21.2** DRL in digital mammography from an update of ISTISAN Report 17/33, Padovani et al., ISS, 2020 [6]

| PMMA thickness (in cm) | Equivalent breast thickness (in cm) | DMG in mGy | |
|---|---|---|---|
| | | Acceptable level | Achievable or desirable level |
| 2.0 | 2.1 | ≤1.0 | ≤0.6 |
| 3.0 | 3.2 | ≤1.5 | ≤1.0 |
| 4.0 | 4.5 | ≤2.0 | ≤1.6 |
| 4.5 | 5.3 | ≤2.5 | ≤2.0 |
| 5.0 | 6.0 | ≤3.0 | ≤2.4 |
| 6.0 | 7.5 | ≤4.5 | ≤3.6 |
| 7.0 | 9.0 | ≤6.5 | ≤5.1 |

DGM (AGD) values for mammography proposed by European guidelines, for different thicknesses of the dosimetric PMMA (poly-methyl-methacrylate) phantom
Achievable or desirable level: optimised dose value
Acceptable level: considered as guard level, and understood as DRL

tral axis of the beam. In its measurement, scattered radiation is not considered. The factor *g* takes into account a standard breast with 50% glandular tissue, uniformly compressed, and is based on thickness and HVL (Chap. 7). *c* corrects for non-standard glandularity and thickness. *s* evaluates the different anode/filter combinations, and thus the *spectrum* used (Chap. 7).

For a standard breast, defined as 4.5 cm in thickness after compression, with: (a) a gland/fat ratio of 50:50; (b) an outer portion of adipose tissue surrounding the central area on all sides; considering (c) 60 cm from the source, the average glandular dose should be as shown in Table 21.3.

In the case of tomosynthesis, another conversion factor, *T*, is added for projections view acquired at angles other than 0 (Chap. 20).

The breast, however, does not really correspond to the 50:50 model. Furthermore, the distribution of fibro-glandular tissue is not homogeneous, and changes significantly in the same person, as age advances, and in the same age range, even more significantly among women.

*AGD therefore only gives an indication of the radiation risk during exposure in mammography: it is an estimate and not a true physical quantity.* Above all, the model used does not take into account individual **radio-sensitivity** and **radio-susceptibility** factors. They have been proven to be directly related to the risk of carcinogenesis from breast exposure to X-rays.

However, safety guidelines rely on the AGD to measure *DRLs*. The European Union introduced the concept of **Diagnostic Reference Levels (DRLs)** in 1997, emphasising the need for their use in 2013, pursuant to the 2013/59/Euratom Directive [13]. This directive establishes basic safety standards relating to protection against the

**Table 21.3** Average glandular dose, desired and acceptable level, in Europe and in US (MQSA)

| Average glandular dose AGD desired level for FFDM |
|---|
| 2 mGy/projection (in Italy and some other European states) |
| **Average glandular dose AGD acceptable level (DRL) for FFDM** |
| 2.5 mGy/projection (for *MQSA*—see Chap. 24—it is 3 mGy/projection) |

dangers arising from exposure to ionising radiation. It was transposed in Italy by **Legislative Decree 101/2020** (see Sect. 21.5). The Italian **Istituto Superiore di Sanità (ISS)** provided scientific support in the transposition of the directive, precisely with regard to the definition of *DRLs*. These are recommendations of dose levels for biomedical imaging examinations for: (a) standard patient groups; (b) by type of equipment, and (c) in some cases, for specific examinations. *They are not dose limits/constraints for individual patients. They are recommendations derived from standards of good practice*, recommended by authoritative sources such as *IAEA, International Atomic Energy Agency, ICRP* and the *European Commission EC*. These levels should not be exceeded for a standard procedure performed with the desired optimisation and performance quality criteria, for homogeneous groups of patients. DRLs must be periodically updated and constitute the **Basic Safety Standards (BSSDs)** [14] for protection against ionising radiation. Due to the uneven transposition of the directive, the BSSDs are not harmonised in the different European countries. A more appropriate adherence to the BSSDs would, however, require first of all a harmonisation of the overall basic and radiation protection competencies of radiographers in Europe (see Chap. 24).

*DRLs are one of the main tools for optimising radiological examination procedures, as they can be used to identify unusually high doses during diagnostic radiology practice.* Effectively, DRLs are selected on the basis of a percentile point (75%) of the dose distribution (median values) to patients, nationwide, measured with a specific imaging modality. Studies carried out on groups composed of homogeneous patients are then compared with results from large-scale studies and from guidelines published by internationally recognised bodies. *In the event of systematic deviations of exposure from the reference values, corrective and punctual actions (sanctioned in the event of non-compliance) must be implemented.*

*Directive 2013/59/Euratom* makes a distinction between existing, planned and emergency exposures. *In the case of exposures in asymp-*

*tomatic patients (screening), it stipulates that procedures must be part of a structured programme. This part has been transposed in 101/2020, Art. 165, where screening is included in special practices.* Patients must be informed of the dose received, and of the potential harm that could result. In addition, all operators who are involved, radiographers before others since they are the actual dose providers, must be adequately educated and informed about radiation protection (see below) [15, 16].

It should be emphasised that in the breast screening programme, the radiographer is very often the only health professional that the patient encounters, and his or her responsibilities are important (see Table 21.4).

As far as worker radiation protection is concerned, although the dose in FFDM is very low, lower than that delivered with the SF system (Chap. 7), it is still an examination that uses ionising radiation. So, the frequency of exposures in the work shift must be considered. The radiogra-

**Table 21.4** Responsibilities of the radiographer from the radiation protection point of view in the senology department

- ✓ She/he must constantly monitor the dose delivered
- ✓ Ensure that the level of image quality (technical and clinical) remains high
- ✓ Inform those responsible of any change in the performance of the equipment
- ✓ Conduct the required QCs
- ✓ Knowing the dangers associated with the use of ionising radiation, and working to minimise them, while maintaining a high level of diagnostic information
- ✓ Being aware of the consequences of an improperly conducted mammography examination, in terms of quality and dose delivered
- ✓ Take the necessary steps (theoretical-practical courses, refresher courses) to avoid the need for repetitions of projections (see Chaps. 9, 11 and 12), which lead to an increase in the dose delivered
- ✓ Ensuring that the patient is not in a state of presumed or established pregnancy (process of justification and optimisation, see below). To be noted: (1) verification of pregnancy status is not required for mammography, according to ACR practice parameters [17]; (2) the 10-day rule[a] could be safely replaced by a 28-day rule[a] [18]

[a] After the onset of menstruation

pher has to work behind an appropriate shielding (Chap. 24), which allows her/him to protect herself/himself. In the meanwhile, she/he should clearly see the patient and be able to communicate with her throughout the examination [19, 20]. With regard to health and safety in the workplace, for what is not expressly described in Legislative Decree 101/2021, in Italy, Decree 81/2008 applies. See Chap. 24.

## 21.5   Overview of Legislative Decree 101/2020 (2013/59 EURATOM)

**Single text 101/2020 is relative to all sources of exposure**, in transposition to the European Directive 59/2013. It entered into force in Italy on 27 August 2020. Title XIII deals with medical exposures and is composed of 16 articles.

*The greater attention to teamwork and the training of the various professionals involved is to be mentioned among the important innovations. This is although the figure of the Radiographer in Italy is not valued as it should be. Another innovation is the need to give prior information to the patient regarding the risk/benefit ratio of the exam.* The three cornerstones of radiation protection are reaffirmed: the *principle of justification*, of *optimisation* and of *dose limitation* [4].

**Principle of justification**: Medical exposures must directly benefit the health of individuals and the community. In particular, a specific justification is referred to for diagnostic radiology procedures in the field of screening, as outlined above. The justification principle is based on the results of the most up-to-date scientific research, and on European and International guidelines, recognised by the ISS in Italy.

**Optimisation principle:** In Article 158, in connection with the *optimisation principle*, it is recommended that doses should be kept as low as reasonably achievable ALARA, updated to as low as reasonably practicable ALARP. This is while looking for the right diagnostic information, at the same time. The radiographer actively participates in this process (Art. 159, paragr. 8).

**Dose limitation**: For the general population, it should not exceed 1 mSV/year; for workers who are exposed for professional reasons, the limitation is 20 mSV/year. It must be emphasised that *there is no dose limit for the individual patient.* Dose limits only apply to workers and the general population, meaning that *the dose to the patient must be justified and optimised for each type of diagnostic procedure, for each individual case, and that the usefulness of the result prevails over the risk of the absorbed dose.* Justification and optimisation thus become crucial.

1. Art.158, para.1 is about the principle **As Low As Reasonably Practicable ALARP,** which refers to the minimum deliverable dose capable of obtaining sufficient diagnostic information to answer the question;
2. The importance of prior information on the risk/benefit ratio to the patient, and responsibility for performing the procedure is underlined (Art. 159);
3. The complexity of the optimisation process includes (a) the equipment (the *criteria for the acceptability of equipment* must be derived from European and International recommendations); (b) the production of sufficient diagnostic information. This implies that there must be a *clinical evaluation of the result,* Art. 163;
4. The importance of the practical aspects of the technical-sanitary act, including programmes for achieving and maintaining quality;
5. Dose monitoring and review of DRLs.

*In the optimisation process, the radiographer is the most involved operator, for: (1) the production of the diagnostic information; (2) the practical aspects of the procedure to be performed; (3) the monitoring of the dose and compliance with the diagnostic reference levels. The latter, together with the medical physics specialist.*
**Local diagnostic reference levels (LDRLs)** should also be defined, so as to closely monitor the dose in order to contribute to a continuous improvement of the examination procedure and protocol, in the centre where one works.

The *information on the dosimetric data* related to the single examination should be in accordance with the guidelines issued by the country of origin. In Italy, they have not been published. Pending their publication, this information, which shall be described in all reports (including screening reports), consists of the **indication of the dose class** related to the specific examination. This is indicated by the Guidelines for Diagnostic Imaging published in Gazzetta Ufficiale, May 2005 [21]. The **dose classes, from I to IV,** are presented in paragraph 6 of Article 161. The effective dose is correlated with the clinical question: it is intended as an estimate of the risk of stochastic effects of the various organs concerned due to their different radio sensitivity, i.e. the different probability of developing radio-induced neoplasms, and hence, the different risks. *There must be a correct association between examination and dose class.* However, the *provisional diagnosis* is not present in all RIS (Chap. 8) and is absent from PACS. This makes it difficult to implement it automatically in the report. Guidelines on this subject, drawn up by the major scientific associations in the field, were published in Italy in 2020, precisely for the reporting of dose classes [22]. See also Sect. 21.7.

In addition to the implementation of dose classes in the report, special attention is paid to the assessment of exposure in the case of pregnant and/or breastfeeding women (in case they have to take radiopharmaceuticals). *If pregnancy is suspected, screening mammography should not be conducted. In the case of a clinical mammography* (in symptomatic patients, Chap. 6), *the breast radiologist must carefully assess the risk/benefit.* In the case of an established pregnancy, and the risk/benefit ratio considered in any case positive, also in terms of time (the examination must not be procrastinated for the patient's sake), the dose to the unborn child must also be calculated by the medical physics specialist. It must be remembered that in these cases even more than in others, once the procedure has been justified, the optimisation process becomes crucial. Legislative Decree 101/2020 focuses attention on the system approach, i.e. involving all professional figures. Furthermore, the optimisation process must by necessity be continuously refined. As a matter of fact, one of the most important cornerstones of the text, dealt with in Article 162, concerns training on patient radiation protection. This is included in the *CME programme* (Chap. 24) so that specific credits on the subject must represent at least 10% of the total credits foreseen in the 3-year period, for the Italian radiographer (Resolution 12/11/2021, Rome, AGENAS). The crucial importance of the continuing education process in the field is underlined by the ICRP and the European Commission EC (in Article 18 of 2013/59 Euratom).

## 21.6 Key Points to Contain the Dose Delivered to the Patient in Mammography, and Risk Communication

See in Table 21.5 the steps to follow for dose containment. In addition, as already reported (Sect. 21.4), it is to be highlighted that the *only part of the patient's body that receives a significant dose in mammography is the breast. For this reason, the lead anti-x collar should not be worn on the thyroid gland.* This in fact would result in a consequent loss of deep tissue (covered by the collar). Again for the same reason, anti-*x* aprons should not be displayed in diagnostics rooms. They must, however, be available when needed for any carers of patients with particular needs, carers who must not receive any radiation, as no benefit is derived from their exposure.

**Risk communication** is in general an important new feature introduced in Decree 101/2020, Art. 161, and it certainly includes **patient contact shielding,** such as the thyroid collar or the better-known gonad shield. As can be seen from the article on this subject by Hiles et al. [23], *the optimisation that has been made possible by technological progress now makes the use of any type of contact shielding rarely necessary in radiology departments.* In some cases can even have a counterproductive effect: for example, if it

**Table 21.5** Steps to follow for dose containment in mammography

1 Radiographer has to use adequate compression, according to the consistency mobility and thickness of the breast. The action makes it possible to (1) reduce the dose delivered to the patient, and (2) improve the diagnostic information offered to the person reading the images (see Chaps. 9, 11 and 26)

2 Doing mammograms only after an adequate training period, so that the mages produced are of sufficient quality for reading, in terms of tissue extension. This makes additional projections unnecessary to make up for the lack thereof
(The European Guidelines generally indicate 2 weeks of shadowing, which the author points up it must necessarily be customised for each individual trainee)

3 Have a pro-active attitude: in case of a drop in performance, realise it quickly, and resort to refresher and re-training in high quality centres
(In the European Guidelines, however, re-training is recommended every 2–3 years)

4 Having such an anatomical and anatomo-radiographic knowledge as to know how to correct any functional joint impotence, acute or chronic of the patient, limiting or rather eliminating the projections to be acquired in addition to the standard examination (Chaps. 17, 25, 26, 27 and Appendix 1

5 Recourse to the help (when possible) of a colleague in case there is:
    1. Insufficient knowledge of acquisition techniques in non-standard cases, such as breast implant-carrier (Chap. 14), or more or less significant physical and/or cognitive disabilities;
    2. The need to reduce the time interval in which the breast is compressed as much as possible in patients with postural and/or joint difficulties
This minimises the likelihood of producing insufficient images in terms of technical and clinical quality, and improves the level of service quality perceived by the patient

6 Knowing how to build an effective communication relationship that increases patient *compliance*. This leads to the production of high quality mammograms, in addition to the patient's better tolerance of compression. Indeed, the patient's stiffening and her discomfort, including psychic-emotional discomfort, increase the likelihood of movement and the creation of artifacts that force a re-acquisition, and therefore an increase in the overall dose delivered

7  1. Continuous training and updating on patient radiation protection;
    2. Knowing the diagnostic reference levels, in particular the local LDRL diagnostic reference levels, for continuous quality improvement, always considering ALARP

borders the field of view in examinations performed with AEC, it can lead to an increase in the dose delivered. *Mammography is one of those examinations in which it is not recommended to use contact shielding*, either in the FOV or outside it, especially not on the thyroid [24, 25]. It should be mentioned that the weight factor for the breast has been increased (ICRP 103). Th*e tissue weight or weighting factor expresses the fraction of the risk from exposure to ionising radiation attributable to that specific organ.* That for the gonads, on the other hand, has been significantly reduced.

## 21.7 Dose Recording and Dose Classes [22, 26, 27]

*Dosimetric information,* especially for higher-risk imaging modalities (CT, NM, interventional radiology), must be calculated during the procedure, and a **dose report is available** at the end of it. All the parameters that contribute to the dose must be stored in a *repository*, for later evaluation. Direct digital mammograms have an automatic system that calculates and displays the average glandular dose and the entrance surface dose, for each patient. Any accidental or undue exposure must also be recorded and analysed. *A systematic and constant collection of dosimetric data must be made for each examination, as expressed in Decree 101/2020, pursuant to Article 168.* It must be done on computer support, in compliance with the Guidelines *of the Agenzia per l'Italia Digitale.* Dosimetric data of the population exposed for medical reasons should be sent to national registries, anonymised and encrypted. A standardised vocabulary as the one proposed by RSNA, the RadLex®, should preferably be used [27].

There are two procedures for assigning dose classes to the examination:

1. According to the examination itself (automatically through RIS);
2. Via software that monitors the dose (i.e. the allocation is done by a calculation system).

The **nomenclator associated with the *LEAs*** (see Chap. 6) is used to classify radiologic examinations, in Italy. The nomenclator code for bilateral mammography is 87.37.1 and corresponds to dose class I (below 1 mSv effective dose). It is integrated into the RIS.

Various solutions exist for recording dosimetric information, together with other data from the radiologic examination. The software that transfers these data are called **Radiation Dose Index Monitoring Systems (RDIM)**. The transfer can take place with **non-DICOM** instruments, by manual recording, by Optical Character Recognition (OCR). In these cases, the software creates a document that can be read but not transferred. The transfer can also be done by **DICOM and HL7 instruments** (Chap. 8). In this second case, mention may be made of:

1. DICOM HEADER.
2. MPPS Modality Performed Procedure Step.
3. RDSR Structured Dosimetric Report.

**DICOM HEADER:** The *Dicom header* is a text file that contains a lot of information, including dose-related quantities (see also Chap. 8). The information is stored persistently and archived in PACS. This is certainly an interesting feature. However, it cannot be separated from the images, and if these are not archived, the dose-related data would be lost as a result. Furthermore, the dosimetric information is not complete.

**MPPS:** Various information is recorded in the *MPPS*, including exposure time, patient anatomy and exposure parameters. The data are collected independently of the images, but cannot be transferred to external media (CD, DVD...).

**RDSR:** The *Radiation Dose Structured Report (RDSR)* is a DICOM object defined by report templates, appropriate for dose monitoring in diagnostic radiology. It is data that can be created, retrieved and displayed like all other DICOM objects. The *IHE* consortium (Chap. 8) in its *Radiation Exposure Monitoring (REM)* integration profile recommends the use of the structured report. There are various predefined templates of structured report, also for mammography.

**SAFety in RADiological (SAFRAD) procedure** is a voluntary dose reporting system that aims to build a database through which it is possible to define so-called **trigger levels.** These are dose values absorbed especially in fluoroscopy and interventional procedures, which can induce clinically relevant tissue reactions.

## 21.8 Radiographer Training on Radiation Protection [28, 29]

Radiographer training (see Chap. 24), as far as radiation protection is concerned, is deeply heterogeneous in the European states. An interesting study assessed this aspect, the **EURAMED rocc-n-roll** [29]: by means of a Strengths, Weaknesses, Opportunities, Threats (SWOT) analysis, it showed that the biggest problems concern accessibility and content. Both aspects could be overcome by implementing standardised European-wide *online training*, preceded by the training of *trainers*. This last factor was also indicated as one of the most critical. See also Chap. 24.

## 21.9 Radio-Induced Tumours in Mammography [30–34]

Creating **risk models** that correlate with harmful effects is one of the most important tasks of scientific associations dealing with the risk from exposure to low levels of ionising radiation at low LET. It is very difficult to assess the risk of radio-induced cancer in the human population, but the conclusion is that the risk has a linear trend at low, non-threshold doses. Therefore, even exposure to a very low dose can be potentially dangerous. This approach is described with the Linear **No Threshold (LNT) model** [30] that is still the model considered best by IRCP to manage the risk of radiation exposure at low doses and low dose rates. *No dose, no matter how small, is safe and without risk.*

In Table 21.6 description of breast radio-induced susceptibility.

Table 21.6 Radio-induced tumour susceptibility

| Site | Spontaneous incidence | Radio-induced susceptibility |
|---|---|---|
| Breast | Very high | high |

Also interesting is the *bystander* theory, whereby even cells that have not been directly affected by the radiation may manifest adverse events. This would lead to an underestimation of the risk calculated with the LNT model.

The **Life Attributable Risk (LAR)** for radio-induced breast cancer is also indicated and has been calculated by various scholars. Warren, Dance and Young [34] assessed the total risk that a woman may develop radio-induced breast cancer during her lifetime, for her participation in British mammography screening, every 3 years, from age 50 to 71. They used the ICRP 103 model, considering dose and **Dose Rate Effects in Radiation Biology and Radiation Protection (DDREF)** as efficacy factors. DDREF is a factor applied to a risk model that modifies precisely the relationship between dose and risk, depending on level and rate. A *DDREF* greater than 1 implies that low or chronic doses are less carcinogenic than low and acute doses. The number of lives saved through screening, compared with the number of deaths from radio-induced cancers, again in screening, for a DDERF of 1 would be 156:1. For women with very thick breasts (less than 2% of the total population), it would be reduced to 94:1 [34].

*The reduction in breast cancer mortality through participation in a screening programme, especially if it is well structured and staffed by competent personnel, definitely outweighs the negative effects, including radio-induced cancers.*

## References

1. Bregant P, Signoriello M. Normativa e principi di radioprotezione dal D.Lgs 187/2000 al D.Lgs 101/2020: novità e implicazioni PPT. https://www.burlo.trieste.it/sites/default/files/slides-corsi/Normativa_e_principi_di_radioprotezione.pdf

2. Stewart B, Zamora D. Fundamentals of radiation protection: sources, limits, detectors, shielding. University of Washington Medical Center, Department of Radiology Diagnostic Imaging Section, June 26, 2014 PPT.
3. Ricciardi R. Rischio da basse dosi di radiazione ionizzante, Tesi, Università degli Studi di Napoli Federico II, Dipartimento di fisica, anno accademico 2016/2017. http://www.fisica.unina.it/documents/12375590/13725484/2665_RicciardiR_23-03-2018.pdf/3a2c5186-bc09-4d1c-a36e-32f4621c6f8d
4. Connolly J. The interaction of X-rays with matter and radiation safety, revision date 23-Jan-07. https://www.cigs.unimo.it/CigsDownloads/labs/xrdp/manuali_letture/02-Rad-Safety.pdf
5. Vano E, et al. Dosimetric quantities and effective dose in medical imaging: a summary for medical doctors. Insights Imaging. 2021;12:99. https://doi.org/10.1186/s13244-021-01041-2.
6. Padovani R, et al. Livelli diagnostici di riferimento per la pratica nazionale di radiologia diagnostica e interventistica e di medicina nucleare diagnostica. Aggiornamento del rapporto ISTISAN 17/33. Roma: ISS; 2020. (Rapporti ISTISAN 20/22 Rev.) ISSN 2384-8936
7. European Commission European Study on Clinical Diagnostic Reference Levels for X-Ray Medical Imaging EUCLID. Radiation Protection N°195. 2021. ISBN 978-92-76-28565-6
8. Bengt H. Evaluation of absorbed dose and image quality in mammography, Thesis, Lund University Malmö. 2009. https://lucris.lub.lu.se/ws/portalfiles/portal/6225437/1389228.pdf
9. Dance DR, et al. Further factors for the estimation of mean glandular dose using the United Kingdom, European and IAEA breast dosimetry protocol, IOP publishing. Phys Med Biol. 2009;54(14):4361–72. https://doi.org/10.1088/0031-9155/54/14/002.
10. Dance DR, Sechopoulos I. Dosimetry in x-ray-based breast imaging. Phys Med Biol. 2016;61(19):R271–304. https://doi.org/10.1088/0031-9155/61/19/R271.
11. Suleiman ME, et al. Mean glandular dose in digital mammography: a dose calculation method comparison. J Med Imaging (Bellingham). 2017;4(1):013502. https://doi.org/10.1117/1.JMI.4.1.0135502.
12. Baek JE, et al. Radiation dose affected by mammographic composition and breast size: first application of a radiation dose management system for full-field digital mammography in Korean women. World J Surg Oncol. 2017;15:38. https://doi.org/10.1186/s12957-017-1107-6.
13. Council Directive 2013/59/EURATOM. https://eur-lex.europa.eu/legal-content/EN/TXT/PDF/?uri=CELEX:32013L0059&qid=1688231284354
14. ESR. The current status of uptake of European basic safety standard (2013/59/Euratom) requirements: results of a follow-up survey in European radiology departments. Insights Imaging. 2021;12:139. https://doi.org/10.1186/s13244-s13244-021-01078-3.
15. Radiation protection and safety of radiation sources: international basic safety standards No. GSR Part 3, IAEA 2014. ISBN 978-92-0-135310-8.
16. Comitato Centrale sezione aspetti giuridici medico-legali Ufficio Legale Piccioli, Decreto legislativo 31 Luglio 2020, n.101, Federazione Nazionale Ordini TSRM-PSTRP.
17. ACR-SPR Practice Parameter for Imaging Pregnant or Potentially Pregnant Patients With Ionizing Radiation Revised 2023 (Resolution 31). https://www.acr.org/-/media/acr/files/practice-parameters/pregnant-pts.pdf
18. Radiation protection of pregnant women in radiology https://www.iaea.org/resources/rpop/health-professionals/radiology/pregnant-women
19. Radiation protection in diagnostic and interventional radiology optimization of protection n mammography. IAEA, PPT. https://www.slideserve.com/Jims/radiation-protection-in-diagnostic-and-interventional-radiology
20. Radiation protection and quality standards in mammography, safety procedures for the installation, use and control of mammographic x-ray Equipment, Health Canada 2013. ISBN: 978-0-662-46-361-0
21. Gruppo di lavoro ASSR, FISM, ISS E ministero della salute, La diagnostica per immagini, Linee guida nazionali di riferimento, approvato dalla Conferenza Stato-Regioni 28 Ottobre 2004, C_17_pubblicazioni1164_allegato.
22. Raccomandazioni intersocietarie per la comunicazione della classi di dose (DLgs.101-art.161 c.5–6) AIFM AIMN AINR SIRM 2020 https://sirm.org/wp-content/uploads/2021/04/324-Documento-intersocietario-AIFM-AIMN-AINR-SIRM-2020-raccomandazioni-comunicazione-classe-di-dose.pdf
23. Hiles P, et al. European consensus on patient contact shielding. Insight Imaging. 2021;12:194. https://doi.org/10.1186/s13244-021-01085-4.
24. Hiles P, et al. Guidance on using shielding on patients form diagnostic radiology applications. BIR, published March 2020, Bir Registered charity number 215869.
25. The ACR and Society of Breast Imaging Statement on Radiation Received on Thyroid from Mammography. https://bergenimagingcenter.com/the-acr-and-society-of-breast-imaging-statement-on-radiation-received-to-the-thyroid-from-mammography/
26. Belli G, et al. I sistemi di "registrazione della dose" report AIFM n.13. 2016. ISBN 978-88-907973-7-8
27. Ria F, et al. Statement of the Italian Association of Medical Physics (AIFM) task group on radiation dose monitoring systems. Insight Imaging. 2022;13(1):23. https://doi.org/10.1186/s13244-022-01155-1.
28. Laurier D, et al. Area of research to support the system of radiological protection. Radiat Environ Biophys. 2021;60:519–30. https://doi.org/10.1007/s00411-021-00947-1.

29. Rainford L, et al. Education an training in radiation protection in Europe: an analysis from te EURAMED rocc-n-roll project. Insight Imaging. 2022;13:142. https://doi.org/10.1186/s13244-022-01271-y.

30. Della Peruta G. Il modello linear-no-threshold (LNT) in radioprotezione: basi radiobiofisiche e questioni aperte. Tesi. Università degli Studi di Napoli Federico II, anno accademico 2019–2020.

31. Tahiri Z, et al. Evaluation of radiation doses and estimation of the risk of radiation-induced carcinogenesis in women undergoing screening mammography examinations. Biomed Pharmacol J. 2021;14(1):249–55. https://bit.ly/3tapXyZ

32. Raed Mohammed K. Risk of radiation-induced cancer from screening mammography. Thesis. University of Salford, Degree of Doctor of Philosophy; 2016.

33. Ali RMKM, et al. Effective lifetime radiation risk for a number of national mammography screening programmes. Radiography. 2018;24:240–6. https://www.sciencedirect.com/science/article/pii/S1078817418300154

34. Warren LM, et al. Radiation risk of breast screening in England with digital mammography. Br J Radiol. 2016;89(1067):20150897. https://pubmed.ncbi.nlm.nih.gov/27585843/

# Magnetic Resonance Imaging of the Breast BMRI

# 22

## 22.1 Introduction

Mammography is the only method that has been proven to be effective in reducing breast cancer mortality, making it a "near-perfect" screening test for early diagnosis. However, it has, as repeatedly indicated, various limitations in terms of accuracy, and the sensitivity of this test is strongly influenced by *mammographic density* (Chap. 3). *MRI of the breast is a key imaging instrument in the breast cancer patient's journey, when used in an appropriate clinical setting*. Indeed, it has many positive aspects: (1) it does not use ionising radiation, but there is a dose delivered in MRI; see below; (2) it does not require compression of the breast; (3) it has a very high sensitivity, superior to mammography; (4) it is not affected by breast density; (5) it is three-dimensional and multiplanar; (6) it allows the documentation of deep, thoracic tissue, which is not visible with other methods; finally, (7) it produces both morphological information and functional information. Of course, it also has many contraindications, built into the acquisi-

tion modality: (1) it requires the patient to remain in an uncomfortable position for about 15–20 min; (2) it does not have a high spatial resolution, very far from that of mammography, which is below 100 microns; (3) it has a variable level of specificity, which, however, becomes very high if this examination is performed after mammography and ultrasound; (4) it is costly; and (5) it is not as widely distributed as mammography.

For it to be useful, it must be performed according to precise indications. It is placed as a second, or rather third-level examination, as specified by the guidelines *EUropean Society of MAstology (of Breast Cancer Specialists)* EUSOMA [1], *EUropean SOciety of Breast Imaging (EUSOBI)* and *American College of Radiology (ACR)*.

## 22.2 Indications

The main indications are summarised in Table 22.1 [1–7].

© The Author(s), under exclusive license to Springer Nature Switzerland AG 2024
C. Poggi, *Breast Imaging Techniques for Radiographers*,
https://doi.org/10.1007/978-3-031-63314-0_22

**Table 22.1**  Main clinical and screening indications of breast MRI examination

| | | |
|---|---|---|
| 1 | Pre-operative assessment | The staging of breast cancer is based on the loco-regional extent of the disease in the breast and axilla. Tt leads to predictive value for prognosis and choice of treatment options. Combined with mammography and US, MRI mammography has a very high sensitivity |
| 2 | Assessment of lesion size | MRI mammography has greater accuracy in measuring tumour size than other methods (greater congruence with histological results) |
| 3 | Study of very posteriorly located lesions | Very posterior (deep) lesions are more difficult to assess in mammography and frequently also in ultrasound. MRI mammography is a useful method for detecting tumour invasion of the pectoralis major muscle and chest wall |
| 4 | Identification of hidden, contralateral synchronous lesions (also reducing the risk of metachronous lesions[a])<br>[a]Occurring within 6 months after surgery | Particularly in patients with:<br>• Dense breasts, in which the summation artefact can hide lesions<br>• Diagnosis of *infiltrating lobular carcinoma,* which is believed to have a greater propensity for bilateral presentation. Also, due to its specific growth pattern, it may be underestimated on mammography and ultrasound |
| 5 | Suspected recurrence in women with a history of breast cancer | In the event that clinical, mammographic and/or ultrasound findings are inconclusive, but a recurrence is suspected |
| 6 | Positive margins after conservative surgery | It is useful for identifying residual disease and the possible presence of *multifocal and multicentric lesions* (Chap. 5) and therefore for re-excision surgery planning |
| 7 | To monitor patients' response to neo-adjuvant chemotherapy | In cases of patients with large tumours, who are nevertheless referred for conservative surgery, BMRI is a useful instrument for monitoring the response to chemo, in terms of time (early response) and efficacy (complete pathological response or remission). See Chap. 5 |
| 8 | Implant integrity assessment | MRI is by far the method of choice for the detection of breast intracapsular implant rupture |
| 9 | Screening in high-risk women (in addition to mammography) | • BRCA 1 and 2 genetic mutation carriers (and according to American guidelines, their untested first-degree relatives)<br>• Patients who have been treated with chest mediastinum radiotherapy at aged between 10 and 30 years of age (e.g. Hodgkin's lymphoma)<br>• Carriers of *specific syndromes*[a] that are associated with an increased risk of having breast cancer<br>• Patients with a cumulative risk of between 20 and 25% and higher of disease occurrence, as calculated by *risk models*[b] |
| 10 | Problem-solving tool in cases of discrepant findings between us and mammography | The use of the BMRI examination in this case is controversial. However, some studies have shown that a negative result after MRI increases the safety rate when choosing between short-term follow-up and stereotactic biopsy |
| 11 | Cup syndrome (metastatic axillary lymphadenopathy, with unknown primary) | In the event that conventional examinations are not conclusive For lymphadenopathy secondary to anti-COVID-19 vaccination, see Sect. 22.20 |
| 12 | Search for hidden primary in a patient with Paget's disease | In the event that conventional examinations are not conclusive |

[a]LI FRAUMENI, COWDEN, ATM, CDH1, CHEK2, NF1, PALB2, STK11
[b]CLAUS, BRCAPRO, BOADICEA, TYRER-CUZICK

## 22.3 Notes on the Physics of Signal Production (And on the Displayed Image) in Magnetic Resonance Imaging (MRI) [8]

The tissue questioned in MRI is represented by hydrogen atoms, made up of individual *protons*. To obtain a response from these, with which to construct the image, it is necessary to immerse the patient in a *static magnetic field* (which does not vary in time), called **B0**, at high strength. This is in order to induce an alignment of the protons according to the magnetic field lines, with the production of a longitudinal magnetisation **Mz**, sum of the individual proton magnetisations. It is called like that because it is located along the longitudinal plane, which coincides for the scanners generally used in the diagnostic imaging, with the head-to-foot direction of the patient, the *z*-axis.

In itself, B0 is not sufficient to create a signal. It is necessary to send a second *magnetic field, variable in time*, pulsed (off-on), called *B1*, at radiofrequency RF (in the range between 1 and 200 MHz), which produces a transverse magnetisation **Mxy**. The RF impulse, i.e., shifts the Mz in the transverse plane or xy, by a desired angle (**flip angle**). Mz is representable by a vector, with a certain magnitude, and it is reset by the RF pulse. Once the RF pulse is turned off, the system tends to return to its original condition: Mz recovers its magnitude. This is happening through the **phenomenon of relaxation**, which is in turn a magnetic field variable in time capable of inducing the formation of an electrical signal in the **coil** (the receiving antenna), according to *Faraday's law of induction*. The signal is called free induction decay (FID). As the FID is very fast to deplete, and therefore difficult to measure, a creation of its own **echo** is induced, the **FID echo**. This represents the true MR signal, and it is the expression of the tissue response to RF.

### 22.3.1 On the MRI Signal and K-Space

The first problem to be faced when studying the signal produced in MRI is that it is a *sum signal*. It is not clearly understood how the contributions of individual protons can be distinguished. It is an analogue signal, consisting of an infinite number of points: it has to be *sampled*, i.e. transformed into a finite series of digital points (see Chap. 8), in order to be reconstructed and displayed as an image. It could then be assumed, by simplifying it enormously, that each individual digital dot or sample, i.e. a portion of the analogue signal, could be considered the contribution of a single proton.

The second problem to be addressed is that this signal sum does not contain spatial information, i.e. where the emitting protons are located. Without this information, it is not possible to reconstruct **the image**, which **is nothing more than a map of protons**. It requires a series of **spatial coding** operations, carried out by the appropriate switching on of the *gradients* (located in the scanner). These are magnetic fields that vary their strength in a linear and known manner, and for this, they assign to each point of the signal or proton a pair of values in phase and frequency. These two values convey the position of the proton itself along the *x*-axis and along the *y*-axis, horizontal and vertical. The **x y plane** is thus mapped. The proton is said to be encoded in frequency and phase. In contrast, the information along *z* relates to the depth of the slice. This too is identified by means of other encoding operations. Each proton will then be uniquely identified by this pair of values in phase and frequency, *x* and *y*, and each pair is called a **spatial frequency**. This information fills the k-space, which is a storage of *raw data*, i.e. not yet reconstructed into an image. The spatial frequencies are graphically represented by rows in different numbers (the higher the number, the higher the frequency

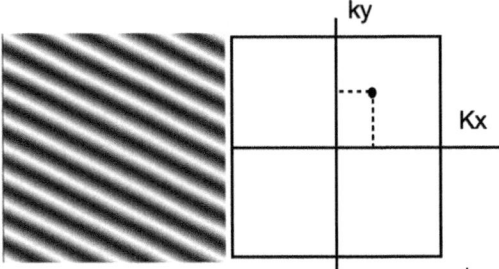

**Fig. 22.1** Spatial frequency and its relative position in k-space for phase and frequency value

value) and different angles (the more the rows are angled, the higher the phase value, or rather the signal phase shift or dephasing). See Fig. 22.1.

Each digital point is also characterised by a third parameter. Since each point represents a portion of the analogue signal, an amplitude value is also associated with each one. This is then transformed into a grey value in the image (Chap. 23). Within the k-space, by convention, the maximum amplitude value of the signal is stored in the centre, where the low spatial frequencies (with low dephasing and frequency values) are located.

Another aspect that is not easy to understand is that there is no relevance between the spatial frequencies of a point, as positioned in k-space, and its position, as a proton, in real space. This is due to how information is stored: each point contributes to the entire image. K-space should be regarded as a row of shelves, one on top of the other, where different information is stored, depending on the position of the shelf. Once combined, all the information will give the image of the object we want to reproduce.

Any object that is to be reproduced in any branch of diagnostic imaging can indeed be represented as a sum of spatial frequencies (Chap. 7). *Spatial frequency is defined as the change in space of the object itself.* Shape and size are described by a small number of *low spatial frequencies*, which convey little change, especially in the case of large objects. They are stored in the centre of k-space, where the maximum signal amplitude, i.e. the maximum information, is located. The edges on the other hand represent the maximum change in space. Inside the edge,

the object is there, and outside, it is not. Edges are defined by a high number of *high spatial frequencies*. We need a lot of them because the change is important and also because high spatial frequencies are associated with low signal amplitude, i.e. low information. They are accommodated in the periphery in k-space.

This is why *high spatial frequencies are related to spatial resolution*, which we have defined as the ability of the imaging system to detect the edges of an object. *Low spatial frequencies are related to contrast*, defined as the ability to recognise a shape relative to the background.

*Therefore, how the k-space is filled affects both spatial and contrast resolution, and not only that, in the displayed image.*

The image is ultimately obtained by applying the inverse Fourier transformation to the filled k-space.

## 22.4  The MRI Signal: Contrast Resolution and Basic Semiotics [9]

The contrast of the MR images is mainly determined by the large difference in tissue relaxation times. This accounts for the high-contrast resolution of this imaging modality.

*The resonance signal is composed almost exclusively of water and fat.*

It is mainly the different percentage amounts of water and fat in the tissue that changes the relaxation times. By relaxation, we mean the phenomenon of restoring the original condition, i.e. the recovery in magnitude or intensity of Mz. This occurs at different speeds. Relaxation is divided into two processes, simultaneous but almost independent. One is called **longitudinal relaxation,** governed by a temporal constant called **T1**. The other is called **transverse relaxation**, with the temporal constant **T2**. Also, T1 and T2 are represented by vectors.

Other aspects count on the semiotics of the signal, e.g. the presence or absence in the studied area of substances with high **magnetic susceptibility.** This is defined as the ability to vary the magnetic

| Signal intensity | Indicated name | How the signal appears | T1 | T2 |
|---|---|---|---|---|
| HIGH SIGNAL | HYPERINTENSE | | SHORT | LONG |
| LOW SIGNAL | HYPOINTENSE | ■ | LONG | SHORT |
| INTERMEDIATE SIGNAL | MODERATELY INTEN-SE (usually related to a predefined tissue) | | INTERMEDIA-TE | INTERME-DIATE |

**Fig. 22.2**   The MR signal: basic principles

field B0 locally. Important is the magnetic susceptibility induced by paramagnetic substances such as the *contrast media CM* generally used in routine examinations. Another factor to consider is the **chemical shift.** It is the difference in **resonance frequency** of the protons found in different molecules. This frequency is proportional to the B0 field, so it should be the same for all hydrogen protons. Depending on the molecule where they are located, however, the electron cloud surrounding them exhibits a varying degree of shielding. Protons will thus perceive a more or less intense B0 value and will therefore have a higher or lower rotational frequency than that of water, known as Larmor. *Fat has a lower frequency than water.*

There are many other factors that affect the signal. Among them is the *diffusion* of water molecules (Sect. 22.16). Also, it counts the number of protons present in the unit mass, called **PD** or **proton density**.

The resonance signal for a flip angle of 90° is given by.

**Signal prop. PD (1-e -TR/t1) e-TE/T2.**

The relaxation is a very complex phenomenon, mediated by the microenvironment in which the studied protons are found. For further information on this regard, please refer to dedicated texts.

## 22.4.1   Extrinsic and Intrinsic Parameters

T1, T2 and PD constitute the so-called **intrinsic parameters**, typical of tissues, which cannot be

modified unless there is a pathological process taking place, or when a contrast medium is administered. The TR and TE parameters are called **extrinsic.** They are modifiable by the operator to obtain a different "weighting" of the sequence, i.e., to emphasise the differences in T1, T2 and PD of tissues (Fig. 22.2). *By sequence, we mean a series of RF pulses, of different types and differently spaced in time, and the appropriate switching of gradients, in order to obtain images with different types of information on the tissues interrogated, according to their T1, T2 or PD.*

High signal is determined by the magnetisation-sum fast recovery, with the gradual reset of Mxy and full recovery of Mz.

*There is no scale of values in MRI that can be compared to that of CT. The signal of the same tissue varies with the sequence and in the same sequence depending on the weighting W. The phenomenon is called rescaling.* In addition to differentiation of weighing according to T1, T2 and PD, it is possible to emphasise only the fluid signal, suppressing fat, or vice versa, or vary the signal by administering a contrast medium.

*The fibro-glandular tissue FGT represents the water signal: Despite this, it appears hypointense in the T2 W sequences;* see Figs. 22.3 and 22.4. The pure fluids have a very long T2, and therefore, the signal should be hyperintense. *FGT is moderately hypointense in T1W sequences,* despite the long T1. This is because the fibrous component prevails.

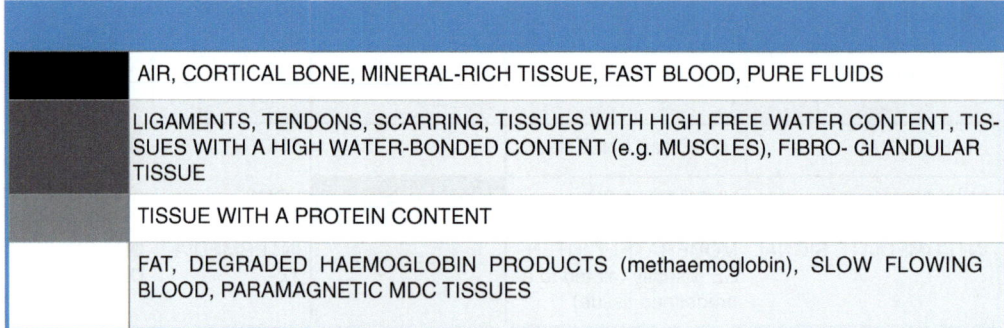

**Fig. 22.3** Contrast variation for morphological sequences T1W

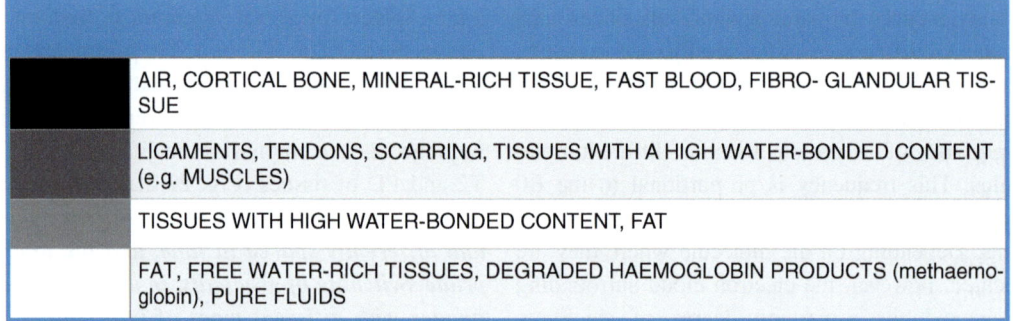

**Fig. 22.4** Contrast variation for morphological sequences T2W

## 22.5 The Basic Principle of BMRI Examination: Neoangiogenesis

The breast is the first organ in which the **process of neoangiogenesis** [10] has been revealed with an MRI examination, by means of the rapid acquisition of a series of images after injection of a *contrast medium (CM)*. This was made possible by technological innovation that made it feasible such a rapid sequence that the *kinetics of enhancement of a lesion* could be observed on the images, after CM administration, practically in real time.

When the neoplastic lesion reaches a certain size, its metabolic demand exceeds that which is physiologically supplied to it by *perfusion*. The tumour demand can be very high. It then induces the release of angiogenic factors in its surround-

ings, with the creation of a newly formed vascular network. This explains the increased enhancement of the malignant lesion compared to healthy tissue, a phase that is referred to as **wash-in.** The newly formed vessels are, however, irregular and leaky, their permeability can be considerable, and this accelerates the release (or wash out) of the CM from the lesion. This is the **wash-out** phase. These two phases are studied in MRI by first monitoring the CM-induced reduction in T1 magnitude and the consequent increase in the signal of the enhanced tissue. Then, the recovery in the magnitude of T1, which, by releasing CM, loses signal intensity (Fig. 22.3 and 22.4). *To be able to study the kinetics of enhancing and washout of the lesion, it will therefore be necessary to have a sequence that is sufficiently fast and T1-weighted.*

## 22.6   Technological and Staff Prerequisites for a High-Quality BMRI Examination [3, 11, 12]

– The static field of the MRI scanner must be at least 1.5 Tesla (T). This is because there is a correlation between field strength and SNR, spatial resolution and temporal resolution (see below). It results in greater diagnostic accuracy. In fact, it is increasingly common for BMRI examinations to be performed at 3 T scanner (in which specific adjustments are made to the sequences also for T1 extension).

– High-performance gradients are needed. This is because it is possible to acquire high-quality images even with echoplanar sequences, used for diffusion studies, which require high levels of technology to be successfully implemented. Not only that, the performance of the gradients is also related to (1) the minimum FOV and minimum slice thickness obtainable; and (2) good field linearity; i.e., the image produced does not show any major spatial deformations of the signal.

– The coil should have at least eight channels, according to the most up-to-date literature.

– 2D sequences must have an in-*plane resolution* of 2–2.5 mm (see Fig. 20.1 in Chap. 20). This is because it is thought BMRI can detect lesions of 5 mm or more [3].

– 3D sequences must have a spatial resolution <1 mm isotropic (0.5 mm desirable).

– Robust fat suppression methods must be applicable.

– *Parallel imaging* techniques of signal acceleration must be available.

– Last but not least, the radiographers performing the examination must have both theoretical and practical training to better manage the scanner at their disposal. An added value is that also she/he works in the mammographic department.

– The radiologist who reports should preferably also be an expert in mammography.

## 22.7   The Protocol According to the European Guidelines [1]

The protocol generally comprises:

1. Accurate centring on the three-plane localiser for positioning the slice packages (called also survey or scout).
2. A TSE T2W morphological sequence, generally without fat suppression, 3D; in axial or sagittal plane.
3. A diffusion-weighted sequence.
4. A dynamic sequence with a series of post-contrast phases (4–6), with robust fat suppression, and high temporal and spatial resolution, in axial or sagittal plane.

### 22.7.1   Positioning the Patient in BMRI [13]

The patient is placed in a prone position, generally in the foot-head direction, although this depends on the design of the scanner. It is, however, the most accepted arrangement for patients. It is necessary to position with great attention, and symmetry is essential, head, neck and chest, but also the hips should be considered. This is to allow mirror reading (comparing the two sides), as in mammography.

The breasts should be hanging freely into the coil, each of them in the centre of the two housings provided. See Table 22.2.

### 22.7.2   Centring the FOV to Launch Acquisition

In the case of acquisition in the axial plane, the slice package must first be placed on the sagittal images of the survey. *The anatomy to be included follows that of the mammography image, from the axillary fossa to just below the IMF.* See Chap. 25 and Annex 1.

**Table 22.2** Positioning the patient in the coil for BMRI examination steps

| | |
|---|---|
| 1 | The breast must be placed in the centre of the coil housing. The field linearity is greatest in the centre, as is the homogeneity of B0. The organ in the centre of the coil therefore and the coil brought to the isocentre |
| 2 | The position of the breasts in the coil is checked by considering all its contact margins |
| 3 | No folds should form in the *IMF* and *intermammary cleft* (see Chap. 3). This is because (1) folds may induce a change in image contrast; (2) the tissue in that area will be compressed, and this may inhibit or slow down the enhancement of a lesion that may be present. Also to be checked the axillary cavity |
| 4 | To obtain symmetry of the chest, it is useful for the head to be rested on a support, via the forehead. The position is uncomfortable, and if it is not possible for the patient to maintain it, it may be decided to have her head rested on the side. Obtaining a perfect symmetry of the chest is more difficult, however. Furthermore, the noise reduction headphones cannot be worn comfortably. Earplugs are then offered |
| 5 | The position of the arms is important. It should be as comfortable as possible, upwards but not too bent, especially the arm connected to the injector. This is because significant bending of the arm could inhibit or in any case slow down the influx of the contrast medium |
| 6 | The symmetry of the patient's body is checked again, from head to toe |
| 7 | The alarm bell is provided, to be used (squeezed) only in the event of an emergency |

As for the inclination of the slice package in the anteroposterior direction on a sagittal localiser image, the guidelines often suggest considering the perpendicularity of the slices in relation to the pectoralis major muscle. The plane passing through the nipple should not be considered at all, since the nipple can be significantly eccentric both with respect to the median sagittal and axial plane. Personally, I believe that the inclination to be considered is along the maximum anteroposterior diameter, in order to optimise the FOV. In the case of acquisitions in the sagittal plane, the package should be placed on the axial images of the three-plane localiser. Again, the position of the nipple should not be considered, but the maximum diameter, in the anteroposterior direction. This is unless there is ductal pathology. In this case, the plane passing through the nipple must necessarily be chosen. *Images in the coronal plane are generally not acquired.* There are two main reasons: the first concerns breathing artefacts, which involve a movement of the chest directed in the coronal direction. The second is anatomical: there are many vessels with an anteroposterior course, and this would lead to their documentation on the coronal plane as foci. That could pose differential diagnosis issues to the reporter.

### 22.7.3 Sequences [14]: The 3D Turbo (or Fast) T2W Sequence

In the centre where I work, it is performed in axial, without fat suppression. The American school prefers acquisitions in the sagittal plane. In some centres, it is performed with fat saturation. *It is actually important that the fat is not saturated in the TSET2W sequence, because the glandular tissue appears hypointense, on the hyperintense fat, and this natural contrast must be exploited.* T2WTSE3D sequence can be performed after the dynamic sequence and then after administering CM. The execution sequence order tends to choose the dynamic one as the first to be performed: this is because it not only allows a lot of information to be obtained, but also requires absolute immobility. The patient is not tired, and the likelihood of moving is reduced. The fact that the 2DT2W sequence is volumetric provides an opportunity to reconstruct it according to other plans, and it is also easier to compare it with the dynamic one.

### 22.7.4 2D TSE T1W Sequence

In the guidelines, the acquisition of a T1-weighted morphological sequence is not mentioned. Priority is in fact given to reducing the overall time of the examination; also, there is a tendency to think that the radiologist already has T1W images, those of the first phase of the dynamic acquired without CM. In reality, however, *the dynamic sequence is not a morphological one*, and it has extrinsic parameters which make it an "imperfect" T1W. It is certainly suitable for a T1 study after CM administration, but much less so without it.

The spatial resolution of this 2D sequence should be around 2.5 mm and, desirably, 2 mm. Such small thicknesses (for medium-performance 1.5 T scanners) require efficient gradients and "tailored" RF pulses, built specifically to achieve a better slice profile. These data, *the minimum slice thickness obtainable in the scanner being worked on, are one of the parameters that must be known by the operator.* The acquisition plan should preferably be the same as that of TSE T2W.

## 22.7.5  3D Dynamic Contrast-Enhanced Sequence (DCE)

It is a volumetric sequence, part of the turbo or fast gradient echo sequence family, with parameters that make it suitable for studying physio-pathological processes. The same anatomical volume is acquired several times, the first one empty (without CM) and the subsequent ones, usually 4 or 5, after CM administration. It implemented *a "robust" fat suppression.* The term robust refers to a process little affected by B1 inhomogeneities, caused by the presence in the imaging volume of tissues with different magnetic susceptibility, i.e., with different permeability to RF pulses.

The dynamic main purpose is to allow the study of the kinetics of enhancement (and wash-out) of the lesion following CM administration. It can be acquired axially or sagittally. It is important for the comparison of the same lesion in the various sequences that the acquisition plane is the same, either axial (CC-like) or sagittal (MLO-like), in all or almost all sequences.

### 22.7.5.1  Shimming
Simply placing the patient in the scanner introduces the greatest source of image noise, the patient, due to her different tissue susceptibility. For this reason, it is necessary, for certain sequences mandatory, to initiate a corrective **shimming** operation. This aims to optimise the homogeneity of B0 in the chosen FOV. It is performed by turning on special coils in the scanner and manually shimming the chosen area. It is worth mentioning again that the error is nevertheless smaller near the isocentre. This means that correct positioning of the breast in the coil, and the positioning of the coil itself at the isocentre of the magnet, is crucial.

**How to Choose the Shimming Volume:** The outlined shimming volume must contain all the tissues to be studied, including the nipples and—partially—the pectoralis major muscle (Fig. 22.5). Therefore, the air between the two breasts must be included. The rectangular box system seems the best system to adopt even at 3 T [15].

**Purpose of Shimming:** To achieve better fat suppression, homogeneous over the whole area.

**How to Implement Fat Suppression with a Chemical Shift-Based Method:** In sequences such as the dynamic one for breast study, fat suppression can be based on the difference in resonance frequency between fat and water. Therefore, when chosen the sequence, a spectroscopic investigation starts automatically, rendering a spectrum that appears in a pop-up window. See Fig. 22.6.

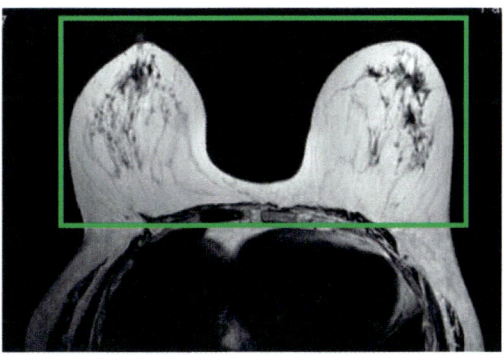

**Fig. 22.5** Shimming volume, in green

**Fig. 22.6** Simplified example of a water-fat spectrum in sequences with fat suppression based on chemical shift: tuning to the water peak

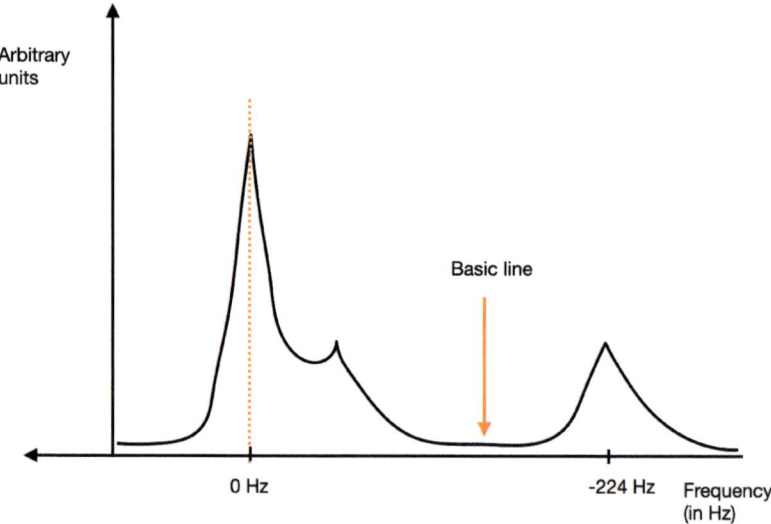

**Table 22.3** Fat water spectrum management in chemical shift-based fat suppression sequence

| Results on spectrum | Accept/refuse |
|---|---|
| The water peak is very low | It is possible for this to happen, the water signal is the fibro-glandular-tissue FGT, which is present in different percentages in each patient. For example, the patient is mastectomised, or otherwise operated on; there are breast implants… |
| Water peak with more than one tip | The presence of jagged peaks, to a lesser or greater degree, is possible. This is baseline noise. It could be acceptable if the principle peak (the water) is well depicted. The tip with the highest frequency should be chosen |
| A third peak appears (as in Fig. 22.6, between water and fat) | In case there are no breast implants (the third peak could silicone, but not in this case, silicone shows a frequency lower than that of fat), it is baseline noise. If it is contained it can be accepted (water and fat peaks must be well depicted) |
| High baseline | The baseline which links water and fat peaks must be low, so to have the two peaks well separated from each other. A high baseline is not generally acceptable |
| Peaks are not well depicted, the baseline is high | *It is not advisable to proceed with image acquisition:* fat suppression would not be optimal. It can happen, e.g., in case of:<br>1. Very large breasts touching the coil;<br>2. Presence of metallic devices<br>It may be useful to redefine the shimming volume, tightening it in antero-posterior direction. Another solution could be choosing the automatic shimming volume |

**How to Proceed:** The operation to be performed is to tune in to the central frequency on which the magnetic resonance scanner works, which is that of water. It is represented by the highest peak (since it has the highest frequency). The scanner will therefore be able to identify exactly the peak of fat, which at 1.5 T is about 224 Hertz (Hz) lower than that of water (Table 22.3). In the Table 22.3 are explained the basic rules to manage the fat water spectrum.

### 22.7.5.2 Outline of the Main Characteristics of the Dynamic Sequence

**Filling the K-Space**

The k-space in this sequence generally has a *k-centric filling order*. This means that the central rows, which are associated with the contrast resolution of the images, are filled first. Moreover, *the filling of the k-space is partial*. This is to speed up acquisition, as in parallel imaging. The fact that the spatial resolution is isotropic (the voxel dimensions are the same in all directions) is an interesting feature for obtaining reconstructions in planes other than the acquisition plane, not so significantly affected by noise. It also features an effective fat suppression method. Fat suppression is in fact related to the k-space filling. The breast is an organ that can have a high sometimes very high percentage of fat: Why is it necessary to suppress it in this sequence? Firstly, because *fat always has a high signal, and this would interfere with the detection of enhancing lesions.* The second reason is explained by the partial filling of the k-space (Fig. 22.7). **The high spatial frequencies,** which we have said are stored at the periphery of the k-space, **are under-**

**sampled.** This means that small lesions, which are practically only edge and are described almost only by the high spatial frequencies, would be lost.

*Suppressing fat in the dynamic sequence therefore allows even small lesions to be discriminated from the background.*

There are many methods for fat suppression. For the dynamic sequence used in the BMRI examination, two systems are generally chosen for their favourable performance characteristics: the DIXON [16] (Fig. 22.8) and the spectroscopic system (based on chemical shift) SPAIR type.

**DIXON:** It is based on sampling the signal at two different TEs. At the first, the signal is such that water and fat are out of phase, and at the second, they are in phase. By means of a calculation in the post-processing phase, the two signals are separated from each other, resulting in a *water* image and a *fat* image (Fig. 22.8). Dixon can be implemented in various types of sequences. There is a three TEs (three points, 3P) version, which allows for the correction of inhomogeneity errors. It is of great interest for the effective abatement of repetitive motion artefacts, such as heartbeat or breathing.

**SPAIR™:** It uses selective spectral inversion pulses for fat suppression; it is not an inversion recovery (IR) sequence. It is very robust system.

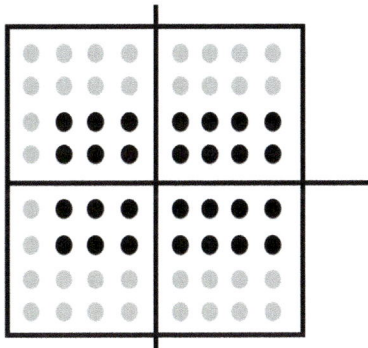

**Fig. 22.7** Simplified representation of partial k-space filling in BMRI dynamic sequence, with undersampling of a large part of the high spatial frequencies (accommodated in the periphery of the k-space)

### Use of Parallel Imaging
*This is a reconstruction technique that accelerates signal acquisition (by reducing steps in the*

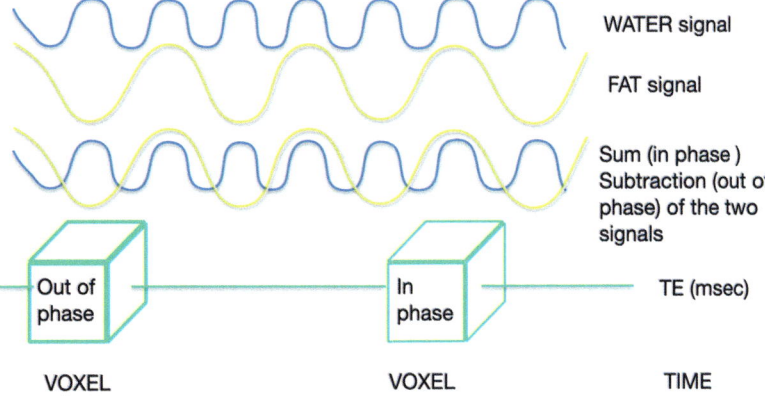

**Fig. 22.8** DIXON method

WATER signal

FAT signal

Sum (in phase)
Subtraction (out of phase) of the two signals

Out of phase    In phase    TE (msec)

VOXEL    VOXEL    TIME

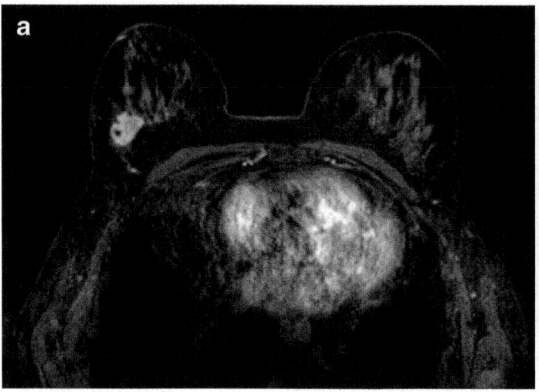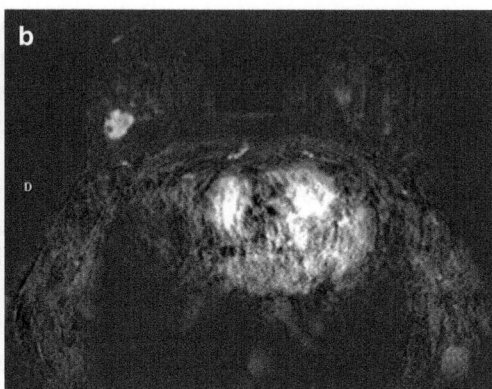

**Fig. 22.9** (**a**) Native dynamic image; (**b**) subtracted image

*phase-coding direction).* Each manufacturer has a different system. Simply put, it is based on the fact that many surface coils are used, connected together in parallel to form a *phased array.* Each of them will produce a different signal depending on the relative position of the coil to the object. In parallel imaging, the signals received from the individual coils are not summed, as is normally the case, but are amplified and processed along separate channels in order to maintain their "identity." The steps along the phase encoding are reduced to accelerate signal acquisition (reduction in scan time TA). This means that the number of spatial frequencies filling the k-space is reduced: undersampling always has a negative impact on the representation of the object. Not only that: *reducing the lines along the phase-coding direction means reducing the size of the FOV in that direction.* This leads to the production of a **wraparound or aliasing artefact**, in which the ends of the object are superimposed on the object itself. One of the main problems of parallel imaging is precisely related to solving this problem. The acceleration factor is generally indicated by the letter **R** (Reduction). With R equal to 2, every other row of the k-space is filled, FOV is halved, and TA decreases. The decrease in the latter is not proportional; in addition to the filled rows, TR and signal averages count.

### The Phases of the Dynamic Sequence: Natives and Subtracts

The first dynamic phase is sent "empty," after the evaluation of the spectrum in case of fat suppres-sion based on chemical shift. The images must be checked carefully to ensure that there were no acquisition problems. The CM is then delivered (see the next section for *timing*), and all the other phases are acquired, one after the other. Images of the dynamic sequence, of all phases, are called **native**. Usually in an automatic way once the last phase is finished, the **subtracted images** are produced. This is a post-processing operation in which the first empty phase is co-registered on the subsequent ones, after CM injection. In these images, the anatomical background is almost completely eliminated (being the same in all phases, including the first one), and only the enhanced tissue is emphasised (CM is not present in the first phase) (Fig. 22.9).

### Duration of the Single Phase in the Dynamic Sequence

This is an important parameter to choose, which is referred to as **time resolution.** According to the English guidelines of the *NHS National Health System* [17], it should be less than 1 min, but preferably less than 45 s. In international lit-erature, however, the most frequently quoted time resolution is 90 s.

*It is important that the duration of the single phase is short enough to be able to intercept the transition phase between enhancement and release of contrast media, at the peak of enhancement.* Making it too short (*having too high a temporal resolution*) means sacrificing spatial resolution, as the two parameters are in antithesis. The choice must take into account

**Fig. 22.10** Timing or synchronisation CM administration and data acquisition

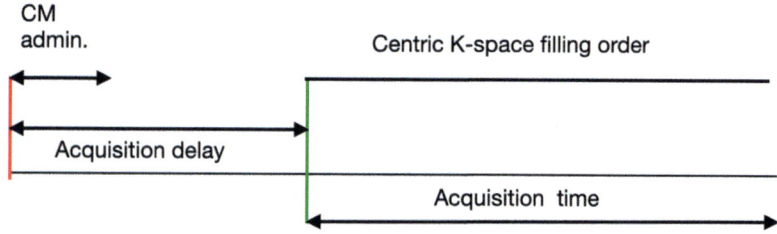

various aspects, such as the characteristics of the sequence and the coil you have, for example, and the scanner.

### Timing or Synchronisation Between CM Administration and Scan Acquisition

The CM used is paramagnetic, in a single dose, 0.1 mMol/Kg of the patient's body. The injection rate indicated in the literature ranges from 2 to 3 mL/s. It is followed by a bolus of 20 mL of saline to keep the bolus of MDC compact, as is the case in CT studies. A dedicated automatic injector must in fact be used. You want to store the arterial phase data in the centre of k-space, which is associated with contrast resolution. To start with data acquisition, and achieving this result, several aspects must be considered (Fig. 22.10):

1. How long does a single phase last.
2. The injection time (which varies depending on the patient's body weight) and the rate (which also varies depending on the patient).
3. How long it takes for the CM to reach the centre of the k-space?

## 22.8   The Abbreviated Protocol and the 4D or Ultrafast Study [18–22]

For some years now, the so-called *abbreviated protocol* in which only two post-contrast phases of the dynamics are acquired has been chosen in many northern European and US centres. Many studies support the results of this approach.

As far as the *4D or ultrafast study* is concerned, a specific dynamic sequence is used. Many phases at very high temporal resolution are acquired (approximately 9–10 s each, but as low as 4 s are described), followed by some conventional 3D phases [20, 21]. This approach allows a lot of information to be obtained and does not require timing calculations, as it is acquired continuously before during and after CM administration. This is especially true according to *radiomics* schemes.

**Radiomics** refers to the extraction of quantitative data from images by means of AI techniques, useful for supporting the decision-making of the reporter [22]. See Chap. 24.

## 22.9   Morphological Post-Processing

The post-processing method used to reconstruct native volumetric images in a different plane from the acquisition plane is called **multi-planar reformatting** or **reconstruction (MPR)**. It is important to remember that reconstructions lead to an increase in noise.

Subtractions are instead reconstructed using another method, the **maximum intensity projection (MIP).** It is a rendering technique in which only the highest signal intensity voxels are projected in the chosen direction, forming a single two-dimensional image. This is then rotated around a chosen axis. MIP is useful for the radiologist, specifically because of the ability to rotate the image obtained in all directions, to assess the real extent of the lesion and therefore its relationship with the surrounding tissues. MRI seems to have the best congruence in size with the real lesion, compared to other modalities, especially in low-density breasts, but with a tendency to overestimate [23, 24]. It is useful for the surgeon in pre-operative planning. These elaborations are easily performed on the image acquisition workstation, but it is preferable to perform and assess them on a dedicated workstation.

### 22.9.1 Functional Post-Processing

The functional data produced by the dynamic sequence are of three types. We speak of (1) a purely qualitative study, through the sole observation of the *time intensity curve (TIC)*; (2) a semi-quantitative one, in which numerical data influenced by the image acquisition technique are extracted. **Wash-in and wash-out maps** are constructed, as well as the TIC, among the data obtained the *TTP, time to peak*, and the *wash-in and wash-out rates;* finally, (3) the truly quantitative approach, which studies the intrinsic *perfusion* tissue property. In the latter two cases, dedicated software is required.

#### 22.9.1.1 Semi-Quantitative Analysis [25–32]

The **time intensity curve (TIC)** monitors the lesion's enhancement behaviour (the change in its T1), this is to say, the variation in signal intensity over time. It is a curve with three time points. t1 identifies the moment at which the contrast medium is administered; t2 is the peak of enhancement and therefore of maximum signal intensity; and t3 represents the lesion's signal intensity in the last phase of the dynamic sequence. Three different trends can be identified in the first part of the curve, called the **wash-in phase** or **initial or early phase:** (a) slow (blue in the figure); (b) intermediate (green in the figure); and (c) fast (red). Point t2 represents the point in time at which the lesion reached maximum enhancement (*peak enhancement*) and where the release of the CM begins. The next stage is **the wash-out or delayed phase**, and this also essentially presents three different trends, as shown in Fig. 22.11.

The slope of the initial curve represents the *wash-in rate*, or enhancement rate, due to the process of neoangiogenesis. It corresponds to the volume of blood that is incorporated into the lesion. The semi-quantitative data that can be

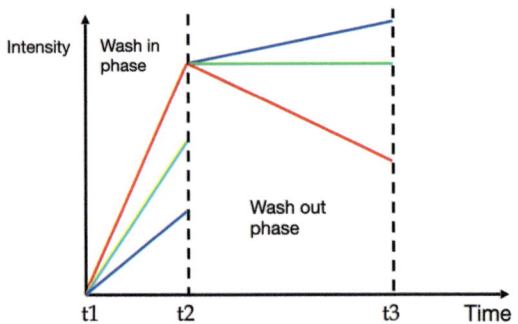

**Fig. 22.11** Three time points TIC, plotting signal intensity values over time after CM administration

obtained are (1) *the time of arrival of the CM* in the lesion (arrival time (AT)), but above all (2) *the time to peak (TTP)*, the time required for the lesion to reach maximum signal intensity (Fig. 22.12). TTP represents the transition to the second part of the curve, whose slope represents the *wash-out rate*, CM release rate, which gives information on capillary permeability.

Passage between the two parts: peak enhancement.

*The late part of the curve is considered the most useful for supporting diagnosis.* In fact, depending on the slope of this part of the curve, three TIC types can be identified (Fig. 22.13), which are significantly associated with different types of lesions, although there is some overlap not only between malignant lesions but also between benign and malignant lesions (low specificity).

The Three different patterns assess how quickly the CM is released.

In the first type, the lesion gains more and more contrast media as it passes from one dynamic phase to the next. In the second type, having reached peak enhancement, this is maintained in the subsequent phases including the last (the lesion does not lose CM, at least not during the time interval studied with the phases of the dynamic sequence). In the third type, having reached peak enhancement, the lesion loses CM, in a more or less accelerated manner. The latter is the one most suspected for malignancy.

A study published in August 2022 in AuntMinnie [30] would indicate *an important sensitivity of the slope of the first phase of the*

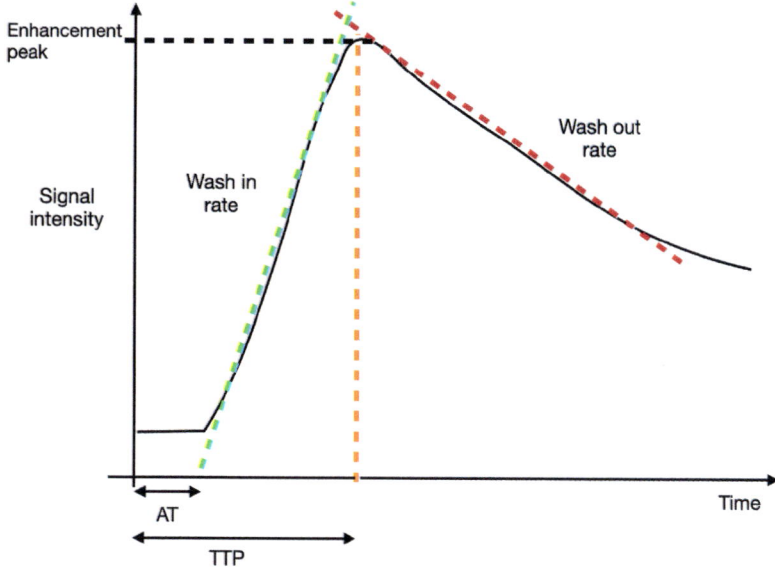

**Fig. 22.12** Semi-quantitative data obtained, assessed on TIC; division into two parts, early (dashed line in green) and delayed (dashed line in red) phases

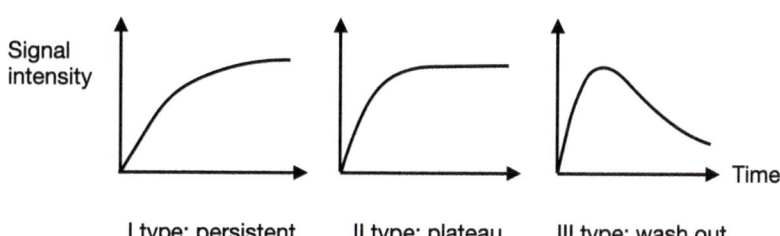

**Fig. 22.13** Types of TIC considering the delayed phase

I type: persistent            II type: plateau            III type: wash out

*curve and TTP for assessing the response of patients to chemotherapy.*

The **semi-quantitative data** are the result of mathematical calculations of the ratio between the signal intensity at the peak enhancement and that of the last phase. As already mentioned, these are data that are influenced by the acquisition technique (hence the term "semi-quantitative") [31, 32].

### 22.9.1.2 Wash-In/Wash-Out Maps and TIC Construction

The first operation that is performed is the so-called *thresholding* or **identification of the threshold value.**

In current display, workstations are done automatically. It is the percentage of variation of the signal in relation to a signal threshold or background intensity, on which to set the processing. Generally, also available automatically, after the

thresholding phase, are the *wash-in and wash-out maps*. Map slices can be viewed along with the native slices of the dynamic sequence and/or with the subtracted ones of the same anatomical level. A colour is assigned to different signal intensity ranges, e.g. the maximum increase relative to the threshold may be associated with red and the maximum decrease relative to the threshold with blue (Fig. 22.14).

However, to my knowledge, there is no international colour code.

### Steps for Generating the Curve

1. **The slice of the phase of the dynamic in which the lesion appears most intense is to be chosen.** It should be in the first or second phase after CM administration. It should be borne in mind that, very often, the breast MRI examination is performed for reasons of surgical planning, and it is already known what

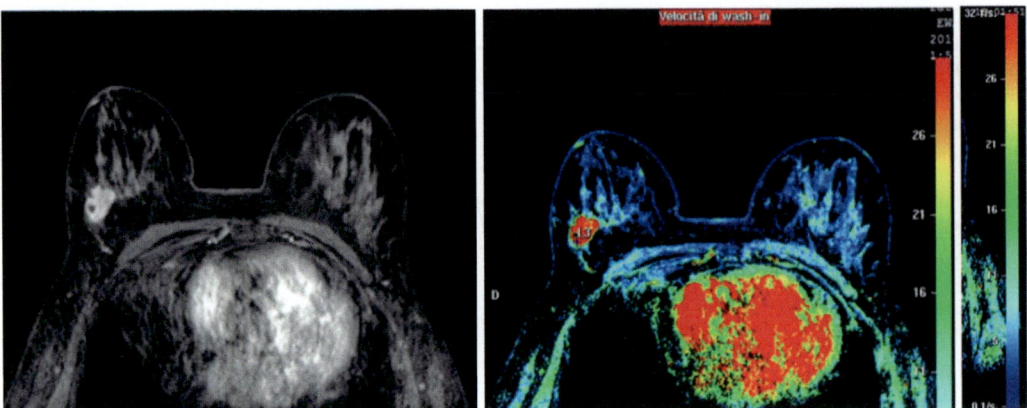

**Fig. 22.14** Native dynamic slice correlated to the same slice in the wash-in map, colour assignment after thresholding

type of malignant lesion it is, and a fast enhancement is expected, at least in most cases. If the behaviour is abnormal with respect to what is expected from the biopsy results, and the maximum enhancement is for example at the fourth or even fifth phase in the dynamic sequence, it could mean that the chosen temporal resolution is too high; i.e., the duration of the phase is too short. In the event that the lesion never turns out to be hyperintense, the causes can mainly be one of two, considering a successful administration of the contrast agent, in patients with standard physiological transit time: either (a) it is a lesion with poor neoangiogenesis or (b) the duration of the phase may be too long, with the consequence of "missing" the enhancement peak.

2. **You select the** region of interest (**ROI**), **to be placed on the lesion to obtain the curve**; several aspects must be considered:

- The **Size of the ROI** First of All. The data in the literature agree that it should be very small, about 3–5 voxels, called "point-like" in some programmes. This is because calculations must be carried out in a homogeneous environment.

- **Where to Place It:** This is a particularly important point to consider. Firstly, the size of the lesion to be studied is assessed: Is it very small? It may be too small to provide enough data to make a curve meaningful. Is it very large? Care must be taken to avoid placing the ROI in the centre of the lesion, or where an absence of signal appears (Figs. 22.14 and 22.15). Neoplastic vertiginous growth in the periphery often causes the starting (central) point to become necrotic, going into hypoxia and die. ***The ROI should always be placed in the periphery of the lesion, even if the lesion appears homogeneous within it***.

- In order to choose where exactly, a ***probing process*** must be put in place, **i.e.** *a search for the part of the lesion that is most active.* You then move the ROI with the cursor, drawing a complete circumnavigation path. The curve is constructed real time at each position where the cursor is moved. A save command is given when a significant curve is seen, i.e. falling within the three types described in Fig. 22.13 (this is not always the case). It is also very useful to compare the wash-in map and the dynamic slice, same level, as presented in Fig. 22.15.

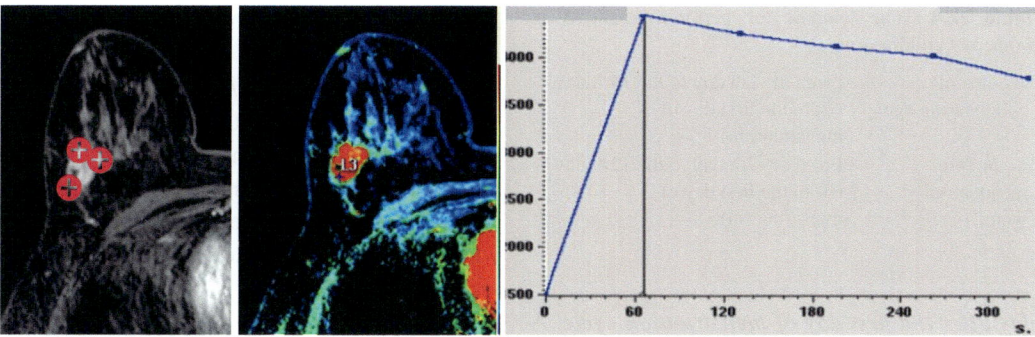

**Fig. 22.15** Probing process to identify the exact location of the ROI and constructing TIC

## 22.10 The Intrinsic Importance of Qualitative and Semi-Quantitative Functional Information Over Morphological: Healthy Versus Pathological Tissue Enhancement, the Dense Breast in MRI [32]

Once, qualitative functional information (through mere observation of the time-intensity curve) was considered much more important than it is today. This was because it was believed that malignant lesions always had a much higher and much faster enhancement than healthy tissue. The latter is referred to in the literature as **background parenchymal enhancement (BPE)**. Similarly, the release of CM from the malignant lesion was thought to be absolutely always different from that of the BPE. In reality, it was later discovered that this is not always the case. Early uptake of healthy tissue is possible; sometimes, it can be as fast and intense as that of pathological lesions. Obviously, this poses a diagnostic problem for the radiologist, similar to that of dense breast in mammography.

*It should be reiterated, however, that breast MRI is in no way affected by breast density* (Chap. 3). It is certainly one of the most interesting advantages of this method. Recently (2022), EUSOBI published new recommendations for the study of dense breasts, which include breast MRI examinations every 2–4 years [33]. There is, however, a **dense breast in MRI**, which is not determined by the amount of glandular tissue but by the enhancement of healthy tissue. Enhancement that may be minimal to marked, concomitant or nearly concomitant to any pathological lesions that may be present. The term **dense breast in resonance** is part of the descriptors included in the standardised ACR BI-RADS® report, in addition to the morphological and enhancement kinetics descriptors. The three types of intensity-time curve described above are part of the last ones.

## 22.11 BMRI in Women of Childbearing Age or on Post-Menopausal Hormonal Treatment: The Time Window

The uptake of healthy tissue is influenced by hormones. They are endogenous in fertile age, exogenous in the case of HRT, in some cases prescribed to peri-post-menopausal patients to alleviate symptoms associated with the decrease and cessation of ovarian activity [34]. See Chap. 2.

**Women of Childbearing Age:** There is a *time window for performing the examination* which must be absolutely complied with for breast MRI, unless an urgency requirement prevails. This extends approximately *from the 7th to the 14th*

**Table 22.4** Time window for performing BMRI in women of childbearing age

| Women of childbearing age | From the 7th day to the 14th day (from the first day of menstruation) |
|---|---|
| Young pre-menopausal women | From the 7th day to the 12th day (from the first day of menstruation) |

*day after the first day of menstruation cycle*. A slight fluctuation from that can be found in the literature. However, it is 1–2 days at most. A time window is when the examination can, and preferably should, be performed. The days that must be avoided are those of the luteal phase (after ovulation), which corresponds to a proliferative phase of breast tissue. *Especially to be avoided is the early part of the luteal phase,* in which progesterone production reaches a peak. It is precisely progesterone that is responsible for the production of foci that eagerly take contrast, sometimes not bilaterally, which can therefore pose a differential diagnosis problem for the reporter. *In the case of young pre-menopausal women, it is recommended to reduce the time window to the 12th day* (Table 22.4).

Luteal phase foci can be so prominent that breasts are dotted throughout their full extent. They are then called "Christmas tree-like." Foci from hormonal influence are also called *unidentified breast objects (UBO)*.

**Women Taking HRT (see Chap. 2):** Theoretically, the breast MRI examination should not be performed, due to enhancement of healthy tissue by HRT drugs. If there is no requirement for urgency, again theoretically, a cessation of 4–6 weeks should be planned before performing the examination. The assessment is made by the radiologist. It should be emphasised that the overall evaluation and therefore the calculation of the risk-benefit ratio for each individual patient is done within the MDM (Chaps. 5 and 6). The radiologist plays in it a fundamental role, and so should the radiographer, as she/he is responsible according to her/his professional profile for the production of biomedical images of high diagnostic quality.

## 22.12 Patient Preparation [35]

It is a *multistep and multi-professional process*, from the administrative staff where the examination is accepted (and scheduled in advance), to the radiographer who positions the patient in the scanner and produces the images, to the doctor who reports on them. Responsibility matrix is shown in Table 22.5.

The patient should be asked to undress completely and provided with an open apron in front.

With R responsible, C is to be consulted.

*The collection of historical data is an important task of the radiographer* (Chap. 16): it is also in MRI. A form to be filled out is suggested, through which data can be analysed for (a) an epidemiological study; (b) monitoring of the proper functioning of the scanner and coil, (c) monitoring the sequences used for this specific examination, (d) verifying patient-related artefacts, and (e) monitoring the specific hardware and software functionality.

In addition to the form proposed in Fig. 22.16, there is a third part for the radiologist's and radiographer's notes (presented in its entirety in Annex 3). This data collection has among its fundamental objectives that of identifying any contraindications to the examination and the patient's compliance with the indications received. The patient's signature is required on the informed consent to the execution of the examination and the administration of the CM. It is important to verify anti-allergy prophylaxis compliance, if required, and prior fasting of at least 4–6 h. This consent must be countersigned by the radiologist in charge of the session.

*Each step in the preparation process must be carefully checked by all team members. The aim is to avoid in every possible way adverse event due to lack of supervision.*

**Second Look US:** This is a widely used procedure internationally. A suspicious finding seen on MRI, which one wants to see again on US exam (to eventually biopsy it), is not so easy to find. This is due to the different patient positioning, prone in one and supine in the other [36]. An

**Table 22.5**  Patient preparation: responsibility matrix

| Actions | Secretarial staff | Radiologist | Radiographer | Nurses |
|---|---|---|---|---|
| Reception | R | | | |
| Welcome | | | | R |
| Evaluation of the documentation in the patient's possession in order to ensure her safety | | R | C | C |
| Clinical information | | R | | |
| Information about the examination | | | R | |
| Collection of historical data | | | R | |
| IV preparation | | C | | R |
| Sequence protocol selection by provisional diagnosis | | R | C | |
| Carrying out the examination | | C | R | |
| Risk-benefit assessment of the examination | | R | C | |

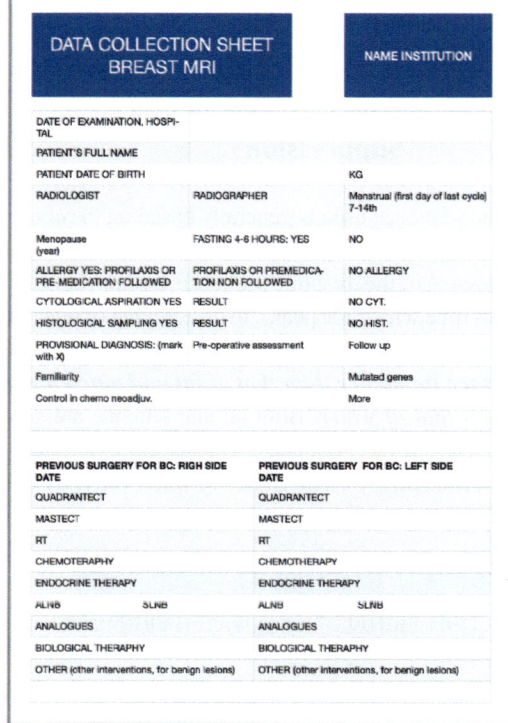

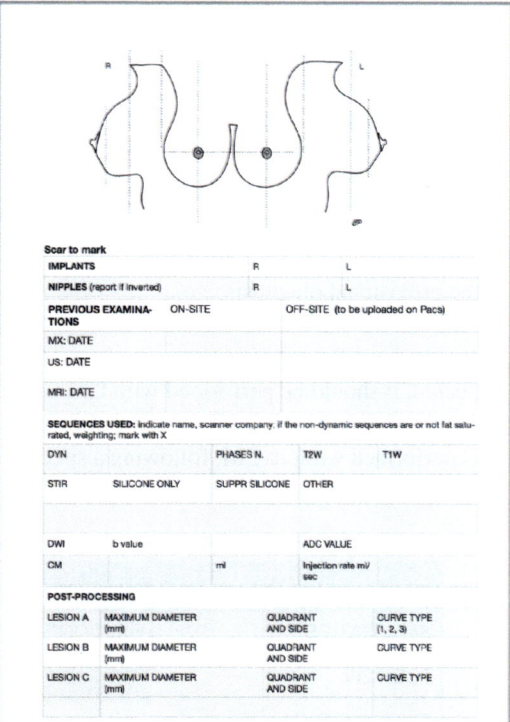

**Fig. 22.16**  Proposed data collection sheet for breast MRI examination in the project MONI.STANrmMAMMO 2020. Present in Annex 3 in its entirety

interesting method to better correlate findings detected in MRI is the DBT-VAB (Chap. 20), using the CC projection approach, to be compared with the axial MRI view, as recently suggested by Urtasun Iriarte et al., RSNA 2023, and mentioned by AuntMinnie [37].

## 22.13  Contraindications to Electronic Devices [38, 39]

Contraindications to BMRI examinations are common to all MRI examinations, for which reference should be made to dedicated texts.

I would mention those due to certain devices, such as the hormone-emitting *intrauterine device (IUD),* which appears to have systemic effects; i.e., it may affect the accuracy of the examination (Sect. 22.11). The *expander* (Chaps. 5 and 14) may have a magnetic marker. This generally makes it an outright contraindication. It may also be marked as **MR conditional**; i.e., the patient may do the examination, taking specific precautions (see Sect. 22.19.1). The patient undergoing expander insertion, while waiting for the definitive implant, receives special documentation on whether it is possible to have an MRI examination, and if so, which RF dose limit is compatible. *Any documentation dealing with safety must in any case be checked against up-to-date and reliable guidelines.*

## 22.14  Indications and Study Protocol for Patients with Breast Implants [40–43]

It is divided into two types of studies, depending on the provisional diagnosis:

1. If a lesion of the breast parenchyma is suspected, it should be performed with CM.
2. If only implant integrity has to be assessed, it is performed without CM, following a specific protocol.

*Magnetic resonance imaging is by far the most sensitive image modality for implant imaging* and required for the report of implant rupture in medico-legal issues (as in the case of PIP implants) [41].

### 22.14.1  Protocol

1. TSE T2W 3D.
2. Sequence with silicone suppression.
3. Sequence with silicone signal only.
4. STIR (optional).

In Fig. 22.17, silicone signal presentation in different sequences.

### 22.14.2  Sequence with Silicone Suppression

The sequence used is generally based on the chemical shift. Consequently, as in the SPAIR™ suppression of the dynamic sequence, a *graph* appears, this time with three peaks, to be accepted or rejected (Table 22.6). *Silicone has a somewhat lower resonance frequency than that of fat and much lower than that of water.* Both fat and silicone are suppressed in this sequence. *The image that is produced is therefore an image of water only.*

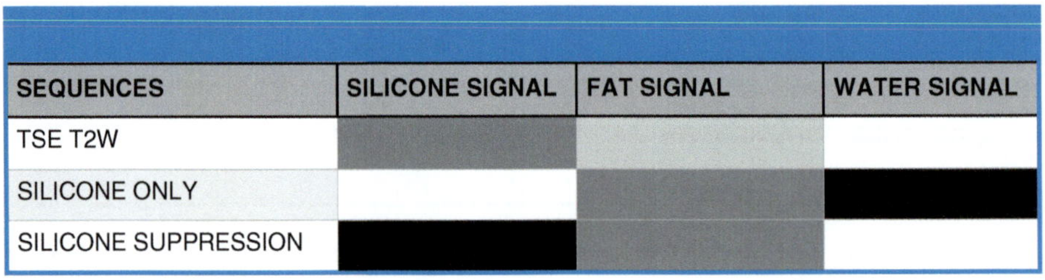

| SEQUENCES | SILICONE SIGNAL | FAT SIGNAL | WATER SIGNAL |
|---|---|---|---|
| TSE T2W | | | |
| SILICONE ONLY | | | |
| SILICONE SUPPRESSION | | | |

**Fig. 22.17** Silicone signal in different sequences

**Table 22.6** Water/fat/silicone spectrum management

| Spectrum results | Acceptability/to be rejected |
|---|---|
| Very high silicone peak and very low water peak | Possible, in the case of a patient with double implant, and with a low percentage of FGT: acceptable |
| Fat peak not depicted | Due to the proximity of the two frequencies, the fat peak can almost completely disappear at high silicone signals: acceptable |
| Silicone peak not depicted | Obviously to be rejected. It may be necessary in some cases to manually adjust the silicone frequency (if this is feasible on the available scanner) |

To Be Noted: The resonance frequencies of fat and silicone are similar. That is why there may be doubts of whether silicone is really suppressed, which is useful when diagnosing siliconoma. Since the T1 of silicone, meanwhile, is very different (much longer) than T1 of fat, inversion recovery (IR)-type silicone suppression sequences have been proposed. They have an interval time TI calibrated to the two different T1s of fat and silicone.

There are also software programs that allow *manual adjustment to the actual frequency of the silicone*, of that individual patient, of that individual breast implant. They are usually associated with spectroscopic sequences [44].

### 22.14.3 Sequence with Silicone Only

This is a dual IR sequence, with two TIs for water and fat suppression.

### 22.15 Risks Related to the Use of Paramagnetic Contrast Media (CM) and Alternative Protocols

The paramagnetic gadolinium-chelated contrast agent has very interesting characteristics [45–49]:

- Does not pass the intact blood-brain barrier (BBB or HEB haemato-encephalic barrier).
- It has an immediate effect.
- Very few proven adverse reactions.
- Great stability.

For some years now, it has been hypothesised that it may remain in the human body for a long time and accumulate on the vascular walls. It has also been associated with *nephrogenic systemic fibrosis (NSF)*, leading to skin thickening and fibrosis. The cases would appear to be related to patients with severe renal problems, and large volumes of CM are administered. The concern would especially affect those patients, such as BRCA-mutated patients, who have to undergo the examination once a year. For this subgroup of patients, macrocyclic GBCA is recommended. The *European Medicine Agency (EMA)* discontinued the use of linear GDBA, except as hepato-specific. It also pushes for a reduction in dose [48], which could be achieved with substances of high relaxivity [49]. The use of this examination is considered by both the FDA and much of the literature to be indispensable, in particular for those patients who have very dense breasts and negative mammography, on suspicion of a lesion. Alternative protocols which do not involve the use of CM have been developed, considering mainly women who have major contraindications to contrast media. These include a diffusion study.

### 22.16 Diffusion Study in MRI [50–57]

*The study target is the diffusive motion of water molecules in organic tissue.* This is a random movement, the trajectory of which varies continually due to the successive collisions of the water molecules themselves with the molecules that make up the tissue being studied. **Diffusion coefficient D** is defined as that parameter expressing the freedom of movement of the water molecule. The higher D is, the freer it is to move. It is an isotropic diffusion, that is, with the same probability of occurring in all directions. In organic tissues, however, we must speak more precisely of **apparent diffusion coefficient (ADC)**. It is an anisotropic diffusion, in which certain directions are favoured over others. *The study target is extracellular diffusion. Studying it provides information about tissue, its cellularity, and microstructure.* This is because, as shown in Fig. 22.18, the random trajectories, with (very fast) time, end up filling the plane and outlining its structure.

### 22.16.1 Diffusion-Weighted Imaging (DWI) Study

The study of diffusion is performed by turning on two specific gradients, which can be accommodated in various types of sequences. Mainly

**Fig. 22.18** Diffusion allows the microstructure of tissue to be studied

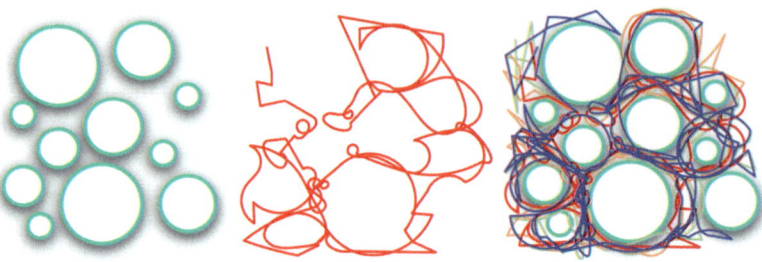

**Table 22.7** DWI images and related maps

| Image $b$-value $= 0$ | Image resembling a heavily weighted sequence in T2 |
| Image $b$-value $\neq 0$ | DWI: diffusion in the three directions of space is considered, which is then summed up |
| ADC map | Indicates average diffusivity |
| eADC map | Exponential |

**Fig. 22.19** (**a**) Diffusion in healthy tissue; (**b**) in the presence of toxic oedema; and (**c**) where there is an increase in cellularity (see text)

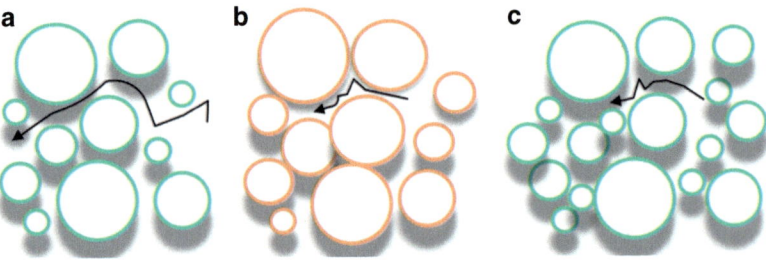

*echoplanar EPI* and also *single-shot SE* (™ PHILIPS) are used. Diffusion weighting is obtained by varying three parameters characterising these gradients: (1) their amplitude; (2) their duration; and (3) the time distance between them. Together, they constitute the **b-value** parameter, measured in s/mm². The b-value should be considered as the TE in morphological T2W sequences. The higher it is, the higher the diffusion weighting. A comparison is then made between the resonance signal obtained with the diffusion gradients off, b-value equal to zero, and the signal with the gradients on, with b-value other than zero.

**In the DWI sequence, two types of images are obtained.** From these, two maps are derived, in post-processing and generally automatically, according to a pixel-by-pixel calculation (Table 22.7).

*The Effect of Diffusion on MRI Signal: It knocks it down, so diffusion is displayed as hypointensity on DWI images.*

Extracellular diffusion will be prevented or at least restricted, when (1) the cells in a tissue undergo *toxic oedema*, which is an event that expresses the first cellular distress. It presents itself with swelling of the cells (Fig. 22.19b); (2) there is an increase in cellularity (Fig. 22.19c). This is called *diffusion restriction, and it is expressed on DWI images as hyperintensity.*

**ADC Map:** It has a contrast that looks like the negative of DWI images: the diffusion is represented as hyperintense. From this map, quantitative information can be derived, i.e. the numerical value of ADC, expressed in $10^{-3}$ mm²/s.

**How the Image of the ADC Map Looks Like:** The so-called *solarised pixels,* determined by the mathematical calculation, are observed. ADC is in fact the logarithm of a very small value, which in this map is converted into a very large value.

**eADC Map:** The contrast is the same as DWI images. The advantage of this map is that it has no T2 weighting. This can be useful for determin-

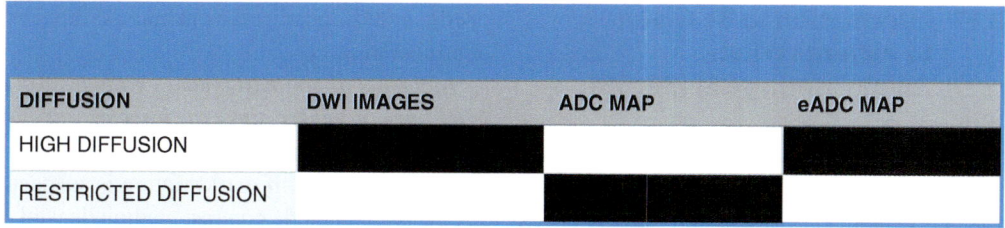

**Fig. 22.20** Signal semiotics comparing high and low diffusion in DWI and maps images

**Table 22.8**  Some of the ADC values reported by EUSOBI, using $b$-value = 800 s/mm$^2$

| Diffusion level | How the lesion paper on ADC map | ADC range of values |
|---|---|---|
| From very low to low | From very hypointense to hypointense | $\leq 0.9 \times 10^{-3}$ To $1.3 \times 10^{-3}$ mm$^2$/s |
| From high to very high | Not so hypointense or not detectable; hyperintense | $1.7–2.1 \times 10^{-3}$ to $>2.1 \times 10^{-3}$ mm$^2$/s |

ing whether there is a *T2 shine through artefact* (Sect. 22.18.2).

Signal semiotics in high and low diffusion in Fig. 22.20.

### 22.16.2 Diffusion in BMRI

The study of the breast with DWI has not yet been standardised. The literature still reports a wide variability of results, especially with regard to numerical estimates of ADC. In fact, DWI is not present in the standardised BI-RADS® report, but is present in the PI-RADS (for prostate studies). Despite this, it should be said that it is acknowledged that numerical estimation of ADC is sensitive to tissue microstructure and cellularity. Therefore, the study of DWI images and numerical ADC assessment is thought to improve the reporter's ability to characterise the lesion.

**DWI Execution Timing in the Protocol:** The DWI should be performed before the CM is administered. This is because it could influence the results, especially the numerical calculation.

**Which B-Value to Choose:** In the BMRI examination, a high or medium-high b-value is used, between 800 and 1000 s/mm$^2$. High b-values can increase the specificity of DWI, since they correspond to a greater weighting in diffusion. ADC, however, tends to decrease (artificially). EUSOBI conducted a study published in European Radiology in 2020, in which 800 s/mm$^2$ is recommended as b-value [54]. See Table 22.8.

**Numerical ADC Estimates:** There are actually no standardised *cut-off* values, between those that characterising malignant lesions and those indicating benign lesions. Malignant lesions are associated with low ADC values.

**How to Calculate the Numerical ADC Estimate:** The lack of standardisation of these estimates is largely influenced by the lack of standardisation of the procedure by which the estimate is obtained. The first step concerns the choice of the size of the ROI; as already reported for the TIC construction, it should be chosen small (three voxels), so as to avoid as far as possible fat. Including it leads to considerable noise. Second step to be considered is as follows: where to place it: it should be chosen the most hypointense part of the lesion in the ADC map (which represents the most active lesion area). It corresponds to the most hyperintense part of the DWI images and on the natives of the dynamic sequence.

## 22.17 Information to Be Given to Patients When Administering CM [38, 58]

The patient safety profile, taken from the historical data collection, should be firstly assessed (see Sects. 22.12 and 22.13); second, a cross-check (by the radiographer, radiologist, and nurse) of the patient's compliance with the required preparation should be done. Another of the radiographer's responsibilities is to provide the patient with full information on what may happen when the CM is administered (via an automatic injector). It is necessary to explain to the patient that:

1. A cold or wet sensation may be felt at the injection site.
2. It is not the same as with CT scan, the patient should not feel the typical hot flush associated with the iodinated contrast medium used in that modality.
3. If, however, the patient feels burning and pain at the point of injection, on the arm connected to the injector, the radiographer should be alerted by pressing the emergency bell. The examination should be interrupted on suspicion of a CM extravasation. In this case, the examination must be rescheduled for another day.

*Giving preventive information on what the patient can expect from the CM administration is crucial to avoid her from flinching or moving. This often makes the examination impossible to interpret.*

### 22.17.1 Contrast Medium Extravasation in MRI [58, 59]

This event is less frequent on MRI than on CT. This is mainly due to the much smaller volumes of CM administered. However, it is more frequent in women than in men, depending on various aspects. The vessels are smaller and deeper in women than in men, with the thickness of the subcutaneous layer being greater. The likelihood of overflow increases with (1) advancing age, (2) as the injection rate increases. Besides, it depends on (3) the diameter of the needle and of the access vein and (4) the site of administration.

*Incidents of contrast media extravasation on MRI have increased since the injector was used, but are still rare and with few serious complications.* Despite this, if extravasation is suspected, i.e. the paramagnetic contrast medium leaked out of the blood vessel, the examination should be stopped immediately.

## 22.18 Artefacts in MRI

An artefact is the visualisation on the reconstructed image of something that is not present in the real object. Object which we would like to reproduce instead as faithfully as possible.

Artefacts are due to a great many factors, and a discussion of them is beyond the scope of this text. Therefore, only a few of them, not all well recognisable, that appear most frequently in breast MRI examinations, will be addressed. Solutions will also be offered.

### 22.18.1 Most Frequent Artefacts in BMRI Examination and Their Solution [60–62]

In an extremely simplified manner will be dealt with artefacts due to:

1. Patient movement.
2. Magnetic susceptibility due to the presence of metal devices.
3. Touching of the breast in the coil.
4. Type I chemical shift.
5. Type II chemical shift.
6. Shimming volume too small or incorrect.
7. High noise in MIP image reconstruction.
8. High noise in MPR reconstructions.
9. Incorrect choice of examination time window.
10. Artefactual enhancement of the nipple-areolar complex (NAC).
11. Parallel imaging.

A specific paragraph is dedicated to artefacts in DWI (Sect. 22.18.2) for the most frequent artefact see Table 22.9.

**Table 22.9** Most frequent artefacts in BMRI and their solution

| Artefact type | How it is displayed | Explanations and solutions |
|---|---|---|
| Movement of the patient | – If moderate: May not be noticed on morphological and dynamic images, where it may present itself as a low lesion enhancement<br>– If elevated: Visible in all sequences, as blurring, important quality degradation especially visible in subtraction images (double contour...)<br>– On the subtracted images, A hyperintensity appears following the skin edge | – Provide sufficient information to the patient about the need to maintain the position for the entire examination, even when there is no noise. Words of motivation should be used<br>– Suggest her to breathe lightly<br>– Examination must be as short as possible<br>– The patient must be comfortable<br>In order to understand whether it is an artefact or not, the patient must be carefully studied in person, to check there is no real reason for skin uptake |
| Movement of the patient at contrast medium arrival | The lesion may appear with a double band, hypo and hyper intense, at one of its margins, in the subtraction images | This is the artefact due to the failure of co-registration between mask (pre-CM phase) and later phases, caused by the movement (jerking) of the patient on contrast medium arrival. It should be explained exactly what the patient should expect in order to avoid it (Sect. 22.17) |
| From magnetic susceptibility due to the presence of metallic devices<br>From magnetic susceptibility due to the presence of metal clips (post-bioptic, see Chap. 18)<br>From needle passage for recent biopsy<br>By magnetic susceptibility for presence of magnetic marker in the expander | Signal loss+ blooming+ eventual signal flare in peripheral FOV<br>Blooming = the artefact makes larger in size the device that produced it<br>Signal flare = signal increase by summation of more signals)<br>Signal flare<br>Loss of signal at trajectory<br>Significant signal loss that can affect the entire side | Metal has a magnetic susceptibility, i.e. an ability to locally alter B0. It is more or less high depending on the device characteristics, size and its relative position in the field<br>For the morphological study, robust sequences such as TSE (FSE) can be used or using the DIXON system (see Sect. 22.7.5, fat suppression)<br>In the event that the clip is located in the armpit, the artefact may present itself as an enhancing lymph node:<br>– Check the patient's history (has the patient undergone surgery?)<br>– Compare with other sequences to see if it is artefactual or not<br>As in US, it may be possible to see the path of the needle<br>– Check the patient's history<br>An artefact that must not be seen in any image (not even in the survey), because its presence must be identified beforehand by data collection |
| From magnetic susceptibility in port | More or less important signal loss associated with peripheral hyperintensity | The impact of the artefact is easily managed iconographically, so much so that if the doctor and nurse deem it compatible, it can be used for CM administration (patients undergoing chemo tend to have veins that are difficult to access) |
| Breast compression from coil support | Signal flare + breast compression<br>Contrast alteration | In the case of very large breasts, the parts in contact with the coil may induce both spatial and contrast signal alterations (generally hyperintensity). Compression may prevent or in any case slow down the CM uptake by the lesion that may be present in the area. ***Very large breasts are an important contraindication*** |
| Chemical shift of type I | Presence of two bands, one hyperintense and one hypointense, at the boundary between water-rich and fat-rich tissues, where there is an interface with voxels where both tissues are present, along the frequency encoding direction | It can only be seen in spin echo sequences, along the direction of frequency encoding, being a frequency error of the scanner. The scanner only recognises the frequency of water<br>By finding both tissues in the voxel, and assigning each proton frequency value a precise correlated location, the fat proton signal is shifted, being thought of as "water in the wrong place" |

(continued)

**Table 22.9** (continued)

| Artefact type | How it is displayed | Explanations and solutions |
|---|---|---|
| Chemical shift of type II | Presence of black bands at the boundary between tissues rich in water, and in fat, where there is an interface with voxels where both tissues are present | It is only seen in gradient echo sequence<br>It depends on the destructive interference between fat and water signals in voxels that contain both. They are deleted (black band appears). It can be seen in both directions. It depends on the TE if sampling is done when the water and fat signals are out of phase. The width of the black band (in pixels) depends on the width of the receiving band (BW). The wider it is, the less important the artefact is, but the noise increases |
| Dishomogeneity of fat suppression in dynamic sequence MPR image noise | Fat suppression fails or is otherwise dishomogeneous in the FOV | Modifying the shimming volume, including the nipples and pectoral muscle, could help<br>Check that there are no metal devices or major folds of breast tissue in contact with the coil<br>It is important that dynamics acquisition has a high spatial resolution in plane, and preferably isotropic, to improve the quality of reconstructions |
| MIP image noise | Insufficient contrast between lesion and vessels in relation to background | There are several aspects to consider:<br>1. Constructed images are always noisier than the ones directly acquired<br>2. If the natives are of low quality, the reconstructed ones will have even lower quality<br>3. Try reconstruction using the TARGETMIP technique (of the entire volume of slices, remove the first and last slices, which carry noise and poor information) |
| Early and important BPE enhancement | Early enhancement of the healthy tissue conceals any lesion taking CM | May possibly be due to wrong execution time window |
| NAC enhancement (nipple-areola complex) | Not only the nipple enhances (normal), but also the areola, in an accentuated manner | In order to be able to tell whether this is an artefact or not, it is necessary to observe the patient live, and to verify that no erosion and/or inflammation of the NAC is in place |
| From parallel imaging | Depends on the type of parallel imaging implemented in the scanner | Possible reduction of the acceleration factor (resulting in increased scanning time) |

## 22.18.2 Artefacts in DWI Images [50]

There are many of these, associated with the sequence used, which is generally the echoplanar EPI. We can talk of (1) *Nyquist ghosts,* due to undersampling resulting from the use of parallel imaging (but not only that); (2) artefacts from chemical shifts due to non-effective fat suppression; (3) artefacts from magnetic susceptibility in the presence of metal and at points where there is a strong gradient; i.e., there is the transition between tissues with very different susceptibility (e.g. air/tissue); and (4) artefacts from *eddy currents*, which lead to spatial and contrast distortions of the signal, also of considerable importance. A very important aspect of spatial

signal distortions concerns the exact positioning of the ROI on the lesion, which is why it is not always an easy task.

**Eddy Currents:** *Eddy currents* are currents induced by rapidly changing gradients and RF pulses. The two of them are time-varying magnetic fields that can produce electric current according to Faraday's law.

In turn, however, since the electric current produced is variable, it produces variable magnetic fields, which oppose to what created them.

**Solutions:** DWIs are sequences that require advanced technological prerequisites in order to be successfully implemented. As far as eddy currents are concerned, the solutions are preventive:

1. Gradients must be shielded (with secondary coils).
2. Gradients should have a special design (pre-emphasis).
3. There are post-processing corrections that effectively correct spatial non-linearities and phase and/or frequency shifts due to eddy currents.

This does not only apply to EPIs, but also to other sequences, including those used for MRI spectroscopy. Among other things, these choices also point in the direction of an improvement of overall patient safety (see Sect. 22.19).

**T2 Shine Through Artefact:** It is a very important artefact of DWI. It can increase the signal of a lesion and "mimics" a diffusion restriction. It is important to keep in mind that DWI images are not only diffusion-weighted, but also T2-weighted (a lot, due to the presence of the additional gradients that increase TE, the time in which the signal is sampled).

**Solution:** In order to assess whether it is an artefact or not, one must compare the DWI images with the map images, especially with the eADC, which is not T2-weighted.

**T2 Black Out Artefact:** It could be found where there are lesions or tissues in the FOV being studied, or findings of any sort, characterised with very short T2. Examples are metal or blood extravasation. The images will then present a contrast alteration caused by this artefact. The calculation of the numerical estimate from the ADC maps will not be reliable.

## 22.19 Overview of Dosimetry in MRI, the SAR

The dose delivered to the patient undergoing MRI examination is not from ionising radiation. The responsible practitioner is, however, always the radiographer. The biological effects from *electromagnetic fields (EMFs)* are thermal effects from the Joule effect, from RF, and from eddy currents (Sect. 22.18.2). It can lead to stimulation of the motor end plate, and in extreme cases, to cardiac fibrillation.

*The dosimetric unit in MRI is the specific absorption rate (SAR). It is used to calculate the temperature rise or, more precisely, the energy deposited in the studied tissue by the RF pulses, per unit of mass.* SAR is measured in watts per kilogram (W/Kg) and is proportional to the electrical conductivity of tissues. This is higher in those with a high water content (high free ions concentration). It is low in fat and cortical bone, for example. Metal, on the other hand, is extremely conductive (thanks to free electrons).

In reality, SAR calculation is very complex and inaccurate.

We know that:

1. Body size matters: the more robust the patient, the higher the SAR delivered.
2. SAR is proportional to resonance frequency squared. Since frequency is proportional to B0, the SAR delivered at 3 T is higher than that at 1.5.
3. SAR is proportional to flip angle-squared. This means that sequences using a 180° refocusing pulse train, such as TSE, will have a high SAR.
4. SAR is proportional to the *duty cycle.* It is the percentage of time that RF is sent out of the total duration of the sequence. Sequences that are short in duration and send a lot of RF pulses, such as EPI, develop a high SAR.
5. The physiological state of the patient counts. If she/he has a fever, the induced temperature rise will be more dangerous.
6. The temperature of the magnet room counts (it must be monitored).
7. The humidity of the magnet room counts (it must be monitored).

### 22.19.1 What to Do in Patients Who Are More Sensitive to SAR Because They Carry Implantable MR-Conditional Devices [63, 64]

In the case of an MR-conditional device carrier, the documentation in the patient's possession should be checked. The acceptable SAR limits in terms of B1 intensity (RF) are in fact indicated. In case the limit is 2 microT; see Table 22.10.

In general, the following sequences have a high SAR: TSE, IR, and GRE with very short TR, and those sequences which send saturation pulses (for fat, for example).

#### 22.19.1.1 Some Systems to Reduce SAR

- Reducing the flip angle of refocusing pulses (which are at 180°). It may, however, lead to loss of SNR.
- Reducing the turbo factor in TSE (FSE), especially in TSE T2W. To be noted: the turbofactor (echo train length (ETL)) is related to the effective TE and thus to the weighting of the sequence. A drastic lowering would change the contrast substantially.
- Switching to low SAR. The procedure for selecting low SAR varies between manufac-turers. On Philips scanner in the contrast package, SAR MODE. On Siemens scanner, the SAR INFORMATION table must be opened and the acceptable B1 is selected.
- In GE, e.g., the width of the RF pulse cannot be changed. The above-mentioned parameters can instead be changed.

Two types of RF pulses with low SAR have been implemented. The one called variable-rate selective excitation (VERSE), has a pulse with a specific "screwed" design. This reduces the amplitude of the gradient associated with the pulse. It may, however, be necessary to consult the medical physicist to assess the individual case, to calculate the SAR of each sequence. It may be a solution to perform the required examination in patients with MR-conditional devices, breaking it into two, on different days.

To finish, some examples from a BMRI examination are presented in Figs. 22.21 and 22.23 and Figs. 22.22 and 22.24; ROI positioning and TIC in Fig. 22.25.

**Table 22.10** Executable sequences with MR-conditional device compatible up to B1 ≤ 2 microtesla: a: sequences to be used without or with minimal modifications; b: sequences to be used with major modification; c: sequences that are not to be used

| Sequence type | Philips | Siemens | GE |
| --- | --- | --- | --- |
| Sequences to be used without or with minimal modifications | | | |
| Volume interpolated spoiled GRE | Thrive | Vibe | LAVA-XV |
| EPI | EPI | EPI | EPI |
| Cube | Cube | Cube | Cube |

| Sequence type | Philips | Siemens | GE |
| --- | --- | --- | --- |
| Executable sequences with MR-conditional devices, with major modifications | | | |
| FAST SPIN ECHO | TSE | TSE | FSE |
| Short TAU inversion recovery | STIR | STIR | STIR |

| Sequence type | Philips | Siemens | GE |
| --- | --- | --- | --- |
| Sequences that are not to be used with MR-conditional devices | | | |
| Single shot fast spin echo | Single shot TSE | HASTE | Single shot FSE |
| Unspoiled GRE/steady state free precession | Balanced FFE/T2 FFE | FISP/TRUE FISP | SSFP/FIESTA |

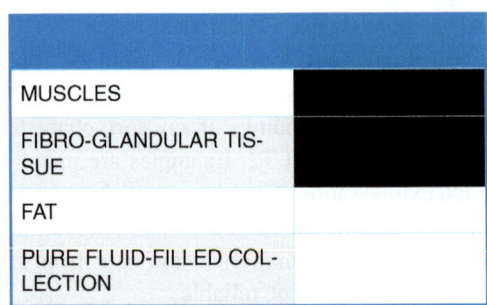

**Fig. 22.21** Basic BMRI signal semiotics in T2W morphological sequences

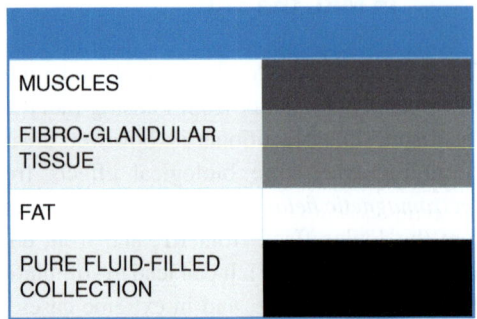

**Fig. 22.22** Basic BMRI signal semiotics in T1W morphological sequences

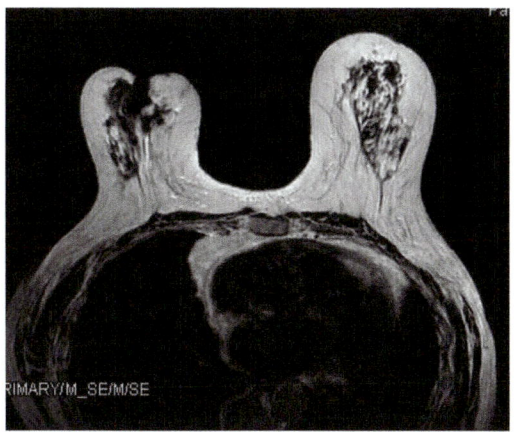

**Fig. 22.23** MRI signal basic semiotics in T2W morphological sequences

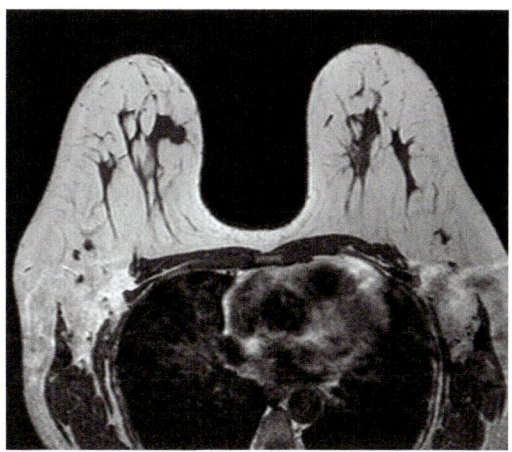

**Fig. 22.24** MRI signal semiotics in T1W morphological sequences

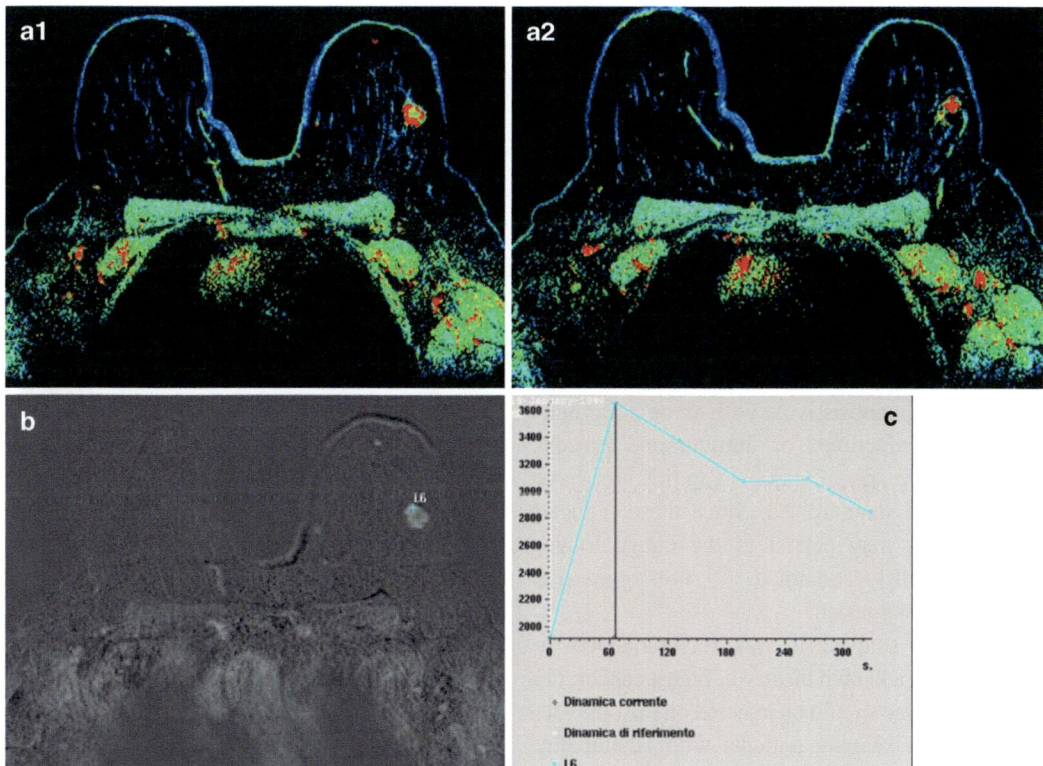

**Fig. 22.25** ROI positioning on highly inhomogeneous lesion; (**a1**, **a2**) wash map in different slices; (**b**) subtracted slice, corresponding level to **a1**; (**c**): TIC of the lesion, with "jagged" tail, due to processing of inhomogeneous data

## 22.20 Effects of Anti-COVID-19 Mass Vaccination on BMRI Images

The implementation of the mass vaccination programme to accelerate COVID-19 disease control produced a number of transient side effects, some in common with other vaccine types. In particular, *axillary adenopathies* have been found much more frequently than in the past in patients undergoing breast MRI examinations. This evidence is well documented in literature around the world. It consists of an axillary lymph node enlargement, ipsilateral to the arm in which the vaccine was administered. It may be accompanied, much more rarely, by axillary oedema.

The data seem to indicate that the lymph nodes affected are more likely to be at levels 2 and 3. They are deep and sometimes undetectable on MRI and appear more frequently after administration of the mRNA vaccines. They seem to induce a very high immunological response compared to other anti-SARS-CoV-2 vaccines. The presence of axillary adenopathy, observed among others in all imaging modalities, includes diffuse thickening of the lymph node cortical and usually appears within 1 month after administration. Recent research on the subject revealed that a subgroup of patients had thickened lymph nodes up to 4 months after the second vaccination. A differential diagnosis issue with an ongoing neoplastic, or infectious, or autoimmune process may therefore arise. Guidelines in this area have not yet been standardised. Since these induced adenopathies may persist in the image longer than previously assumed, a non-aggressive approach is suggested.

In some studies, it was recommended in patients with a known history of breast cancer: (1) that the vaccine should be injected on the opposite side and (2) keeping patients with adenopathy under observation for a sufficiently long period. At least an interval of 6 weeks, in some studies 12 weeks is indicated, before moving on to the next stage in the *work-up* (biopsy). This is unless there are cases in which breast cancer has already been diagnosed, either in the present or even in the past. In that instance, it is necessary to follow the procedure indicated by the guidelines quickly.

In summary, these aspects must be carefully assessed: (a) the patient's personal history; (b) the concomitant presence of a suspected lesion in the ipsilateral breast; and (c) the time at which the vaccination was carried out [65]. Along the same line are the EUSOBI recommendations [66].

Of particular note is the delay in breast screening in general, across the world, caused by the pandemic. It resulted in a significant delay in diagnosis and a consequent decrease in early-stage diagnosis [67, 68]. The number of patients returned to breast screening is still not as high as pre-pandemic and will require long-term monitoring [69, 70].

## References

1. Sardanelli F, et al. Magnetic resonance imaging of the breast: recommendations from the EUSOMA working group. Eur J Cancer. 2010;46:1296–316. https://doi.org/10.1016/j.ejca.2010.02.015.
2. Schoub PJ. Understanding indications and defining guidelines for breast magnetic resonance imaging. SA J Radiol. 2018;22(2):1353. https://doi.org/10.4102/sajr.v22i2.1353. eCollection 2018. https://pubmed.ncbi.nlm.nih.gov/31754513/
3. Mann RM, et al. Breast MRI: state of the art. Radiology. 2019;292:520–36. https://doi.org/10.1148/radiol.2019182947.
4. Lee CS, et al. Screening guidelines update for average-risk and high-risk women. Am J Roentgenol. 2020;214:316–23. https://doi.org/10.2214/AJR.19.22205.
5. Argus A, Mahoney MC. Indications for breast MRI: case-based review. Am J Roentgenol. 2011;196(3_supplement):WS1–4. https://doi.org/10.2214/AJR09.7213.
6. Christensen DM, et al. Preoperative breast MRI: current evidence and patient selection. J Breast Imaging. 2023;5:112–24. https://doi.org/10.1093/jbi/wbac088.
7. McCarthy AM, et al. Performance of breast cancer risk-assessment models in a large mammography cohort. J Natl Cancer Inst. 2020;112(5):djz177. https://doi.org/10.1093/jnci/djz177.
8. Mlynàrik V. Introduction to nuclear magnetic resonance. Analyt Biochem. 2016;529:1–6. https://doi.org/10.1016/j.ab.2016.05.006.
9. Signal weighting (T1, T2, PD) and sequences parameters: TR, TE, e-MRI. https://www.imaios.com/en/e-mri/nmr-signal-and-mri-contrast/signal-weighting-and-sequences-parameters
10. Frankhouser DE, et al. Vascularity and dynamic contrast-enhanced breast magnetic resonance imaging. Front Radiol. 2021;1:735567. https://doi.org/10.3389/fradi.2021.735567.

11. Rinck PA. Magnetic resonance in medicine a critical introduction, 12th completely revised edition. 2018. ISBN: 978-3-7460-9518-9.

12. Guidance on Screening and Systematic Breast Imaging, Appendix 2. Breast MRI protocol an reporting guidelines. 4th ed. The Royal College of Radiologists; 2019.

13. Yeh ED, et al. Positioning in breast MR imaging to optimize image quality. Radiographics. 2014;34(1):E1–17. https://doi.org/10.1148/rg.341125193.

14. http://mriquestions.com website founded by ELSTER, A.D. (FACR).

15. Hancu I, et al. On shimming approaches in 3T breast MRI. Proc Intl Soc Mag Reson Med. 2012; 20:862.

16. Freitas Lins C, et al. Application of the Dixon technique in the evaluation of the musculoskeletal system. Radiol Bras. 2021;54(1):33–42. https://doi.org/10.15907/0100-3984.20190086.

17. Clayton D, et al. Technical guidelines for magnetic resonance imaging (MRI) for the surveillance of women at higher risk of developing breast cancer. NHSBSP; 2012. Publication no. 68 06ISBN 978-1-84463-067-7

18. Lee-Felker S, et al. Abbreviated breast MRI for estimating extent of disease in newly diagnoses breast cancer. J Breast Imaging. 2020;2(1):43–9. https://doi.org/10.1093/jbi/wbz071.

19. Kwon M-R, et al. Diagnostic performance of abbreviated breast MRI for screening of women with previously treated breast cancer. Medicine. 2020;99:e19676. https://doi.org/10.1097/MD.0000000000019676.

20. Gao Y, Heller SL. Abbreviated and ultrafast breast MRI in clinical practice. Radiographics. 2020;40:1507–27. https://doi.org/10.1148/rg.2020200006.

21. Samreen N, et al. Screening breast MRI primer: indication, current protocols and emerging techniques. J Breast Imaging. 2021;3:387–98. https://doi.org/10.1093/jbi/wbaa116.

22. Hu Q, ct al. A deep learning methodology for improved breast cancer diagnosis using multiparametric MRI. Sci Rep. 2020;10:10536. https://pubmed.ncbi.nlm.nih.gov/32601367/

23. Kyung ANJ, et al. Tumor size measurements with breast magnetic resonance imaging (MRI) in elderly cancer patients: a comparison of Breast MRI with mammography and ultrasound. Iran J Radiol. 2021;18(3):e110817. https://doi.org/10.5812/iranjradiol.110817.

24. Azhdeh S, et al. Accurate estimation of breast tumor size: a comparison between ultrasonography, mammography, magnetic resonance imaging, and associated contributing factors. Eur J Breast Health. 2021;17(1):53–61. https://doi.org/10.4274/ejbh.2020.5888.

25. Agrawal G, et al. Significance of breast lesion descriptors in the ACR BI-RADS MRI lexicon. Cancer. 2009;115(7):1363–80. https://doi.org/10.1002/cncr.24156.

26. Kuhl CK, et al. Not all false positive diagnoses are equal: on the prognostic implication of false-positive diagnoses made in breast MRI versus mammography/digital tomosynthesis screening. Breast Cancer Res. 2018;20:13. https://doi.org/10.1186/s13058-018-0937-7.

27. Kaiser WA. Sign in MR-mammography. Springer 2007. ISBN 978-3-540-73292-1 Library of Congress Control Number: 2007933374

28. Grippo C, et al. Correct determination of the enhancement curve is critical to ensure accurate diagnosis using the Kaiser score as a clinical decision rule for breast MRI. Eur J Radiol. 2021;138:109630. https://doi.org/10.1016/j.ejrad.2021.109630.

29. Rahbar H, Partridge S. Multiparametric MR imaging of breast cancer. Magn Reson Imaging Clin N Am. 2016;24:223. https://doi.org/10.1016/J.MRIC.2015.08.012.

30. Allegretto A. Ultrafast DCE_MRI helps predict breast cancer treatment response AuntMinnie.com staff writer. August 1, 2022. https://www.auntminnie.com/index.aspx?sec=ser&sub=def&pag=dis&ItemID=136572

31. Yamaguchi A, et al. Kinetic information from dynamic contrast-enhanced MRI enables prediction of residual cancer burden and prognosis in triple-negative breast cancer: a retrospective study. Sci Rep. 2021;11:10112. https://doi.org/10.1013/s41598-021-89380-4.

32. Breast MRI Technique. https://oncohemakey.com/breast-mri-technique/

33. Mann RM, et al. Breast cancer screening in women with extremely dense breasts recommendations of the European Society of Breast Imaging (EUSOBI). Eur Radiol. 2022;32:4036–45. https://doi.org/10.1007/s00330-022-08617-6.

34. Barriga-Pooley P, Brantes-Glavic S. In: Lutsenko EI, editor. Normal menstrual cycle, from the edited volume menstrual cycle. IntechOpen; 2018. https://doi.org/10.5772/intechopen.79976.

35. Hansson B, et al. MR_safety in clinical practice at 7T: evaluation of a multistep screening process in 1819 subjects. Radiography. 2022;28:454–9. https://doi.org/10.1016/j.radi.2021.12.007.

36. Youngjean Park V, et al. Second-look US: how to find breast lesions with a suspicious MR imaging appearance. Radiographics. 2013;33:1361–75. https://doi.org/10.1148/rg.335125109.

37. Ward P. Clinical support builds for DBT-guided breast biopsies. December 20, 2023. https://www.auntminnieeurope.com/clinical-news/womens-imaging/article/15660580/clinical-support-builds-for-dbtguided-breast-biopsies.

38. Risk and contraindication breast MRI. https://www.verywellhealth.com/using-mri-for-breast-cancer-diagnosis-and-screening-430311#toc-risks-and-contraindications

39. Brooks L, Harris I. Breast MRI shows IUDs have Systemic effects, RSNA 2021, Newsroom (NOv.27-Dec.2, 2021) 1-312-791-6610 released: November 22, 2021.

40. Wong T, et al. Magnetic resonance imaging of breast augmentation: a pictorial review. Insights Imaging. 2016;7:399–410. https://doi.org/10.1007/S13244-016-0482-9.

41. Fuchs S, et al. Sandwich course of the radiological Society of The Netherland, February 2021. https://radiologyassistant.nl/breast/breast-prosthesis/breast-prosthesis-imaging

42. Moan R. Use MRI to diagnose PIP breast implant ruptures, Dutch say, AuntMinnie. https://auntminnie.com/index.asp?sec=ser&sub=def&pag=dis&ItemID=106790

43. Seiler SF, et al. Multimodality imaging-based evaluation of single-lumen silicone breast implants for rupture. Radiographics. 2017;37:366–82. https://doi.org/10.1148/rg.2017160086.

44. Clauser P, et al. Fat saturation in dynamic breast MRI at 3Tesla: is the Dixon technique superior to spectral fat saturation? A visual grading characteristics study. Eur Radiol. 2014;24(9):2213–9. https://doi.org/10.1007/s00330-014-3189-7.

45. Dapeng H, et al. MRI contrast agents: basic chemistry and safety. J Magn Reson Imaging. 2012;36:1060–71. https://doi.org/10.1002/jmri.23725.

46. Stephan P. Gadolinium use in breast cancer in MRI: weighting the benefits and possible risks. On line updated on March 30, 2021.

47. Sardanelli F, et al. Gadolinium retention and breast MRI screening: more harm than good? AJR Am J Roentgenol. 2020;214(2):324–7. https://doi.org/10.2214/AJR.19.21988. Epub 2019 Dec 4

48. EMA's final opinion confirms restrictions on use of linear gadolinium agents in body scans. European Medicine Agency. EMA/45761/2017. https://www.ema.europa.eu/en/documents/press-release/emas-final-opinion-confirms-restrictions-use-linear-gadolinium-agents-body-scans_en.pdf. Accessed 20 July 2023.

49. Kuhl C, et al. Efficacy and safety of half-dose gadopiclenol versus full-dose gadobutrol for contrast-enhanced body MRI. Radiology. 2023;308(1):e222612. https://doi.org/10.1148/radiol.222612.

50. Partridge SC, Amorssiripanitch N. The role of DWI in the assessment of breast lesions. Top Magn Reson Imaging. 2017;26(5):201–9. https://doi.org/10.1097/RMR.0000000000000137.

51. Wielema M, et al. Region of interest standardization for diffusion-weighted imaging of breast malignancies. EPOS™; 2017. https://doi.org/10.1594/ecr2017/C-2765.

52. Durur-Subasi I. DW-MR of the breast: a pictorial review. Insight Imaging. 2019;10(1):61. https://pubmed.ncbi.nlm.nih.gov/31161458/

53. Dietzel M, et al. Breast MRI in the era of diffusion weighted imaging: do we still need signal-intensity curves? Eur Radiol. 2020;30:47–56. https://doi.org/10.1007/s00330-019-06346-x.

54. Vasmel JE, et al. Dynamic contrast-enhanced and diffusion-weighted magnetic resonance imaging for response evaluation after single-dose ablative neoadjuvant partial breast irradiation. Adv Radiat Oncol. 2022;7:100854. https://doi.org/10.1016/j.adro.2021.100854.

55. Liu L, et al. Correlation of DCE-MRI perfusion parameters and molecular biology of breast infiltrating ductal carcinoma. Front Oncol. 2021;11:561735. https://doi.org/10.3389/fonc.2021.561735.

56. Guidance on screening and symptomatic breast imaging. 4th ed. The Royal College of Radiologists. https://www.rcr.ac.uk/system/files/publication/field_publication_files/bfcr199-guidance-on-screening-and-symptomatic-breast-imaging_0.pdf

57. Baltzer P, et al. Diffusion-weighted imaging of the breast-a consensus and mission statement from the EUSOBI international breast diffusion-weighted imaging working group. Eur Radiol. 2020;30:1436–50. https://doi.org/10.1007/s00330-019-06510-3.

58. Behzadi AH, et al. MRI and CT contrast media extravasation. A systematic review. Medicine. 2018;97(9):e0055. https://doi.org/10.1097/MD.0000000000010055. NIH PMC PubMed Central

59. ACR Extravasation Bullets Points Recommendations to contrast extravasation with Associated Strength of Evidence, ACR. https://www.acr.org/-/media/ACR/Files/Clinical-Resources/Extravasation-of-Contrast-Media%2D%2D%2D%2DBullet-Points-and-Chapter-Text%2D%2D-FINAL.pdf

60. Clauser P, et al. Motion artifact, lesion type, and parenchymal enhancement in breast MRI: what dose really influence diagnostic accuracy? Acta Radiol. 2019;60(1):10–27. https://doi.org/10.1177/0284185118770918.

61. Yitta S, et al. Recognizing artifacts and optimizing breast MRI at 1,5 and 3 T. AJR Am J Roentgenol. 2013 Jun;200(6):W673–82. https://doi.org/10.2214/AJR.12.10013.

62. Ojeda-Fournier H, et al. Recognizing and interpreting artifacts and pitfalls in MR imaging of the breast. Radiographics. 2007;27:S147–64. 10.1148/rg27si075516

63. Safety Guidelines for Magnetic resonance Imaging Equipment in Clinical Use. February 2021 MHRA Crown copyright.

64. Guidance for adjusting MRI scan sequence SAR and B1+rms Values. https://www.mri-q.com/uploads/3/4/5/7/34572113/mri_guidance_-_sar___b1_rms_final_12.23.15.pdf

65. Zuckerman SP, et al. Outcome's of COVID-19 vaccine-related incidental axillary adenopathy in women undergoing breast MRI. J Breast Imaging. 2022;4(4):392–9. https://doi.org/10.1093/jbi/wbac036.

66. Schiaffino S, et al. Axillary lymphadenopathy at the time of COVID-19 vaccination: ten recommendations from the European Society of Breast Imaging (EUSOBI). Insight Imaging. 2021;12:119. https://doi.org/10.1186/s13244-021-01062-x.

67. Mantellini P, et al. Rapporto sui ritardi accumulati dai programmi di screening italiani in seguito a pandemia da Covid-19. Terzo rapporto aggiornato al 31 Dicembre 2020, ONS. https://www.osservatorionazionalescreening.it/sites/default/files/allegati/Rapporto%20ripartenza-12_20.pdf

68. Han X, et al. Changes in cancer diagnoses and stage distribution during the first year of the Covid-19 pandemic in the USA: a cross-sectional nationwide assessment. Lancet Oncol. 2023;24:855–67.

69. Shankarapryan S, et al. Patterns of screening mammography and breast MRI during the COVID-19 pandemic: a retrospective, char-review study. LBI. 2023:277–86. https://doi.org/10.1093/jbi/wdad006.

70. Funaro K, Niell B. Screening mammography utilization in the United States. J Breast Imaging. 2023;5(4):384–92. https://doi.org/10.1093/jbi/wbad0Bibliography.

## Further Reading

Bernstein MA, et al. Handbook of MRI pulse sequences. Elsevier Academic Press; 2004. ISBN-13: 978-88-907973-7-8

Haacke EM, et al. Magnetic resonance imaging-physical principles and sequence design. Wiley & Sons; 1999. ISBN 0-471-35128-8

McRrobbie DW, et al. MRI from picture to proton. Cambridge University Press; 2017. ISBN-13: 978-0-511-34944-7

Stark DD, Bradley WG. Magnetic resonance imaging, vol. 1. 3rd ed. Mosby; 1999. ISBN 0-8151-8518-9

# Ergonomics and Work-Related Musculoskeletal Disorders

**23**

## 23.1 Introduction

*The term ergonomics generally refers to that science applied to the design and arrangement of things that people use, which aims to ensure that the interaction between people and things is as effective and safe as possible*. It is actually an absolutely composite science. It can be divided, but there are various schools of thought, into *physical*, *cognitive* and *organisational ergonomics* [1–4].

**Physical ergonomics** studies the anatomical anthropometric and biomechanical factors of human interaction with systems. Its main contribution is the prevention of *work-related musculoskeletal disorders* resulting from static and dynamic physical activity. Of interest to assess in the context of the work of the breast radiographer are, above all, the repetitive movements of the upper limbs. Anthropometric measurements assess the movement of the body, and therefore, the space needed by the worker. The correct sizing of work spaces is closely linked to their functionality and to safety conditions.

**Cognitive ergonomics**: studies how people perceive, interpret and process the information derived from the instrument they use, and how this leads them to implement actions to achieve the intended purpose. More simply, the aim of this branch of ergonomics is to make human-machine interaction as simple and safe as possible. The design of electro-medical instruments, including the mammographic machine, must therefore be based on cognitive ergonomics with a *user-centred design*. This means building instruments that are highly usable, simple and intuitive, so as to reduce the possibility of error, and make it easier to learn. This approach speeds up and improves the quality of results, since it allows the focus to be on the objective rather than on how to operate the device.

**Organisational ergonomics**: this is a branch of ergonomics that studies how the human factor impacts the other components of the organisation. The healthcare context is extremely complex. Among the factors to consider are the work activity rhythm, the relational climate, communication and teamwork (see Chap. 24).

It could actually be summarised, given the trend towards automation and increasingly widespread digitalisation, that the target of ergonomics is the **study of interfaces** and of the usability of machines. The term "machine" takes a more broadly meaning, i.e. the set of devices controlled by the health operator. The suggested subdivision could then be:

*Hardware ergonomics*: evaluating the human-machine interface;

*Ergonomics of the working environment*: dealing with the human-environment interface;

*Cognitive ergonomics*: concerning the human-software interface;

*Macroergonomics*: assessing the human-organisation interface.

*Ergonomics could therefore be defined as the study and design of complex systems that study the interaction of humans according to various aspects. It is implemented with the collaboration of experts in different disciplines. The approach must therefore be systemic, being the scenario very complex, with the aim of finding rational solutions.*

The ergonomics approach is absolutely anthropocentric. *Man is both beneficiary and reference model of the ergonomic project* (Vallone, cit.) [5]. Since, however, there is no standard man on which to base the project, it is absolutely necessary to analyse who the beneficiaries of the project are, according to various dimensions, anthropometric, physiological, perceptive and cognitive. The financial investment required to follow ergonomic principles has been shown to be not only advantageous from the point of view of operator and user satisfaction, but also economically. For example, it has been noted that an ergonomic environment decreases *turnover.* This is about the worker leaving the workplace, losing her/his professional skills, that maybe the facility itself has helped to create, perhaps from scratch.

## 23.2 The Legal Aspects of Ergonomics

The protection of workers is explicit in Article 38 of the Italian Constitution, and in Article 2087 of the Civil Code. There are no universal ergonomic standards, of course, since the type of work is extremely varied. We refer to reference standards validated by Italian **UNI**, European **CEN** and International **ISO** (see below). Standards for the design of work systems are contained in the 2017 UNI EN ISO 6385 [6]. Social organisational aspects and their mutual interaction are contained in the 2018 UNI EN ISO 10075 [7, 8].

Legislative Decree 626/94, transposing various European directives into Italian law, made the application of ergonomics in the workplace compulsory. It provides surveillance information and training, focusing on the human factor.

*Currently in Italy the standard to refer to for the protection of workers' health and safety in*

*the workplace is the Legislative Decree 81/08.* It talks about psychophysical integrity and how to maintain it.

The standards *European Committee for Standardization (CEN),* and *International Organization for Standardization (ISO),* have been defined for each specific field. The European Commission *Safety and Health Act* (**OSHA**) deals with work-related musculoskeletal disorders (see below).

## 23.3 Ergonomics in the Health Work Environment: Focus on the Breast Division [9–20]

Ergonomics deals with harmonising workers with the equipment they use. So, both the capabilities and limitations of operators must be taken into account. There are many aspects to be considered:

1. What the workplace is like for operators, in many respects;
2. What type of activity and workload (shifts, pace…) is there;
3. How the devices are to be used; what their design is, especially with regard to their appropriateness to the specific task;
4. How usable and accessible the information is, and to what extent, if any, can be modified;
5. What the working environment is like, in terms of temperature, humidity, lighting and noise;
6. What are the physical and psychological characteristics of the individual operator (in terms of height, weight, strength, posture), and the senses, especially sight, hearing and touch;
7. What her/his personality is like;
8. What her/his knowledge, skills and abilities are, and her/his training in the specific field;
9. How experienced she/he is;
10. What is the organisation and what are the social aspects, team structure, supervision and leadership, communication, resources, in the working environment.

An interesting aspect is the fact that not having a say in how work is organised, for example, could lead to lower quality and productivity. In the long run, it could lead to job dissatisfaction, which can increase the likelihood of developing work-related joint diseases.

In this chapter, only some of these aspects will be considered, focusing on the Senology division, deferring a broader and more complete treatment to specialised texts.

### 23.3.1 The Workplace: The Room Where Mammography Is Performed: (1) Size, Temperature and Humidity

*The workplace must first of all be the right size for the task at hand. That is to say the operator can make the movements required to effectively complete her/his task.* The room in which mammography is performed is generally small. The size of the mammographic unit has reduced over time; it is increasingly compact and therefore has a minimal dimension. The area of the room in which mammograms are performed ranges from 16 to 26 m², that is typical for stationary electromedical equipment diagnostics rooms. It is a class 1 FGI, according to the *Facility Guidelines Institute*, a non-profit organisation that develops guidelines for hospital construction. The radiographer's console (with a 1.5 mm lead-equivalent protective barrier), and the patient's changing room (which should be excluded from the minimum size of the area), should also be considered. Being small, there may be **temperature** problems. The mammographic unit dissipates a lot of heat, and to a much lesser extent, so do the computer and the image acquisition monitor. Direct digital detectors in general are very sensitive to temperature changes. In particular, the amorphous selenium of which the detectors are made (Chap. 7) does not tolerate high temperatures. More precisely, *temperature changes from the range indicated by the individual manufacturer, below and above the tolerated limit, can degrade the detector sometimes irreversibly.* This is why the room should have an independent temperature control.

**Humidity** control is also important: (1) both for operator and patient comfort, (2) also to reduce the possibility of electrostatic attraction of dust on the compression paddle and detector.

### 23.3.2 The Workplace: (2) Lighting

Some preliminary information is provided first.

*Photometry* is a branch of optics that deals with the measurement of that part of electromagnetic radiation that is in the visible range for the human eye. It is therefore part of *radiometry*, which deals with the entire spectrum of electromagnetic radiation, a subject that is well known to the professional figure of the radiographer. For a better understanding, it was therefore thought to provide a parallel between photometric and radiometric quantities.

**Luminous intensity** indicates the light emitted in a specific direction. The parallelism is with radiant intensity. It is measured in *candelas (cd),* described as the ratio of the *lumen* (which expresses the eye's standard response to light) to the *steradian* (which is the unit of measurement of the three-dimensional solid angle).

**Illuminance** indicates the amount of light a surface receives. The parallel is with irradiance. It is measured in *lumens per square metre (lux).*

**Luminance of a surface:** the parallel is with radiance. It is the ratio between the luminous intensity emitted towards that surface, which is projected towards the observer (apparent area). It is measured in *cd/m²*. Another unit of measurement for luminance is to be mentioned, the *foot-Lambert* (fL), used in the Anglo-Saxon world (conversion formula: 1 fL = 3.7 cd/m²) [19].

For a correct visualisation of the images on the acquisition modality monitor and on the computer display, the room should be illuminated with artificial light. In mammographic diagnostics, natural light is very seldom exploitable. It should be around 300–400 lux. For the execution of examinations, it is however convenient to decrease it. The *secondary screens* (see below) should have a *low minimum luminance and a high maximum luminance.* The recommended range for 5 MP display workstations is

$0.51–492$ cd/m$^2$ [20]. While the examination is being carried out, the room illumination must be dimmed, considering the need to accurately assess the *light field or active area* (Chaps. 7 and 8). This is important also to avoid compression paddle glare. It is therefore useful to have an electronic device in the diagnostics to adjust the ambient brightness, the **dimmer.** Lighting is now generally provided by low-power LEDs, warm neutrals, between 3000 and 4000 Kelvin. That is, the chromatic properties of the light are assessed, by *temperature* (which is the colour appearance) and the *colour rendering index* (which indicates how much of its natural colour an object illuminated by an artificial light source appears). An interesting aspect, which has not yet been sufficiently studied and above all has not been resolved, is the *glare or reflection of the compression paddle*. It can be very disturbing and requires a careful study of the lighting points in the room, in order to reduce it to a minimum. *It should be emphasised that ambient illuminance can adversely affect the efficiency of the devices in use.* They should include the *review, or secondary displays* as well as the reporting *displays* (see below). The adequacy of artificial lighting is regulated by "good engineering standards," according to EN 12464 [14].

### 23.3.3 The Workplace: (3) The Image Acquisition Monitor, Features

Height (depending on the height of the operator) and the distance of the monitor from the operator, 60–80 cm from the operator's head, should be adjusted. The upper edge should be set at eye level, so that the eyes are slightly tilted downwards. This avoids improper neck and head postures. Monitors should be positioned also to avoid reflection problems (e.g. from ceiling or wall light spots).

*Biomedical displays* [17–20] can generally be classified as *primary* (of the reporting work station), and *secondary*, also called review displays, used (mostly) by radiographers for the evaluation of the images produced. They are associated to the image acquisition modality.

These monitors generally do not follow the same rules as the first ones, which are very precise and rigid. When the characteristics are very far-worse-from those of the primary displays, various problems may arise for the radiographer (see Chap. 16). Acquisition monitors should therefore also have minimum characteristics to be respected, in terms of luminance range and spatial resolution. Some mammographic machine manufacturers cite the recommendation of the ACR that the resolution of image acquisition monitors and that of reporting monitors should be similar. This is especially important when mammographic devices are associated with stereotactic systems (Chap. 18).

The data interface is included in the operating system of the mammographic unit (*browser*), thanks to **web technology**. The RIS is integrated with the PACS (Chap. 8). The display system acquires the image with a given grey scale, which are converted into luminance values. More precisely, the video card contains a LUT that converts p-values into **digital driving levels** (**DDL**) which in turn are converted into luminance values, according to a function characteristic of each monitor. It is not standardised and cannot be modified. For this reason, a special function has been introduced to make the display of images on different devices consistent, the *Grayscale Standard Display Function (GSDF)*. See Chap. 8. GSDF is very important especially in mammography, even though the comparison between examinations of the same patient, in some cases, remains difficult [14].

### 23.3.4 The Workplace: (4) Shelf with Accessories, Furniture Elements in General

The accessory shelf must be at a height (calibrated to a standard operator height) that reduces the need to lift and push forwards the arms and torso and not far from the mammographic machine. The so-called **working triangle** (mammographer—shelf with accessories and the necessary for sanitising—acquisition mode) must be reduced as much as possible.

### 23.3.5  The Workplace: (5) The Position of the Mammographic Unit in the Room, in Relation to Console and Other Furniture

The arrangement of the mammographic unit in the room is also interesting. It has a certain impact on the mammography clinical quality and comfort of the patient. The radiographer must be able to control the patient during acquisition, from behind her/his station, as well as to move around the patient ergonomically. This is also to reduce as much as possible the time interval in which the breast is compressed, passing quickly, without obstacles, from the mammographic unit to the console. The radiographer must therefore be able to participate in purchase decision and approval conference tables of diagnostic imaging equipment.

### 23.4  Physical Ergonomics and Work-Related Musculoskeletal Disorders or of Professional Nature (WRMSDs) [21–26]

**Musculoskeletal disorders (MSDs)** are the leading cause of occupational disease in all countries with advanced post-industrial development. They are a multifactorial and complex phenomenon related to occupational risk. This could induce or aggravate MSDs, which include many inflammatory and/or degenerative lesions. They are caused by (1) biomechanical overload; (2) repetitive strain (short-cycle work); (3) incorrect postures maintained over a long period of time; (4) cumulative trauma; and (5) psychosocial factors. The focus of these paragraphs will be on *short-cycle series activities*, requiring repeated and frequent movements and/or efforts: it is the exact ergonomic description of the job of the breast radiographer, as far as the physical part is concerned. Repeated movements, above all of the upper limbs, typical of mammographers, do not generally induce serious problems.

However, they can be disabling, limiting the operator's suitability for the job. They may lead to her/his eventual removal from the job as breast radiographer, which in some cases may become definitive.

*Repetitive movements of the upper limbs are defined as the repetition of movements that are always the same. They over time can trigger acute inflammatory processes and tend to become chronic. They affect shoulder, elbow, wrist and hand.* **ISO STANDARD 11228-3** [27].

Various aspects contribute to the onset of these processes. To be included:

1. The imbalance between the effort required and the functional capacity of the operator. This in turn depends on many personal factors, such as age, gender, psycho-physiological conditions and personal history of previous disorders, and lifestyle;
2. Organisational factors and relationships with colleagues and managers in the workplace;
3. The absence of practical training and education in the ergonomic field must certainly be considered in the overall assessment of the risk of onset and/or worsening.

Another aspect to be taken into account, especially in this post-acute phase of the Sars-CoV-2 pandemic, is *mental fatigue*. Dr. Samuele Marcora (currently full professor of Sport Science at the University of Bologna) has proposed a psycho-biological model of physical ergonomics. It is thought for athletic-type activity, which can however be transposed to the healthcare reality, in the writer's opinion. Mental fatigue determined by prolonged cognitive efforts can have an impact on performance comparable to muscular exhaustion [28].

Recent studies would show a clear link between psychological variables and, for example, cervicalgia or lumbago. Stress, depressive symptoms, anxiety and poor sleep quality could play a role at the intraspinal level and at the medulla oblongata, which could manifest itself in distant *hyperalgia* [29]. **Hyperalgia** is defined as the accentuation of the ability to feel a painful stimulus.

*MSDs are also called cumulative trauma disorders (CTD), repetitive strain injuries (RSI), for the upper limbs only, or more generally work-related musculoskeletal disorders (WRMSDs). They are defined as acute and chronic disorders of muscles, tendons and nerves, caused by repeated exertion and rapid movements made over a prolonged period of time.* They are therefore not "accidents," but a wide range of phenomena involving pain, reduced movement or loss of sensation. The European Union has published recommendations to standardise the diagnosis of WRMSDs and define risk factors. Obviously, they vary extraordinarily depending on the type of work (ICD-10, see below).

## 23.5 The Movement of the Human Body: The Joints

The movement of the body is enabled by the interaction between the skeletal and muscular systems. That is to say, by the *joints,* which hold two or more bony surfaces in contiguity. To study a joint kinematically, its range of motion or *excursion* is measured. The possible movements, which allow its direction with respect to the coronal, sagittal and transverse planes are:

CORONAL or FRONTAL PLANES: *lateral flexion, abduction and adduction, supination and pronation*;

SAGITTAL PLANES: *flexion and extension*;

TRANSVERSAL (or HORIZONTAL) PLANES: *rotation;* for the shoulder, abduction and adduction are also on the transverse plane.

The direction of the movements is also indicated by the axis around which they occur: LONGITUDINAL or VERTICAL AXIS: *torsion and rotation movements*; *prone-supination movements in the case of hand and forearm*; TRAVERSAL AXIS: flexion *and extension movements*; SAGITTAL AXIS: *abduction and adduction movements.* See Table 23.1.

*The majority of movements are not monoplanar, but three-dimensional. Therefore, involving several planes become difficult to describe.*

**Table 23.1** Movements according to planes and axes around which they occur

| Terminology | Definition |
|---|---|
| Flexion | Movement consisting of the bringing together of two body segments, with a reduction in the angle between the distal end of one and the proximal end of the other, contiguous |
| Extension | Movement consisting in moving two contiguous body segments apart, increasing the angle between the distal end of one and the proximal end of the other |
| Hyperextension | Extension above the standard position |
| Abduction | Lateral movement away from the midline of the body or sagittal axis |
| Adduction | Medial movement towards the midline of the body |
| Rotation | Movement performed by a body segment in trunk to its own (longitudinal) axis; also applies to the trunk |
| Pronaution | Internal rotation (segment facing downwards) |
| Supination | External rotation (segment facing upwards) |
| Ulnar deviation | Bring the V finger closer to the ulna |
| Radial deviation | Bring the first finger closer to the radio |
| Protraction | In this case, it means the anterior translation of the neck and head |

### 23.5.1 Hand-Forearm

*Forearm pronation* means a rotational movement in which the hand and part of the arm are rotated so that the first finger points towards the body. *Forearm supination* means an outward rotation (the first finger points away from the body). *Dorsal flexion of the hand is* a hyperextension of the wrist towards the dorsal side of the forearm. *Palmar* flexion is a flexion of the wrist towards the palm and the ventral side of the forearm. This is an extreme simplification, as pronation and supination movements can be in different planes, and this depends on the position of the shoulder.

### 23.5.2 Hand First Finger

Being positioned at 90° with respect to the other fingers, it makes the hand capable of grasping objects and imparting force to the grip. It also allows them to be manipulated and immobilised. This is a focal point to be considered in the biomechanics of the breast radiographer.

### 23.5.3  Foot

In the case of the *foot, pronation* is rotation of the sole of the foot outwards. S*upination* is rotation of the sole inwards. *Plantar flexion* is a movement that decreases the angle between the sole of the foot and the back of the leg. *Dorsal flexion* decreases the angle between the back of the foot and the leg. The toes move closer to the tibia.

A simplified model or diagram was used f*or the representation of the positions assumed by the mammographer.* It is called *STICK* and is depicted in Fig. 23.1, in a neutral anatomical position.

A study was done about the incongruous positions assumed by the mammographer in her/his work routine, and the duration of them, expressed as a percentage of the total working time or cycle. Four anatomical segments were considered:

1. The arm in relation to the shoulder (flexion, extension and abduction);

2. When the elbow is involved (arm-forearm flexion-extension, forearm prone-supination);
3. When the wrist is involved (flexion-extension and radial or ulnar deviations);
4. The hand (whose grip type is considered).

JGIO68, cit. [30].

## 23.6  Performing the CC Projection from a Biomechanical Point of View

After the reception in the patient's room, we proceed to the historical data collection. Although this part represents a small portion of the time dedicated to each examination, it must be considered in the overall ergonomic calculation (see Sect. 23.3). Also, the seat must be congruous, with the possibility of modifying its height from the floor to accommodate radiographers of different height. Once the data collection is finished, the examination is sent from the worklist to the acquisition modality, and we proceed to its execution.

**Fig. 23.1** Simplified diagram of the joints that allow movement of the human body, in an anatomical or neutral position, standing upright, fingers outstretched and feet forward. STICK model, see text

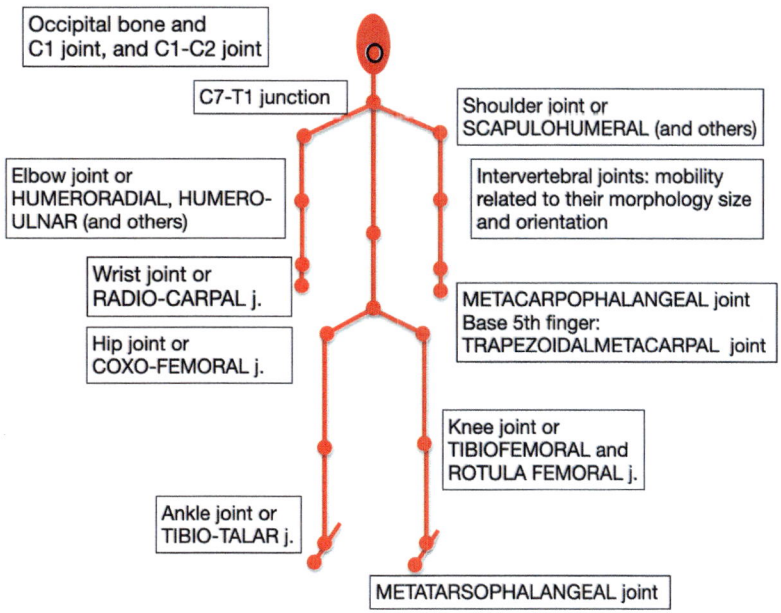

For the preliminary procedure to the examination, see Chap. 16; for the performance of the examination step by step, see Chap. 9.

Here listed is a subdivision into *tasks* of positioning in an ergonomic sense [21–26, 31–33]:

- *The patient is in front of the mammographic unit,* shoulders relaxed. Her posture is corrected if necessary, chest and hips on the same line. The radiographer is on the patient's medial side, perpendicular to her, see Fig. 23.2a–c. Neck flexed laterally, and head and neck *protraction*. This in in order to coordinate vision with movement, throughout the examination, overcoming the impediment given by the mammographic unit and the patient herself;

- *The patient's shoulders are wrapped up to that of the side under examination, which is to be pushed downwards,* as clearly visible in Fig. 23.2b, h, i. *The arm is raised, either at the same height or higher than one's own shoulders in a neutral position,* if the patient is taller than the radiographer. This is a position which, by the way, must be maintained for almost the entire examination. Dynamic or static actions involving the elevation of the arm in flexion or abduction even at shoulder height alone can induce problems in the shoulder joint itself. This is just for only 10% of the total cycle, according to literature on the subject [30]. The required flexion-abduction of the radiographer's upper limb is important and considered to be at risk (because of the wide angle of excursion). The radiographer's elbow is flexed. The wrist is equally flexed, fingers sometimes spread apart. A downward thrust is impressed, which may require some force if the patient has joint problems or is generally tense and stiff (Fig. 23.2h, i);

- *The breast must be lifted* with the palm of the other hand, forearm supinated, inserting its fifth finger deep into the IMF, finger abducted. Breast is lifted until the axial plane is parallel to the sensitive plane. The movement of maximum supination requires a high involvement of the elbow joint (Fig. 23.2e). The wrist is flexed and in lateral deviation. The grip of the hand is at "spoon" (palmar grip) [33];

- *The detector is raised to the appropriate height for the patient,* generally using the

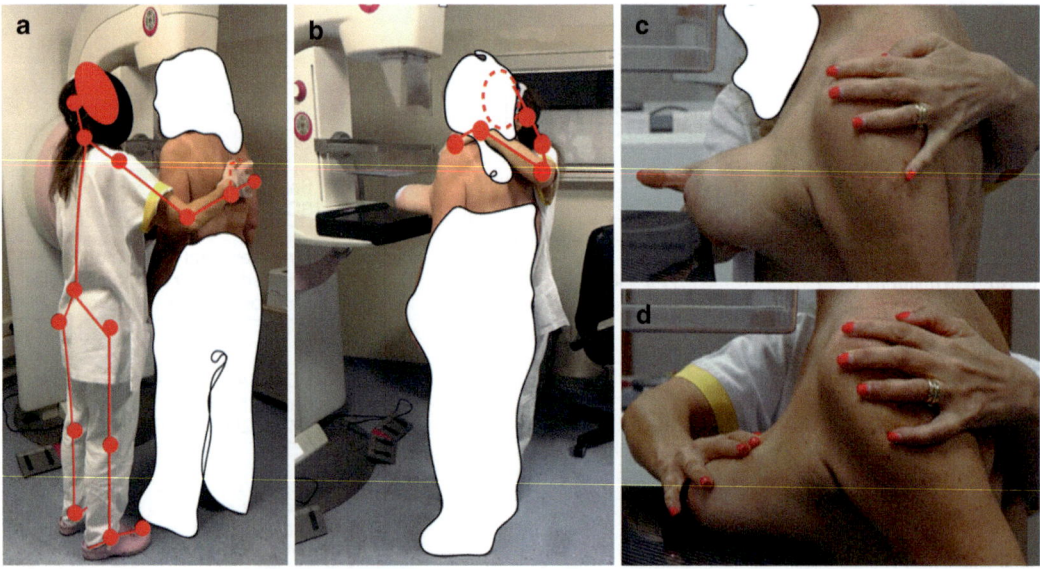

**Fig. 23.2** (**a**–**j**) Some positions assumed by the radiographer performing CC projection. Stick model. See text. (**k**–**m**) Radiographer biomechanics, CC projection, standard examination, stick model. See text and preceding and following pages. Note also the posture assumed "at rest" by the operator, during image acquisition, with neck protraction, pathological kyphotic posture and posterior tilt of the pelvis (bringing the hips forward), see Chap. 26

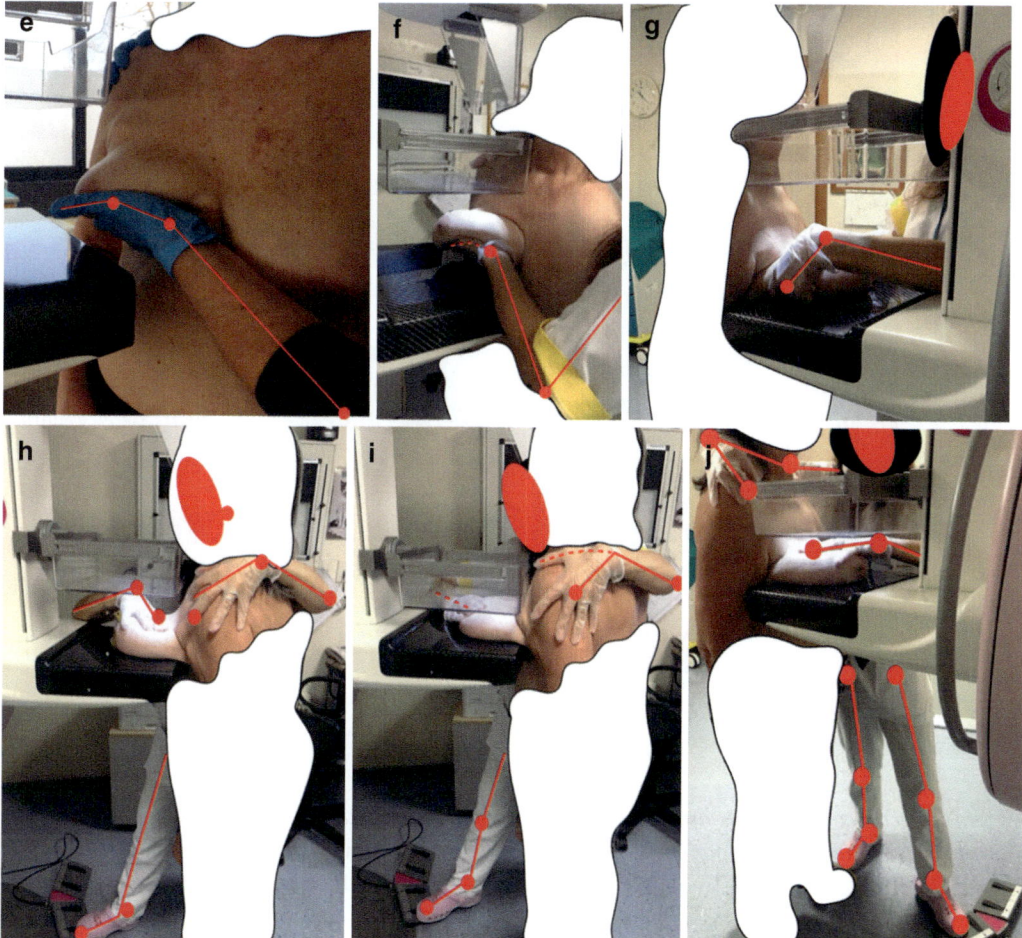

**Fig. 23.2** (continued)

pedal control. This must be brought close to radiographer, so that she/he does not have to move too far away from the neutral position. *The foot is in dorsal flexion, pressing* via *the metatarsophalangeal portion.* The knees can be flexed, the lower limbs spread apart, to achieve better balance. The weight is in any case distributed unevenly;

- *The breast is further lifted, and brought well forward,* Fig. 23.2f. Wrist is flexed and in radial deviation. This particular task: *lifting the breast*, is indicated by much of the relevant Anglo-Saxon literature as being the one with the highest risk, to the elbow, wrist and first finger. Consideration must be given to: (1) the size and weight of the breast being studied and therefore the overall muscular effort required;

(2) the strength and size of the radiographer's hand (Fig. 23.2e, f);

- *Placing the breast on the detector* is an essential step, Fig. 23.2h, i, j. It must be carefully controlled and monitored. To do so, radiographer's neck and head must be rotated and extended. Often the torso must also be rotated and flexed, in order to maintain a view of the breast. With the other hand the patient is shown how to move the other breast out of the FOV, Fig. 23.2k;
- Some radiographers use the *two-hand manoeuvre to bring the breast forward,* Fig. 23.2g. In this case, we speak of a palmar grip exercised by both hands;
- Other radiographers, including the writer, use their own bodies to push the patient's torso

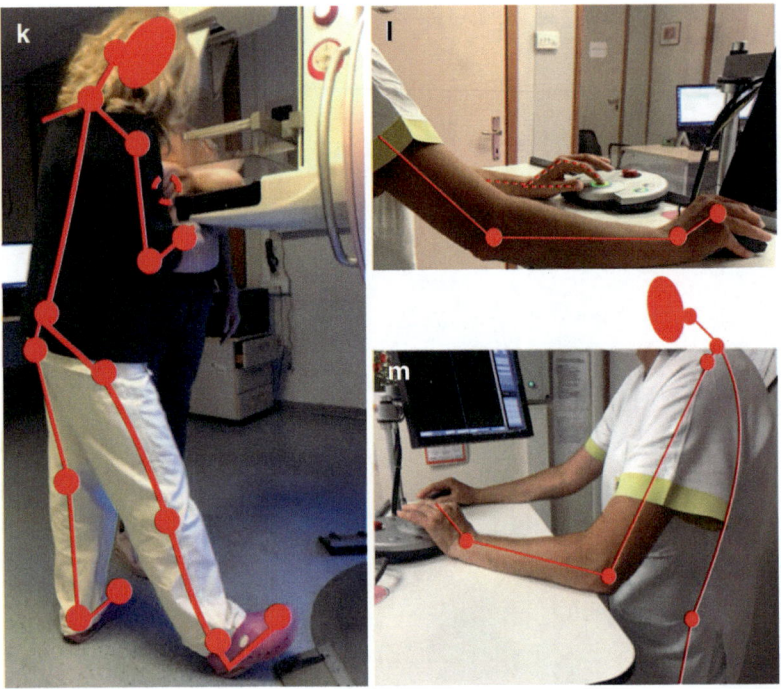

**Fig. 23.2** (continued)

forward. *Direct pressure is applied anteriorly with the arm around the patient's shoulders,* Fig. 23.2i. The operation requires a certain amount of force, depending on the patient's cooperation. It is significant if the patient has stiffness problems at the cervical level. It is therefore in general always requested in dealing with kyphotic patients (see also Chap. 26). *Rotation of the torso, bending of the knees*;

- *The breast must be stretched forwards,* Fig. 23.2i, j, to eliminate any skin folds that may form, and to bring the deep upper tissues further forwards. *Stretching must be done by exerting a certain amount of pressure directed towards the detector and anteriorly, with the fingers not spread.* If the radiographer's hand is small, this is not an easy task. *Hand pronated, wrist deviating first radially then ulnarly,* Fig. 23.2j. *Elbow semi-flexed, shoulder in an intermediate position between flexion and abduction, at an angle that varies according to the patient's height*;

- *One begins to compress,* Fig. 23.2h–j, using the pedal control: *foot in dorsal flexion and*

*pelvic balance, knees flexed.* The lateral and inferior folds are stretched out using the free hand, with fingers together. A blunting directed superiorly and inferiorly respectively is to be done. A fair amount of force is imparted to the movements. T*he grip is called precision grip or pinch grip.* It is characterised by fine movements of the fingers, and it can only develop about one-fourth of the total prehension force of the hand. This is why it is considered to be more risky than other grips;

- It is quickly *checked, neck and head rotated and extended or flexed depending on the height of the patient and the radiographer. The torso is rotated and flexed in coordination with the visual monitoring of the breast.* Also to check the achieved compression value. Usually, it displayed either at the base of the mammographic unit or at the height of the detector support. So the consequent neck-head movements are to be considered. The additional pressure of the foot worsens the already unequal distribution of weight between lower limbs;

- *One moves quickly to the imaging acquisition workstation.* Its position must be as ergonomic as possible, according to the criteria listed in the first paragraphs. The modality monitor must be positioned at the right height, as must the table. The table must not be too high to avoid the elevation of the shoulders, nor too low, so as to *allow the elbow to rest and avoid excessive muscular activity in the proximal segment of the upper limb.* The acquisition button, or buttons, is/are pressed, avoiding always using the same finger, Fig. 23.2l. We could think of alternating the finger for example with the palm of the hand (immediately anterior to the wrist), or, when possible, using the pedal acquisition mode;
- See also static posture, Fig. 23.2m.

## 23.7 Performing the MLO Projection from a Biomechanical Point of View [21–28, 31, 32]

- The patient is in front of the mammographic unit, shoulders relaxed, with the body positioned at an angle of 45–50° to the detector, chest and hips on the same line. The radiographer is behind the patient, Fig. 23.3a, b, if his height and that of the patient allows it. Otherwise, more medially. *The breast to be studied is picked up with two hands.* First the deep lateral tissues are pushed forward, with one hand. Then *the whole breast is picked up with the other, with a pinch grip* (first finger in front and the other four behind, Chap. 9). Pinch grips are characterised by the opposition between the first finger and the distal joints of the other four. This grip is the one intrinsically more at risk from a biomechanical point of view;
- *The radiographer guides the patient forwards towards the detector,* with *a firm grip of the patient's ipsilateral arm, immediately in front of the armpit. This is until it rests on the upper profile of the detector, as far forwards as possible,* with palmar grip, Fig. 23.3c, d. The muscular effort is sometimes very important. To this must be added the exercise of an effective communication (Chap. 24), with words of explanation and request to do only the required movements, without moving the feet or turning around. The force exerted also requires a stable position of the radiographer's whole body. *Knees flexed or very flexed* in case the patient is small in height and the mammographer tall. *Head-neck flexion rotation and protraction,* Figs. 23.3e and 23.4;
- You move towards the patient's arm. If necessary, you bring the arm Fig. 23.3f, g (grip grip)

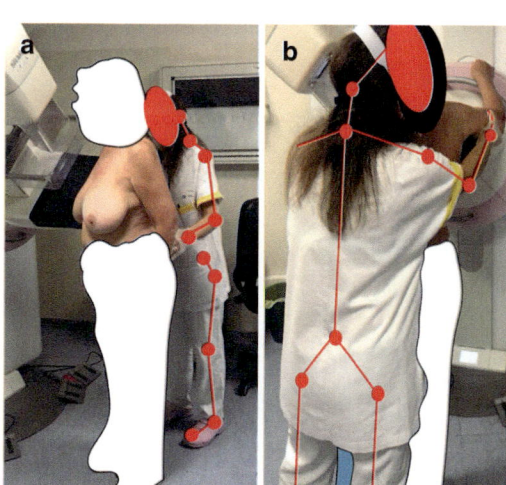
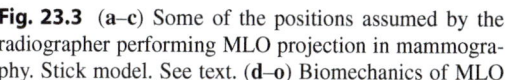
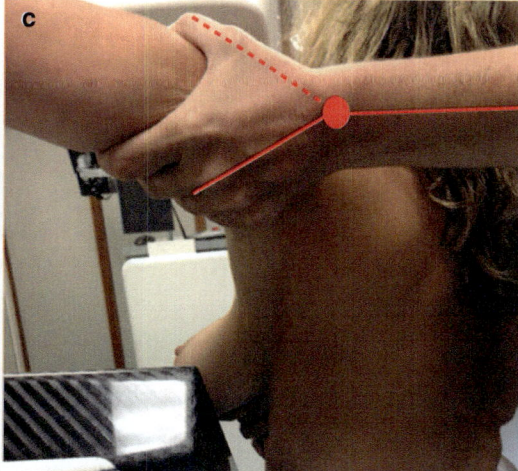

**Fig. 23.3** (**a–c**) Some of the positions assumed by the radiographer performing MLO projection in mammography. Stick model. See text. (**d–o**) Biomechanics of MLO projection, standard examination, Stick model. See text. (**p–s**) Biomechanics of MLO projection in mammography, see text

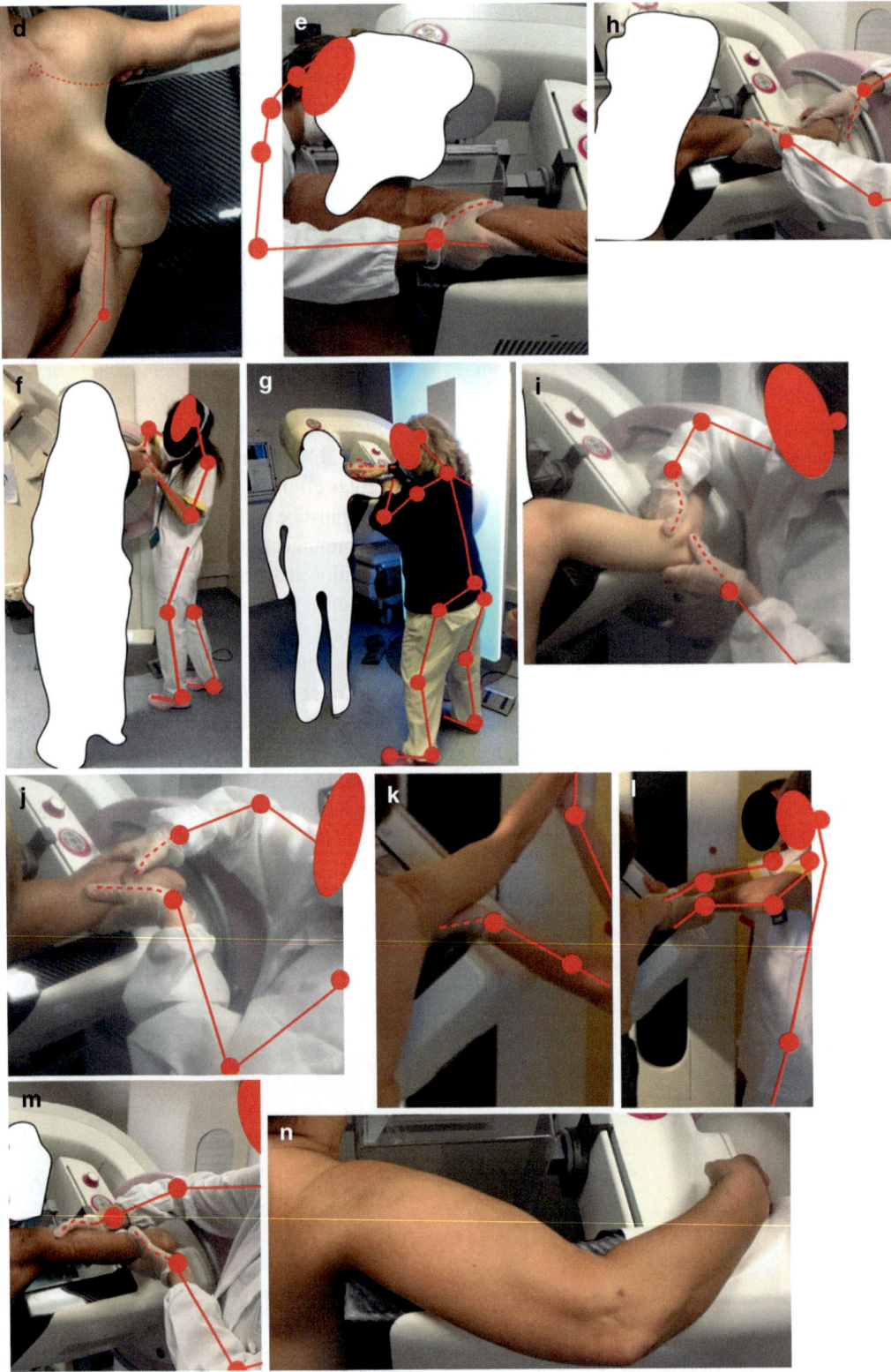

**Fig. 23.3** (continued)

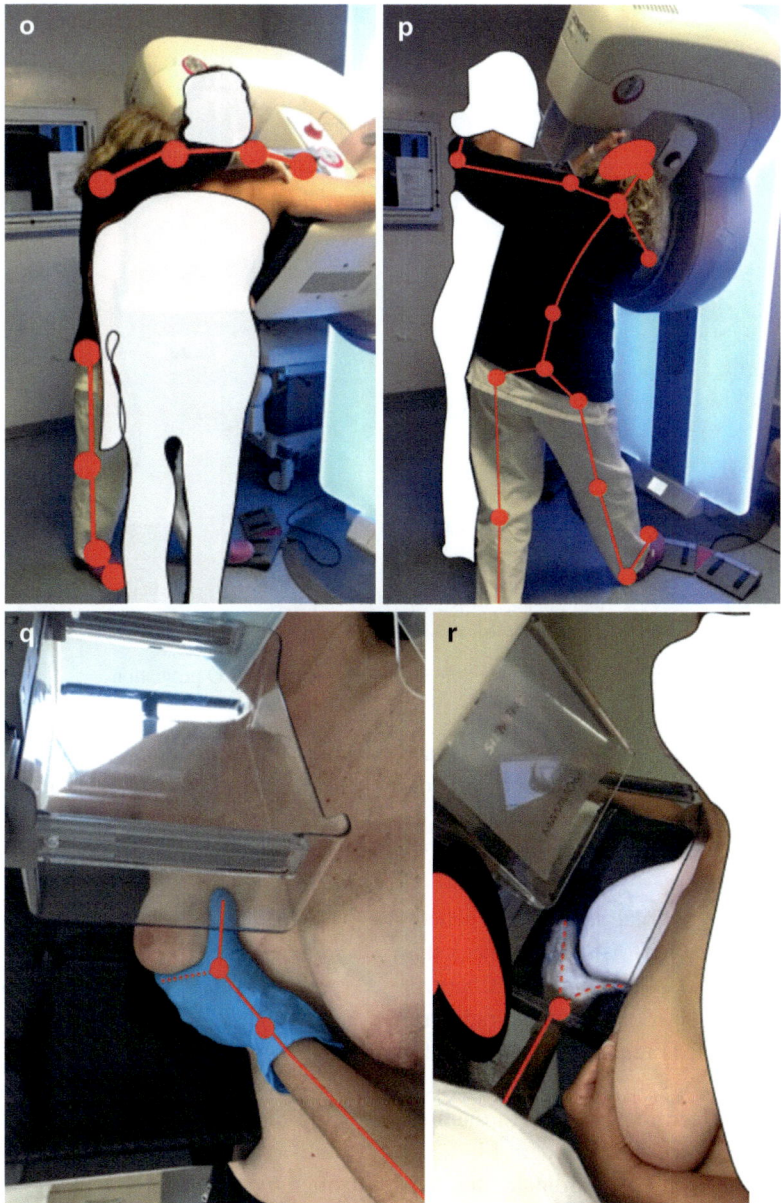

**Fig. 23.3** (continued)

further forward. T*he first rotation of the arm is done* (Poggi method) *directed superiorly and anteriorly, using the two hands,* Fig. 23.3k. Shoulder elbow wrist and hand engagement. The grip is a palmar-type;

- The *second rotation of the arm, with the* shoulder stationary, is done, *directed superiorly and posteriorly* (see Chap. 9 and Fig. 9.5c). Again using both hands, fingers

together, the patient's arm is extended downwards and forwards. Elbow flexed and the patient's hand relaxed, Fig. 23.3h–j, m, n. The grip is a palmar-type. The position assumed and the force exerted to lengthen the patient's arm impacts the wrist and shoulder joints, with possible *subacromial conflict or impingement.* This is happen when the arm is lifted a great deal in relation to the trunk. As a conse-

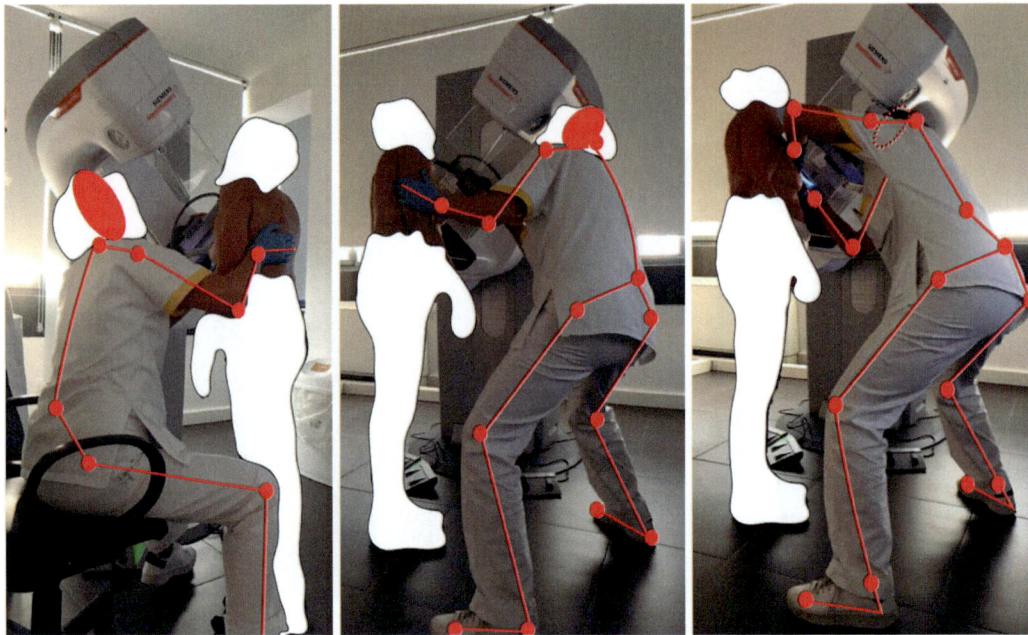

**Fig. 23.4** The seated radiographer, compared with the standing position, MLO projection

quence, there is a narrowing of the space between the head of the humerus and the acromion, where the tendons of the cuff run;

- The result sought with the two rotations is shown in Fig. 23.3o;
- We return to the medial side of the patient, Fig. 23.3p–s. *The breast is lifted* to check that no folds have formed behind (see Chaps. 9 and 17 on this subject). About the radiographer's position: it is recommended to sit for performing this phase of the MLO projection. This is to avoid incorrect postures of the lumbar and cervical spine and shoulders, Fig. 23.4;
- All movements must be co-ordinated for constant visual monitoring of the correct progress of the examination. This may require *extension and twisting of the neck. The pinch grip* [33], Fig. 23.3r, is *retrieved.*
- The patient is asked to rotate her hips (and feet) towards the device;
- *The breast is stretched upwards and anteriorly* (UP&OUT manoeuvre, Chap. 9). When possible, this manoeuvre is done with two hands, especially dealing with very large breasts, and that is more feasible if the radiographer is seated. Stretching out requires firm

pressure of the breast towards the detector, as well as upwards and anteriorly. Load is posed on the shoulder elbow and wrist joints, and on the first finger;

- *One begins to press (using the pedal control),* Fig. 23.3p, q. A *smoothing out any posterior folds, at the IMF,* is done. It is used the small *pincer manoeuvre* (Chap. 9), *first and second fingers together.* This is a precision pinch grip. The fingers slide in front of and behind the IMF, with vertical downward direction;
- In order to keep the breast clamped in place until compression fixes it, the *first finger is* often *hyperabducted* as in Fig. 23.3s;
- Care is taken when passing the compression paddle over protruding bony parts. If necessary, the tissue is moved superiorly and posteriorly (upwards and backwards). This is to decrease the discomfort of the compression itself. This is done, if the radiographer is seated, *by raising the free arm. The free hand reaches the patient's sternum and shoulder. The other holds the breast. T*he upper limb is *above the* shoulders, often above one's head. This increases the biomechanical risk score. If the MLO is performed standing, the risk

depends on the height of the patient and the radiographer, Fig. 23.4;

- Once the breast has been blocked and checked that there are no anatomical parts of the patient that can project onto the image, one *moves quickly to the console. The acquisition button is pressed* (see same task in CC), Fig. 23.2l, m.

## 23.8  MSDs in Mammography, Damage Stages and Related Pathologies

The **cervical spine** must certainly be considered at biomechanical risk due to the need to flex the neck laterally and extend/flex it in the sagittal plane, and protrude it, in order to (1) monitor with the sight the exact positioning of the breast on the detector; (2) globally evaluate the anatomy of the patient avoiding the head of the mammographic unit. The risk of localised or diffuse MSDs may also affect the **thoracic-lumbar spine,** and this is especially true considering the increasing average age of health operators, not only in Italy, and the possible increase in BMI. The need to bend the thoracic-lumbar spine, leaning forwards and rotating the torso, involves a shift of the force of gravity to the front of the rachis. It induces a flexion that is counteracted by the muscles of the back. The greater the inclination of the trunk, the greater the load on the muscles.

The need to bend the knees in case the operator is tall and the patient short, for performing the MLO projection, certainly also poses a risk for MSDs: the **knees** must therefore be included in the radiographer risk valuation in a Senology Department.

*The greatest risk, however, is borne by the upper limbs. This is due to the work with the arms raised, away from the body, and higher than shoulder level. In some cases, they are above the head, with the wrist deviated, and the first finger abducted. All of this require a significant use of force (***i.e. the biomechanical effort required to perform the action)***.* This risk obviously increases with (1) the *frequency of repetition* (see also Sect. 23.11); (2) possible *stereotypy*

(identical repetition of the same movement); (3) *incongruous postures,* if they are maintained for a long time.

The synovial fluid contained in the tendon sheaths may, due to repeated movements, not be produced in sufficient quantity for its function, that is preventing friction. This can lead to the onset of an *inflammatory process.* The repetition of inflammatory episodes can then result in the formation of fibrous tissue and thus the chronicisation of the pathology. Inflammation of the sheath of the tendon is generally called **tenosynovitis.** It is associated in the specific case of the breast radiographer, precisely with the repetitive movements of the wrist. One speaks of **bursitis** if there is an inflammation of the serous joint bursa. Its function is to perform a lubrication for the sliding of tendons and muscles with respect to the bones. This is done in particular at the level of the knee, elbow or shoulder. Bursitis can be caused by repetitive movements and the pressure exerted on the joints. We speak of **spondylitis** if the inflammation is at the intervertebral discs. The term **tendinopathy** is used when tendons are affected, e.g. at the *rotator cuff* (shoulder joint). **Epicondylitis** is the term used when the inflammation includes the area between the bone and tendon insertion *(insertional tendinopathy).* Again, this is linked to repetitive extension movements of the fingers and wrist and at the elbow. The pain may extend to the forearm.

**Stages or degrees of damage that can be considered**: *mild, moderate, severe* [20, 32]. This subdivision is necessarily very schematic, so the symptoms suffered may not fit into it precisely. The first degree is characterised by a dull pain or unpleasant sensation, episodic, reversible. In the second degree, the recurrent pain is more frequent than in the first stage. It could be experienced during the working day, but may recur outside of work. Swelling of the affected area may be observed. This stage is also reversible, but would require a period of rest from those movements that induced the problem. In the third stage, pain, fatigue and weakness may be felt even when the operator is at complete rest. Generally, the damage is no longer reversible *(evaluation models,* see below).

### 23.8.1 The Most Common WRMSDs of Breast Radiographers

These pathologies can be cited among the most common among breast radiographers, in order of frequency, as deduced from the literature [22, 23]. It should be considered also that they are difficult to diagnose, at least at an early stage. Because of this, they are often underestimated by the operators themselves.

*European and WHO ICD 10 recommendations* were considered for the associated acronyms [34]:

1. **De Quervain Syndrome ICD-10-M65.4 (Radial Styloid Tenosynovitis)**: affects the tendon sheath of the first finger. It causes intense pain in the wrist and base of the first finger, especially in the flexion-extension movement, on the radial aspect of the wrist. It is the most frequent of the overload disorder affecting the wrist;

2. **Carpal Tunnel Syndrome ICD-10-G56.0**: is a neuropathy that manifests itself by pain and tingling in the hand and sometimes in the arm. It is due to the median nerve compression by the inflammatory process. It is the most common peripheral neuropathy, and the literature shows significant evidence of a correlation between this pathology and repetitive movements. Women are affected more frequently than men. The pain associated is on the palmar aspect of the hand. This usually includes the first three fingers and part of the fourth;

3. **Cervicalgia ICD-10-M54.2**: it is a spinal pathology, sometimes associated with the arm, *cervico-brachialgia*. The pain is felt at the nuchal level. It can be superior or inferior (up to the shoulder blades). it is a very common pathology, multifactorial, linked for example to: (1) genetic factors; (2) the coexistence of lumbago; (3) previous traumas; (4) prolonged postural postures in flexion of the head and neck. Much literature shows that repetitive work with continuous arm and hand involvement places a load on the neck and shoulder muscles;

4. **Pathologies of the Rotator Cuff (ICD-10-M75.1)**: a malfunction of the rotator cuff is involved. Its inflammation results in joint instability and pain in the lifting and rotational movement of the arm. The shoulder is a complex joint: the *rotator cuff* is made up of the tendons of four muscles, which wrap around the humeral head and give it stability. The joint surface, the glenoid fossa, is small and shallow, which is why the shoulder itself has poor stability. It is a common pathology whose frequency increases with age. The pain worsens during the night. It is also associated with work that requires repeated arm movements above the shoulders and head;

5. **Lateral Epicondylitis (ICD-10-M77.1) or Insertional Tendinopathy of the Extensor Muscles of the Wrist**: it is an inflammation at the insertion point of the extensor muscles of the forearm and wrist. It gives pain in prone-supinated movements. The literature on the subject shows strong evidence of a correlation between repetitive movements of the upper limbs and posture, and this pathology;

6. **Acute Lumbalgia (ICD-10-M54.5 low back pain or lumbago)**: the lumbar spine does not allow ample rotation, but in the event of sudden twisting movements, an acute contracture of the related muscle segment may occur, leading to a sideways tilt of the spine. In addition to personal predisposition, lifestyle (such as not exercising to keep the muscles relaxed and stretched) and BMI must be considered;

7. **Bursitis of the Knee ICD-10-M70.50, or Gonalgia (knee pain) in General**: bursitis is one of the most common causes of swelling and pain in this joint. *Gonalgia* is a multifactorial condition. It can occur as a result of repeated flexion movements of the knee during work.

To the aforementioned pathologies must also be added:

1. **Tenosynovitis (trigger finger, ICD-10-M65.3)**: this is a swelling in the tendon sheath of the flexor muscles of the fingers. It

causes pain during flexion and extension movements;

2. **Adhesive Capsulitis (ICD-10 M75.1 frozen shoulder)**: a condition characterised by pain and marked limitation of joint movement in all planes. It has a multifactorial aetiology, sometimes post-traumatic or resulting from other shoulder pathologies.

This latter pathology or in general pathologies affecting the cervical spine and shoulder are also very common among patients presenting for mammographic screening, in an increasing percentage over the last 2 years.

For some time now pathologies such as *osteoarthritis or arthrosis* have no longer been considered a simple cause of ageing. The aetiology is much more complex, various other factors must be considered, including psycho-social ones. Stiffness of the neck-shoulders area, and a greater difficulty in collaborating with the radiographer were in fact noted in the last 2 years of work activity. Even if this is not supported, to date, by experimental data, it would anyway pose an interesting research question, considering, for

example, the impact of the Sars-CoV-2 pandemic, lockdown and psychological-emotional health.

See Table 23.2 for a summary of the risks and symptoms of the most common MSDs of the breast radiographer.

## 23.8.2   Risk Measurement

Risk can be measured according to the **ASSESSMENT OF REPETITIVE TASKS model (ART)** [35]. In this model, three grades are considered, by filling in a questionnaire. The low level is indicated with the colour green, the medium risk with yellow. In this case, the assessed task must be closely monitored. The high level is indicated with red and requires immediate corrective action. It is a system that aims to identify significant risks and reduce their level. Another model to mention, used by National Institute Insurance Against Accidents at work (INAIL), in Italy, is the **INDEX OCCUPATIONAL REPETITIVE ACTION (OCRA)** [36, 37]. In this model, an analysis is first made with the mapping of the work reality;

**Table 23.2**  MSDs, risk factors and symptoms

| MSD | Risk factors | Symptoms |
|---|---|---|
| De Quervain syndrome | Repeated movements in extension/flexion and rotation, as well as high muscle engagement grips | Pain at the base of the first finger, possible swelling in the same area; difficulty in movement of the first finger and wrist when a gripping action with the hand is involved |
| Carpal tunnel syndrome | Repeated movements with deviated wrist | Pain, tingling in fingers, even at night, numbness and weakness in grip |
| Cervicalgy | Incongruous posture maintained for a long time, repetitive movements of the neck and shoulders and generally of the upper limbs | Tension in the neck area, pain that sometimes radiates to the arm |
| Lateral epicondylitis (elbow) | Repeated wrist and forearm movements, in flexion-extension and rotation, as well as incorrect postures | Pain, possible swelling, numbness and tingling, which may also involve one or more fingers |
| Lumbalgia | Incorrect postures leading to muscle contractures | Pain, stiffness in the lumbar region |
| Tendinitis/ tenosynovitis | Repeated wrist and shoulder movements | Pain, swelling, more or less significant inability to use the joint, burning sensation |
| Rotator cuff pathology | Repeated movements of the upper limbs above shoulder height and above the head | Dull pain in the shoulder, disturbed sleep, arm weakness, difficulty moving the arm posteriorly |
| Knee bursitis | Repeated work requiring bending of the lower limbs on hard surfaces | Pain in place, swelling and sensitivity to simple touch, which feels warm to the touch (due to inflammation) |

then a secondary analysis is made on the workplaces that were found to be medium or high risk. The questionnaire concerns the ratio between the number of actions performed with the upper limbs in the total cycle. Any lack of recovery time is also taken into account, as well as various other factors, including the worker's posture.

The compilation of these models is referred to other specific texts on the subject. The biomechanical risk assessment followed in this text is a qualitative one: it was done thanks to a brain storming between the author, expert breast radiographer, and the expert physiotherapist Paola Bagnoli. Siria Giovannini, a recently graduated physiotherapist, author of a thesis on work-related musculoskeletal disorders, also participated.

## 23.9 Specific Ergonomic Tips for Positioning and Compression

**General Ergonomic Recommendations**

1. The room in which mammograms are performed must be the right size for the service to be rendered (*fit for purpose*). Also to be considered the workflow;
2. To reduce work-related MSDs, the *work triangle* must be reduced;
3. Operators need to be trained so that they become aware of and can apply safety strategies, and know how to correct their postural errors where necessary;
4. The activity, i.e. the technique of conducting the mammographic examination, for positioning and compression, must be taught by an accredited centre. The tutor or trainer must be also aware of the associated ergonomic strategies;
5. Observing the work of more experienced colleagues certainly helps;
6. The activity must vary, even introducing periodic micro-breaks;
7. The activity must also be adapted and customised to one's physical and psychophysical characteristics. Adaptation must be based on scientific evidence and recommendations by expert physiotherapists, workload being equal;
8. Training must include a conscious use not only of the mammography device(s) at hand, but also of the various devices. That is to say, the associated computers, and related programmes. This reduces stress and increases job satisfaction, with the positive effects highlighted in Chap. 24;
9. Signs that could indicate the onset of MSDs should by no means be underestimated, neither by the practitioner nor by the physician. The different subjective perceptions of pain/discomfort should also not be underestimated;
10. The practice of asking for help from an experienced colleague, whenever possible, should be sought. This is especially when performing examinations on difficult patients with significant motor disabilities. In the case of a patient in a wheelchair, it is recommended that the examination is always performed by two radiographers.

**Specific Ergonomic Recommendations for the Mammographic Exam**

1. Before the examination, make sure that the pedal control for compressing and moving the detector up and down are positioned correctly, so that the lower limbs do not have to be extended, and unbalance the weight between them;

2. Stand as close to the patient as possible, also so that you do not have to move your arms far from your body;

3. In the case of a very short patient and a tall radiographer, the MLO projection should be done with the radiographer seated. This is because the biomechanical risk for both the neck and the lumbar spine become unacceptable. The same recommendation comes from the English guidelines for mammographers, which talk about the *seated radiographer*, Fig. 23.4;

4. In the case that the radiographer is short, and the patient tall, it is convenient to have the patient sit for the CC projection. This is to avoid stress on the radiographer's shoulders and neck. The operator may even have to stand on her/his tiptoes [26];

5. Avoid abducting the first finger to hold the breast up in the MLO projection. It is better to use the joined finger hand at all times. It may be helpful to hold the breast up in position until the breast is completely blocked with compression using the knuckles;

6. It is important not to always use the same finger to press the exposure button. One may choose to press through the base of the hand, or otherwise keep the wrist in a neutral position to avoid MSDs. There is the possibility of equipping the mammographic unit with an acquisition pedal. In this case it would be useful to alternate;

7. A table of the movements required to perform the two standard projections, such as those listed in Tables 9.2 and 9.4 should be available for less experienced radiographers. It should also be correlated with a description from an ergonomic point of view, as proposed in this Chapter, both for understanding the risk and for reducing it.

## 23.10 Recommended Exercises to Minimise the Risk of Occurrence of MSDs in the Mammography Room

The onset of repetitive work disorder is gradual, with a cumulative effect. It is correlated to: (1) the frequency of action; (2) excessive use of force; (3) incorrect and stereotyped postures and movements; (4) the absence of breaks and micro-breaks for recovery. Exercises are proposed to be done regularly and during work breaks (in the absence of contraindications). They are proposed by Paola Bagnoli, physiotherapist, Upper Limb-Hand Surgical Rehabilitation referent, and Siria Giovannini (physiotherapist). They include *relaxation* and *activation*, which prepare the muscle for lengthening, and *stretching*, which reduces muscle tension and improves joint mobility. They should be performed slowly, without forcing. The perceived sensation should only be one of slight tension. Figure 23.5a–q show the exercises proposed.

**Fig. 23.5** (a) Relaxation activation and stretching exercises proposed for the breast radiographer. Siria Giovannini, in her physiotherapy thesis on WRMSDs, supervisor Paola Bagnoli, expert physiotherapist. (a) Neck Relaxation: while sitting with your torso straight, without the support of the backrest, place your index and middle fingers on your chin. Push your chin back, always looking forwards without bending your head down. Hold the position for a few seconds. Repeat ten times. (b–g) Relaxation activation and stretching exercises proposed for the breast radiographer, Siria Giovannini, in her thesis (supervisor Paola Bagnoli). (b) Activation: perform ten repetitions of the following movements: extension and flexion. (c) Activation: ten repetitions also of right and left rotation. (d) Activation: ten repetitions of left and right tilts. (e) Stretching: back straight, one hand grasps the edge of the chair. Bring the other hand to your temple and carefully pull your head in the direction of your shoulder. Hold for 20 s and repeat two times on each side. (f) Shoulder-Arms: Relaxation: assume this position while breathing deeply for a few minutes. Relax your shoulders and arms. (g) Arm-Shoulders Activation: back straight, alternately stretch one arm towards the ceiling and the other towards the floor. Repeat ten times on each side. (h–l) Proposed exercises for breast radiographers (Siria Giovannini, Paola Bagnoli). (h) Activation: arms outstretched with the palm of the hand facing forwards, stretch them downwards while slightly pulling the shoulders back. Hold the position 20 s and repeat two times. (i) Stretching: bring one arm towards the chest, outstretched and in line with the shoulder. Bring it as close to your chest as possible by pressing at elbow height with your opposite arm (with your wrist). Hold for 20 s and repeat two times. (j) Shoulders-Arm Stretching: bring your hands behind your head with your fingers intertwined: slowly drop your elbows towards the floor so that the weight of your arms can increase the flexion of your head. Hold the position for 20 s and repeat two times. (k) Stretching: keeping the torso straight, bring one arm behind and with the other hand grasp the wrist and stretch back. Hold for 20 s and repeat two times. (l) Arm-Wist-Hand: Activation: Hold the position shown in the photo with hands joined, without forcing. Rotate hands and wrists outwards and then inwards, returning to the starting position. Repeat the sequence ten times. (m–q) Exercises suggested to reduce the biomechanical risk for repeated limb activity, to minimise/prevent the occurrence of musculoskeletal disorders in breast radiographers (Paola Bagnoli, Siria Giovannini, Cristina Poggi). (m) Forearm and back of the hand resting on the table with fingers flexed into a fist, open the fingers one at a time and then close them one at a time, returning to the starting position. (n) Stretching: extend the arm with the palm outwards and the fingers towards the floor, grasp all four fingers with the other hand. Pull the fingers towards you without forcing them. Remain in this position for 20 s, and repeat two times on each side. (o) Open and stretch your fingers on the table and gently pull your first finger in the opposite direction to your index finger. Remain 15 s and repeat three times per hand. (p) Activation: from a sitting position, hands on knees, inhale by bringing the pelvis forward, arching the back, then exhale by performing the opposite movement (pelvis back, arching the back). Perform the sequence slowly and repeat five times. (q) Relaxation: standing upright, keeping your feet firmly on the floor and with your hands on your hips, bring your pelvis forward. Hold the position for a few seconds, then return to the starting position. Repeat five times

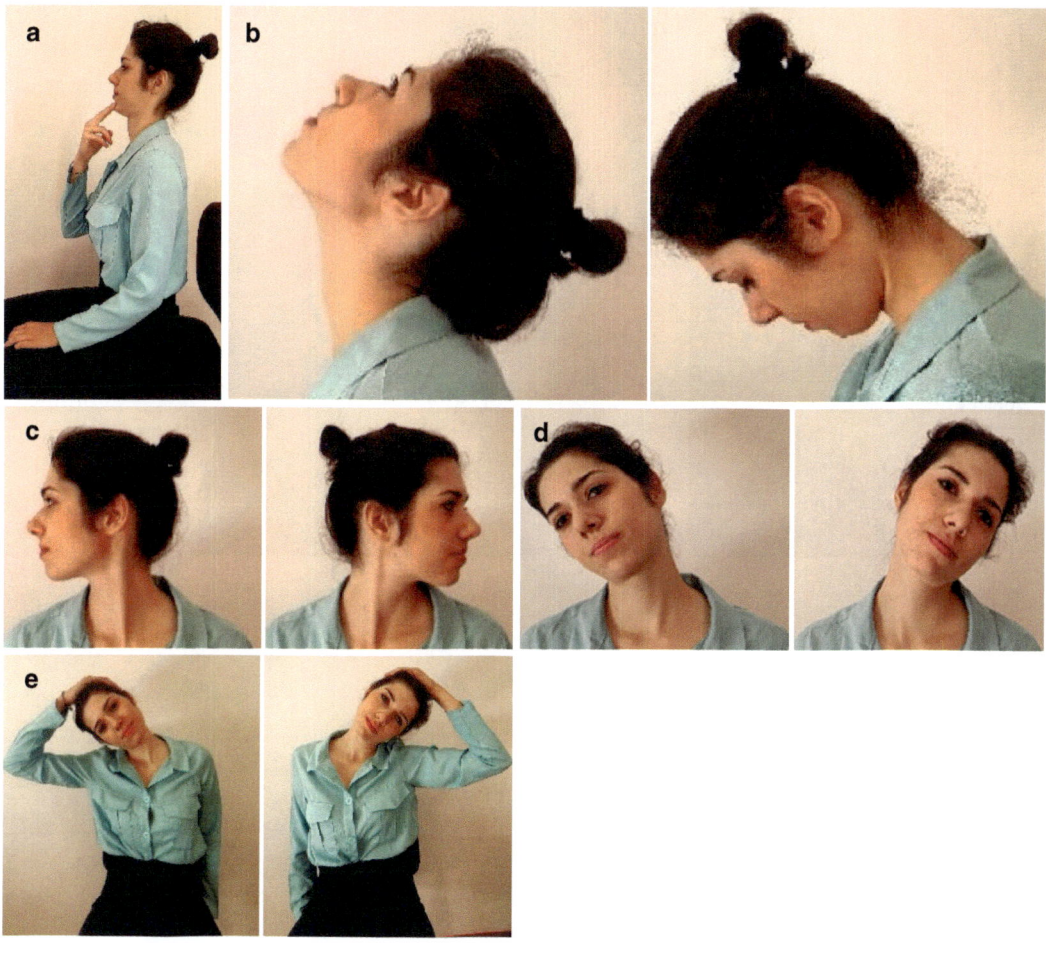

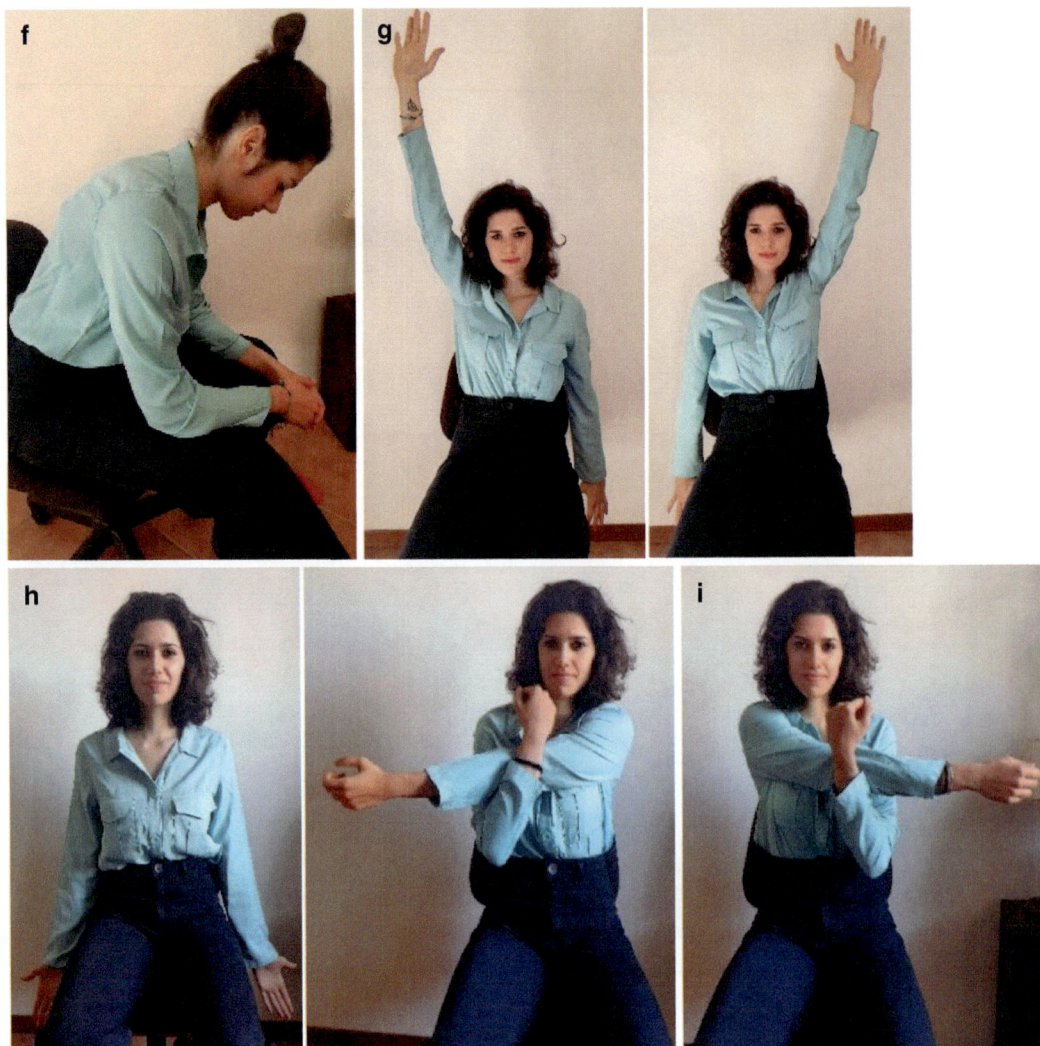

**Fig. 23.5** (continued)

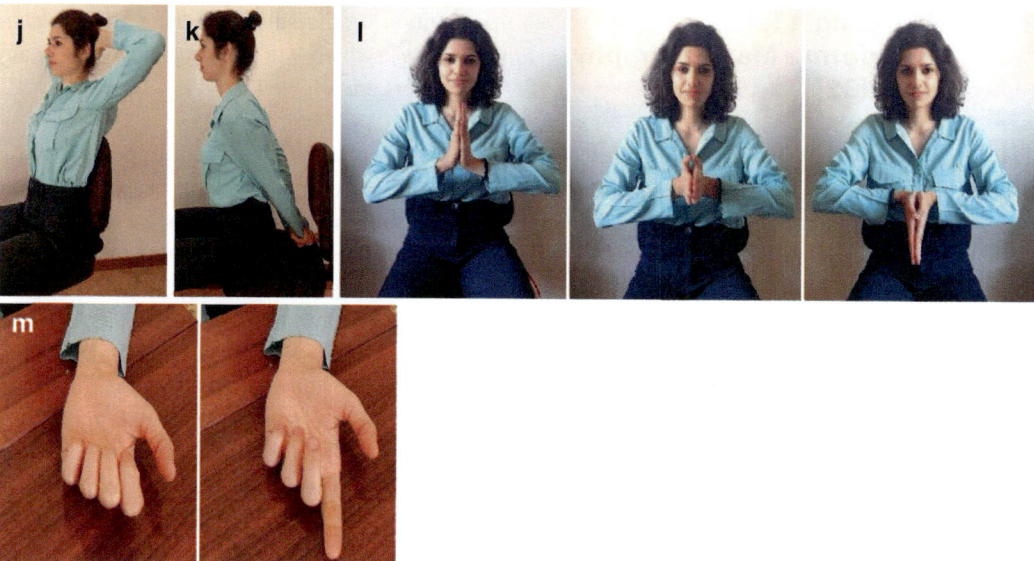

**Fig. 23.5** (continued)

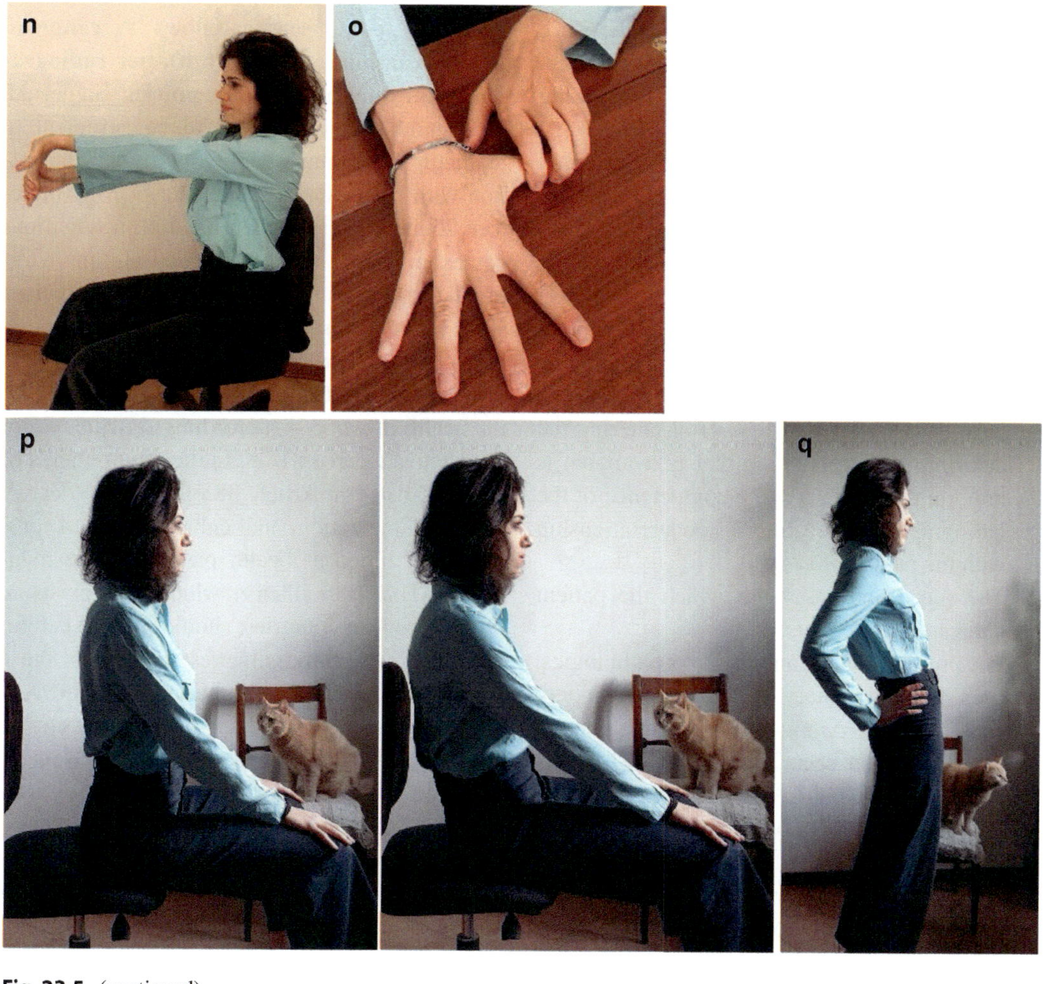

**Fig. 23.5** (continued)

## 23.11 How Long It Takes to Perform a Mammography Exam [32]

This is not an easy subject to deal with. However, it certainly affects the likelihood of developing work-related musculoskeletal disorders, since the risk of the movement leading to a problem depends heavily on the number of repetitions of the movement. Doing a mammogram takes a time that is difficult to define depending on multiple factors. Among them:

1. Surely the most accidental is the competence and experience of the breast radiographer (and her/his personal attitude towards the job);
2. The available mammography machine counts a lot, for usability and response efficiency;
3. Also important is the room in which the examination is performed, in terms of size and comfort. Important in general is all the work environment, including the waiting room. This is because it can affect working ergonomics;
4. The type of mammography to be performed counts, whether screening, follow-up or symptomatic (see Chap. 6);
5. The cooperation or compliance of the patient is crucial;
6. The time to collect the data and to explain how the programme works, in the screening or clinic realm, especially if it is the first time, must be considered. The ease of entering the data into the programme that is available is important; and so, it is the competence of the radiographer in creating a good relationship with the patient;
7. The speed and ease with which the patient undresses also counts;
8. The presence of: (**a**) any patient's pathologies, even if only transitory; (**b**) her state of anxiety and ability to *cope* with it, are to be considered. The latter seem to be worsened in this post-pandemic phase, precisely for the level of tolerance to pain or simple discomfort. It could be also due to the need to wear facial masks, having to assume more uncomfortable positions to avoid related artefacts. To be

mention on the subject is the *post-pandemic fatigue*, which—in varying degrees—many workers are affected by.

**An average time of 10–12 min per patient is suggested.** Taking into account: (a) possible exceptions to the average giving an examination to patients with special needs; (b) the time needed at the beginning of the session for warming up the mammographic unit; (c) the quality checks; (d) breaks and micro-breaks for the operators; (e) the change-of-shift-report; (f) data collection, etc. **For a 6-h shift**, in a centre with good ergonomics of the workplace, and experienced radiographers, a programme comprising a total of **25 examinations/shift/radiographer** is thus composed.

A range must be considered **in screening**, given the fluctuation often present between one day and the next, but generally related to the weekend, and to seasonal flows. A **range of 20–30 examinations/shift (6 h), per radiographer, per mammographic unit** is suggested. This number is considered to be sufficient to maintain good image quality, and good interaction with individual patients. Considering therefore 25 examinations per shift, four acquisitions per examination, without considering any additional projections, **the repeated movements in a shift will amount to 100**. This certainly has an impact that should not be overlooked. In Italy the "**competent doctor**" is in charge of monitoring the health of workers, according to Article 25 of Legislative Decree 81/08. In the requirements of the role, listed in Article 38 of the same decree, the implementation and enhancement of programmes aimed at health promotion are mentioned. This surveillance, which also exists in other European countries, should include careful investigations and possible rest periods for those workers who report the symptoms listed above, at an early stage. That is, in the fully reversible phase.

In this sense, *it is the worker her-himself who can request a medical examination by the competent operator, in the presence of WRMSDs, so that a possible judgement of temporary unsuitability for the job can be made.*

# References

1. Mozzi V. Ergolean: quando ergonomia e Lean Manufacturing integrano il management e la sicurezza aziendale, Tesi in tecniche della prevenzione nell'Ambiente e nei Luoghi di Lavoro. Università Politecnica delle Marche. anno accademico 2017–2018. Last access January 2020.
2. Pozzi B. Mente e corpo: sinergia perfetta per una migliore prestazione sportiva, Tesi, corso di laurea in Scienze e Tecniche psicologiche. Università di Padova. anno accademico 2021–2022. https://thesis.unipd.it/handle/20.500.12608/30236.
3. Human factors and ergonomics. Common risks from human factors. NHE. https://www.hse.gov.uk/human-factors/top-ten.htm.
4. Koirala R, Maharjan K. Cognitive ergonomics on employee wellbeing: a literature review. J Econ Concerns. 2023;13(1):93–106. issn online: 2705–4802. Published by NECS, Nepal, downloaded from researchgate.net/publication/370654307.
5. Vallone MR. Human centered design: sviluppo di un metodo per la valutazione oggettivo del confort posturale degli arti inferiori, Tesi di dottorato. Università degli Studi di Salerno' 2014–2017. https://elea.unisa.it/handle/10556/2587.
6. UNI EN ISO 6385. https://www.certifico.com/normazione/214-documenti-riservati-normazione/organismi-normazione/documenti-iec/3103-iso-6385-2016-principi-ergonomici-nella-progettazione-dei-sistemi-di-lavoro (version in English available).
7. Centro Italiano di Ergonomia. https://www.centro-ergonomia.it/norme-ergonomia.html.
8. Todaro N. Il carico di lavoro mentale INAIL; 2022. https://www.inail.it/cs/internet/docs/alg-il-carico-di-lavoro-mentale.pdf?section=attivita.
9. Breast screening mammography: ergonomics good practice. NHS; 2018. https://www.gov.uk/government/publications/breast-screening-ergonomics-in-screening-mammography/.
10. Considerations-when-designing-a-mammography-suite, posted by Guest Contributor on Jul 9, 2019. Last access Dec 2022.
11. Gale AG, et al. Ergonomic assessment of mammography units. NHSBSP equipment report 0708. 2007.
12. Hayward C. Sizing imaging and procedure rooms. https://blog.spacemed.com/.
13. Langland B, Burlingame B. The 2018 FGI guidelines PPT, health care design HCD expo + conference 2017, Session E-94 Orlando. https://www.fgiguidelines.org/wp-content/uploads/2017/11/E94_HCD2017_A_New_Class_Act.pdf.
14. Ciconi A. Illuminazione delle workstation di refertazione radio-diagnostica, Applicazione di un sistema di illuminazione innovativo, Tesi di laurea magistrale in Ingegneria Edile. anno accademico 2012–2013. Università di Pisa. https://core.ac.uk/download/pdf/19203764.pdf.
15. Picture archiving and communication systems (PACS) and guidelines on diagnostic devices 2nd edition 2012 Board the the Faculty of Clinical Radiology. The Royal College of Radiologists.
16. Picture archiving and communication systems (PACS) and guidelines on diagnostic devices, 3rd ed. 2019 Board the Faculty of Clinical Radiology. The Royal College of Radiologists.
17. Report AIFM. Sistemi per la visualizzazione delle immagini mediche, Porcello per i controlli di qualità N.9. *AIFM*. 2013. ultimo accesso 27 Nov 2022.
18. Compliance requirements for ionizing radiation apparatus uses in diagnostic imaging, part 1-mammography. EPA; 2020.
19. Compton K, Oosterwijk H. Requirements for medical imaging monitors (part 1). https://otechimg.com/publications/pdf/wp_medical_image_monitors.pdf.
20. Strudley CJ, et al. Mammography cancer detection: comparison of single 8MP and pair of 5MP reporting monitors. Br J Radiol. 2018;91:20170246. https://doi.org/10.1259/bjr.20170246.
21. Taylor-Phillips S, et al. Mammography workstation design: effect on mammographer behavior and the risk of musculoskeletal disorders. In: Sahiner B, Manning DJ, editors. Medical imaging 2008: image perception, observer performance, and technology assessment. Proceeding of SPIE 6917, 69171G.
22. Musculoskeletal disorder in mammography a guide to tackling the issues in the workplace, 1st ed. SOR. isbn:978-1-906225-07-0. https://www.sor.org/getmedia/060920d7-5099-4bb4-84b6-0a65d5d6241b/sor_msd_mammography_guide.pdf_1.
23. Vibberts M. The strain of being a mammography technologist. The voice of Beekley medical; 2019. https://blog.beekley.com/the-strain-of-being-a-mammography-technologist. Last access Oct 2023.
24. Sommerich CM, et al. Collaborating with mammographers to address their work-related musculoskeletal discomfort. Ergonomics. 2016;59(10):1307–17. https://doi.org/10.1080/00140139.2016.1140815.
25. Costa S, et al. Mammography equipment design: impact on radiographers' practise. Insight Imaging. 2014;5:723–30. https://doi.org/10.1007/s13244-014-0360-2.
26. Cernean N, et al. Ergonomics strategies to improve radiographers' posture during mammography activity. Insight Imaging. 2017;8:429–38. https://doi.org/10.1007/s13244-017-0560-7.
27. ISO 11228-3:2007. https://www.iso.org/standard/26522.html.
28. Marcora S. Psychobiology of fatigue during endurance exercise. In: Meijen, editor. Endurance performance in sport. Routledge. pp. 15–34. https://www.researchgate.net/publication/332783788.
29. Kaseminasab S, et al. Neck pain: global epidemiology, trend and risk factors. BMC Musculoskeletal Disord. 2022;23(1):26. PMC article. https://doi.org/10.1186/s12891-021-04957-4.

30. JGIO68, G, L'analisi e la valutazione delle posture incongrue e della stereotipia. https://www.slideshare.net/Jgio68/allegato-3-posture.

31. Rinella D. Body mechanics for mammography technologists. https://docplayer.net/14427220-Body-mechanics-for-mammography-technologists.html.

32. Gale AG, et al. Ergonomic assessment of mammography units. HHSBSP equipment report 0708. 2007. https://assets.publishing.service.gov.uk/government/uploads/system/uploads/attachment_data/file/442792/nhsbsp-equipment-report-0708.pdf.

33. Gashette R, Lauwers T. Grip & pinch strength in relation to anthropometric data in adults. HSOA J Orthop Res Physiother. issn:2381-2052. https://doi.org/10.24966/ORP-2052/100039.

34. IDC-10 Version: 2019. https://icd.who.int/browse10/2019/en.

35. Assessment of repetitive tasks of the upper limb (the ART tool). Health and Safety Executive HSE INDG438 published 03/10. https://www.hse.gov.uk/pubns/indg438.pdf.

36. Godderis, L., et al., European Agency for Safety and Health at work, alert and sentinel approaches for the identification of work-related diseases in the EU-Publication Office. 2019. https://data.europa.eu/doi/10.2802/869066.

37. ALLEGATO 1-b INAIL, lo strumento per la mappatura del rischio da sovraccarico biomeccanico degli arti superiori: la checklist OCRA. https://www.inail.it/cs/internet/docs/allegato-1-b-linee-guida-lombardia-pdf.pdf?section=attivita.

# The Evolution of the Radiographer's Educational Path: EBP and Communication Skills in the Mammography Room

## 24.1 Introduction

The evolution of radiological science and practice has been very fast in recent years. This has required an adaptation of the radiographer's education path, which unfortunately remains profoundly different among the states of the European Union. It must be said that, for many years, there have been attempts at cooperation aimed at harmonising education. The *International Society of Radiographers and Radiological Technologists (ISRRT)* has published documents describing the role, skills and responsibilities of the radiographer since 1995. It should be emphasised that the university system in Europe was made homogeneous thanks to the **Bologna process** [1] in 1999. It was promoted by the main European states, for the free movement of students, which set out to achieve the *European Higher Education Area* [2] by 2010. The goal was moved to 2025 at the Gothenburg summit. The nations that joined the Bologna process ratified the *Lisbon Convention on the Recognition of Higher Education*, elaborated by the European Council and UNESCO. However, there are still unresolved problems.

## 24.2 Radiographer's Education in Europe, UK and United States

In almost all European countries to practise as a *radiographer* is required a 3-year university degree, or a Bachelor's degree, equivalent to level 6 *European Qualification Framework (EQF)* [3]. There are some distinctions. In Germany, the radiographer practises after obtaining a 3-year technical diploma, which can be obtained after secondary school. It is the same in Spain, where it lasts 2 years. In Estonia, a level 7 EQF (master's degree) is required to work in ultrasound and radiotherapy [4, 5]. In the United Kingdom, the degree is 3–4 years although there is *apprenticeship*, i.e., a way in which it is possible to practise the profession before graduation under supervision [6].

In no European country is there a specific training path to work as a *certified breast radiographer*, which is present in the UK [7]. It lasts 2 years, after graduating to work as a radiographer, and it also allows them to obtain skills to report. This expansion of the role of the radiographer, or rather, *mammographer* in this case,

© The Author(s), under exclusive license to Springer Nature Switzerland AG 2024
C. Poggi, *Breast Imaging Techniques for Radiographers*,
https://doi.org/10.1007/978-3-031-63314-0_24

should not be surprising: *by its very nature, the radiographer is an image evaluator as well as an image producer* [8]. Our profession is educated to identify what is physiological in an image and then to recognise what is not (which deviates from it); to understand which image is useful for diagnosis and which is not. Traditionally, the report is the responsibility of the radiologist; in some countries, the chronic shortage of radiologists has led to the inclusion of interpretation and reporting among the tasks of radiographers. This trend is also indicated in the recent **European Federation of Radiographer Societies (EFRS)** *White Paper* [9] on the future of our profession. However, in the UK, where this expansion of the role has been in place for many years, some ideological barriers have been identified on the part of the radiologists.

In the United States, there is a Bachelor's degree, lasting 4 years; it is although not required to practise as a *Radiologic Technologist*. About half of all RTs choose the 2-year *Associate of Applied Science* program. On the other hand, there is a very precise training path to become a *mammographer RT(M):* first of all, 40 h of training and 25 mammography examinations must be performed under supervision, according to the *Mammography Quality Standard Act (MQSA)* criteria. A further 8 h must be spent in other image modalities that still concern the breast, followed by another 75 mammographies. It is then necessary to do at least 175 every 2 years (in addition to the 25 MQSAs). This pathway allows for certification as a specialist [10–12]. There is an examination that accredits and certifies the skills acquired, to be repeated, by the *American Registry of Radiologic Technologists*. The Registered Technologist Mammographer is indicated with the acronym RT(M). Interesting is the cycle of monitoring and validation of competences, according to MQSA and American College of Radiology (ACR) rules, which foresees various types of inspection, also random, on the quality of the image produced. It was recently updated in 2023 [13].

In all countries, the **recommendation for continuing education is strong,** *Continuing Professional Development (CPD)*, in terms of number and type of credits.

## 24.3   The Legal Evolution of Radiographer Educational Path in Italy

The radiographer educational path has been a long one and is still evolving. A brief section is summarised below, starting with the reform of the university system Law No. 341 of 1990. Thanks to this law, the degree courses were created, replacing the special purpose schools for technical health professions established in 1982. In implementation of Law 341/90 is another important legislative decree, No. 502 of 1992. In this, the discipline of healthcare is profoundly renewed, with the fundamental shift from the logic of the job description to that of the professional profile, pursuant to Article 6, paragraph 3. There is a novelty in that the job market, that is to say the *National Healthcare Service (SSN),* is entrusted with the role of identifying the needed professional figures and the university system the task of training them. The regulations concerning the identification of the figure and relative professional profile of the *TSRM (or TRMIR, radiographer)* date back to Ministerial Decree *DM 746 of 1994*. It focuses on the responsibility for acts within its competence, and above all, *the radiographer is identified as the only figure (together with the radiologist) capable of understanding what damage can be caused to a patient in the event of incorrect iconography.* In Law No. 42 of 1999, the designation of *auxiliary health profession* disappears. That is, we move to a regulated profession, linked to the professional profile, in which the type of service is defined; the operator is then given broad autonomy and responsibility. With Ministerial Decree 509 of 1999, the teaching autonomy of universities was reorganised; the so-called training tree was introduced, 3 years for the bachelor's degree and 2 years for the specialist degree. *Formative credits* were defined. Law No. 251 of 2000 reforms the profiles of the nursing, technical, rehabilitation and prevention health professions, as well as the midwifery profession, all of them with reference to the *Code of Ethics* (drawn up for radiographers in 2004). Management positions are only open to those who hold a *specialist degree*, which with Ministerial Decree No. 270 of 2004 is called *master's degree.*

The **Crediti Formativi Universitari (CFU)** are defined, which correspond to 25 h of student commitment. They are intended both for personal study and for laboratory, internship and frontal teaching activities. 1 CFU corresponds to 1 European Credit Transfer and Accumulation System.

**Bachelor's degree**: provides general theoretical–methodological preparation and theoretical–operational professional skills: 180 CFU.

**Master's degree:** after the bachelor degree, provides advanced training to perform highly qualified professional activities: 120 CFU, for skills of the following types: management, training and research.

With Law No. 43 of 2006 *Provisions on health professions [...] and delegation to the government for the establishment of the relevant professional orders*, the *colleges* are transformed into *Orders* (for radiographers in 2018). In Article 6, the coordination function is established. The figure of *specialist is* also indicated, as she/he who holds a professional specialisation master course. With Law 3/2018, the prerequisites of 43/2006 are realised, at least in part. The figure of the specialist is not yet delineated, pending the definition of the educational plan at the national level.

There are a total of 30 health professions in Italy (at the time of publication); radiographers are part of the technical health professions in class 3A. Professional activities, the exercise of which is only permitted by law following registration with an order, are regulated, intellectually ordered professions. Orders have as their main function to guarantee the competence and professionalism of their members to the citizen. That is why they each form and publish their own register, reviewed periodically, repressing abuses and providing opinions on professional disputes.

The deontological obligation of continuous training is also affirmed, as is the implementation of new knowledge. The administrative management of the **Continuing Medical Education** program lies with the **National Agency for Regional Health Services** [14].

## 24.4  Online and Communication Training

Another extremely interesting aspect, which cannot be addressed by editorial choice in this text, is **online training**. Having become a compulsory necessity in the pandemic era, it has strongly impacted the education of all health professionals, including radiographers, who were unable to carry out training as well as attend classes, in person. *Online resources have therefore become indispensable*. Proof of this is the project started in the United Kingdom, by Hogg, P. and Holmes, K. [15], and was made available worldwide on chest X-ray examination. It was about performing and reporting SARS-CoV-2-induced disease. The *EURAMED* project [16], see Chap. 21, also highlighted the need to produce online courses, in this case radiation protection. The possibility of providing teaching by a European group of experts, complementing that of individual nations, could solve the perennial lack of qualified trainers. However, attention must be drawn to the fact that not only learners but also teachers had to adapt to the new reality. From what can be deduced from the literature, it was essential to: (1) have expert professionals available for the creation or implementation of platforms suitable for the purpose and (2) enlist those who could create high-quality content and provide the possibility of interaction and real, comfortable use of content by students. That is to say, a high platform usability. Especially, *asynchronous lessons* were welcome for the possibility of repeatability.

In Italy, the Ministerial Decree of February 2009 defines the descriptors of the learning objectives at first and second levels:

1. Knowledge and understanding
2. Applying knowledge and understanding
3. Communication skills
4. Learning skills

*Among the knowledge, skills and competences required to practise our profession, there are also those on communication.* We are talking not only about communication between health professionals and patients, but also between professionals themselves. In an increasingly complex and multidisciplinary system, this become essential, even more so in the pandemic and post-pandemic phase.

Health professionals are required, with regard to communication skills, to be *able to effectively balance listening and observing what the patient is communicating and to dialogue effectively with patients, colleagues and co-workers*, cit. Ministry of Health, 2015 [17]. This type of competence, surprisingly, is not yet adequately implemented (in the author's opinion) in the course of study of a large part of the healthcare professions, in Italy. It is a problem that already existed in the pre-pandemic phase.

## 24.5 Radiographer Knowledge, Skills and Competence

The achievement of the radiographer qualifying degree should confer the acquisition of: (1) professional or disciplinary, *knowledge*; (2) *competence*, understood as the ability to use knowledge, personal, social and/or methodological skills in professional development, responsibility and autonomy; (3) *skill*, ability to apply knowledge in a cognitive and practical sense (use of logical thinking and the manual dexterity to use methods, materials and equipment), cit. EQF radiographers, 2018 [18].

Performing a technical-sanitary act requires a significant practical preparation, also to solve more or less complex and unpredictable problems that may arise in everyday activity. The type of teaching offered in Italian universities shows some deficiencies in that regard, in the face of a good or even excellent theoretical preparation.

## 24.6 Evidence-Based Practice (EBP)

It is defined as **Evidence-Based Medicine**, later to become **Evidence-Based Practice (EBP)** due to its extension to all healthcare professions, a cultural movement that has spread internationally. It is driven by various phenomena, which have determined a progressive crisis of the historical models, such as: (1) the increasingly important complexity in health matters and therefore the difficulty of keeping up to date; (2) the limited transfer of scientific results into daily work practice, with the result of having a wide professional variability; (3) the greater degree of user awareness and (4) the explosion of the Internet for health information. *EBP is a "didactic mission," which involves identifying one's own knowledge gaps, searching for the best available evidence, critically evaluating it and integrating it into the decisions made in one's work activity* (cit. GIMBE, an independent foundation founded in Italy for research, training and scientific information [19]). It means evaluating over time how effective and efficient the first steps were, so as to constantly improve. The author, with her educational offer, aims to base the improvement of the performance of the breast radiographer precisely on this.

## 24.7 Radiographer's Communication Skills

The **communicative competence** is one of those required of the radiographer and is mentioned in the EFRS documents for EQF level 6 (Sect. 24.2). A very summarised table on basic knowledge, skills and competences on communication, according to EQF, is presented in Table 24.1.

**Table 24.1** Basic knowledge, skills and competence in communication, EFRS

| Basic knowledge | Basic skills | Basic competence |
|---|---|---|
| Theory and practice on communication | Identification and understanding of how to communicate effectively | Communicate verbally (and in written form) and interact in a multidisciplinary, multicultural and/or international environment |
| Verbal and non-verbal communication strategies | Use appropriate professional terminology | Communicating with other professional groups |
| Communication and respect for patients, health personnel, other professionals in the team | With the various figures outside the health personnel | Instructing, teaching and/or guiding staff and students to develop their skills |
| | Communicating effectively with patients and other health professionals regarding radiation protection, procedures… | |

Adapted from European Qualifications Framework (EQF) reference document: radiographers, 2018 [18]

## 24.8 Importance of Communication Skills for Mammographers

The role of the radiographer dedicated to Senology, or *mammographer*, is not yet well defined in Italy. It could be said that she/he is responsible for the production of mammograms that are of high clinical quality, easy to read for the radiologist, for extension and stretching out of the acquired tissue and satisfaction of the acquisition geometry parameters. See Chaps. 9–12, 25–27 and Annex 1. In Italy, there are no degree courses in Senology as in UK, or certifications qualifying the breast radiographer for practical and theoretical competence that are recognised on a national basis, as is the case of USA, for example (see Sect. 24.2).

Communication skills are particularly important for this specialised branch of radiology for many reasons:

1. Breast cancer is a high incidence cancer disease and therefore has a high social impact.
2. It is incredibly complex at a biological level and therefore requires major scientific studies.
3. If not detected at an early stage, it could have an unfavourable prognosis. Although mammography is the best method to increase the chances of survival, it is not always sufficient.

4. It is difficult to treat, especially some subtypes (Chap. 5).
5. It has an incredible impact on a psychological level, because it compromises aspects of identity in the role of a woman and in the couple's relationship.
6. It requires a synergic and multidisciplinary intervention for the rehabilitation pathway, especially in cases of non-conservative treatments.

Although the absolute majority of patients who respond to the invitation within the screening program are healthy, the disease is well known. The burden of anxiety is often felt by the patient. *In fact, patient anxiety is internationally regarded as one of the main harms of mammographic screening* [20]. The relationship established between the breast radiographer and the patient plays a fundamental role in how the overall experience will be perceived. Many studies can be cited in the literature that point out how much this relationship influences adherence to the program itself [21–24].

## 24.9 Definition of Communication: Strategic Communication

There are many definitions of communication. *Communication* can be said to be a *complex relationship between people, through which one creates a connection with another, making them to participate in a content* [25–36]. The Greek–Latin etymology of the word is interesting; it speaks of sharing. The more modern meaning is passage, transfer and transmission. Transmission, however, is typical of hierarchical structures; it presupposes that there is no influence between the interlocutors.

Communication is information; one of the purposes is that the recipient of the message gets extra knowledge. Providing information to patients is indeed relevant and one of the most important tasks for all health professionals. However, *communication is not only informing.* Underlying the *transactional communication* model is the sharing of part of one's own representation of reality, made up of personal ways of thinking, experiences and interests, which each person creates over time. There is the need to find points of contact, considering that there is always *noise* in the transfer of the message, and it may sometimes take on meanings very different from those intended by the sender.

The elements that come into play in communication are listed in Table 24.2.

Communication is a dynamic process, made up of exchanges, in which interlocutors are both senders and receivers. Communication contains a **content aspect**, the message, the data, the information and a **relationship aspect**, which defines the interconnection between the interlocutors, i.e., how the data itself are transmitted. Thus also how it is to be interpreted. It is also called *meta-communication*. It is necessary to try to get the message across correctly and for it to be understandable. That is, the **channel**, which is the means of expression, and the **code**, which is the type of language, must be carefully chosen. Both must be accepted and known by the interlocutors.

*There are three channels: the verbal, the non-verbal and the paraverbal or paralinguistic. That is: what is said (the content, the data and the message); how it is said (using the body) and how the message is delivered (using the voice).*

Non-verbal communication can complement, reinforce or regulate verbal communication, but

**Table 24.2** Elements that come into play in communication

| Sender/transmitter | The party initiating communication, producing a message, encodes it and transmits it |
|---|---|
| Receiver/recipient | The subject receiving the message, receives it, decodes it, understands it and interprets it |
| Message | What is communicated and how it is done; it must be translated into signs and senses, using a code |
| Channel | Communication route, means by which the message is channelled: the most commonly used is sound waves that carry the sound of the voice through the air means of expression |
| Code | Set of conventional, socially recognised rules by which the message is produced and interpreted; interlocutors must use the same code to produce and interpret the message |
| Feedback | • The sender receives verbal and non-verbal signals from the receiver <br> • The sender perceives the message she/he is producing <br> • Checking and adjusting the issued message |
| Noise | Communication disorder |
| Ridondance | Repetition of the same information in different ways |

it can also contradict it. People generally tend to trust non-verbal communication more, also because it is more difficult to simulate. They certainly trust non-verbal communication more, especially when they notice that there is no convergence, i.e., there is a high degree of contradiction between the two channels. Healthcare personnel do not receive formal training in communicating with patients in Italy, and this is particularly surprising, even for radiographers, who are believed to have a less deep, and certainly more episodic, relationship with the patient than nurses, for example. Instead, effective communication, or more precisely, *strategic communication, which defines a specific set of interaction modes and tactics aimed at producing desired changes in human behaviour, plays a major role in healthcare.* The objectives to be achieved are those in the interest of the patient, accompanying them toward the desired outcome. This must be done maintaining high levels of motivation and trust between patient and health operator. There must be mutual acceptance, ensuring the highest levels of patient **compliance** (collaboration) in the technical healthcare act, knowing how to manage in the best possible way any unforeseen events and all this always guaranteeing the *appropriateness of the performance*. It is necessary for the practitioner to have the ability to pick up even weak signals from the patient that may indicate negative, but also positive, changes in the relationship. Therefore, it is of paramount importance carefully observing the patient's non-verbal language and checking one's own. This, in fact, increases the ability to obtain the desired outcome. It is a very effective form of "listening," which is especially important for the breast radiographer.

*Patients are obviously different from one another, and therefore there is no universal technique, just as there is no vocabulary of non-verbal behaviour that provides unambiguous meanings.*

## 24.10 The Assumptions and Principles of Strategic Communication

The first assumption for effective communication is the attribution of dignity and legitimacy to one's opinions, emotions and individuality. The operator who is professionally self-confident communicates better than those who are not. This is why the first measure to be taken, strongly advocated in this text, is the implementation of professional development programs: more knowledge and the acquisition of specific skills and abilities increase one's perception of one's own work status and improve job satisfaction. This makes one more confident.

Another assumption is that there is a substantial equality of the communicating parties, so that they can "meet." Therefore, it is indispensable to recognise the identity and dignity of the person, the patient, with whom we talk and legitimise her or his opinions and emotions. This does not necessarily mean always being in agreement or flattening one's responsibilities. The patient–healthcare worker relationship is one in which the

professional is seen to be in a dominant position, and it is the patient herself who gives us cognitive authority by virtue of our specific expertise. It should be noted that this aspect has diminished over the years to the point of being rejected outright in some cases, as we bitterly witnessed when the SARS-CoV-2 pandemic broke out. It can certainly be said that this authority must be increasingly demonstrated and deserved.

*Principle of flexibility*: it indicates the adaptation of the communication strategy to person and context. It requires overcoming the stereotypes that make the health worker perceives the patient as less informed, of a lower socio-cultural level. "It is useless to explain because he/she would not understand." It is not possible to completely overcome prejudices and stereotypes, but being aware of them can help diminish them.

*Principle of parsimony*: messages, as already mentioned, should be as simple and concise as possible and adapted to the patient's language according to the principle of flexibility.

*Utilisation principle*: this refers to the use of the language, attitude and arguments of the recipient of the message, for persuasive purposes. It means accepting the messages sent to us by the patient, without challenging them. *Any confrontation is a danger to effective communication.*

*Principle of restructuring*: *it means guiding a person to change her/his point of view on aspects of her/his experience that are negatively, critically or painfully experienced.* Although this principle seems more pertinent to the doctor–patient relationship, it is actually also present between patient and breast radiographer. It is precisely about overcoming the feeling of pain from compression, or lack of respect for one's own perceptions, experienced in the mammographic room by the patient.

To be able to follow these principles presupposes: (1) a knowledge of the interlocutor, to be able to identify her or his communicative style, which is actually not feasible in a fleeting encounter and (2) to recognise the conscious and unconscious signals that are sent and received. This is feasible, but it certainly requires constant attention to listening on the part of the operator.

*The strategic communicator is, first and foremost, in fact, an attentive listener and observer* cited, Secci and Duo [31].

It is therefore essential to have a basic knowledge and to be able to make conscious use of the three channels.

## 24.11 The Channels

The **verbal channel**, which involves verbal or written language, is the most common mode of communication. It can be very precise and has a much higher complexity than non-verbal communication. It simplifies, analyses and organises reality (which is enormously complex). It is made up of words, it is constantly renewed, and it is controllable. In order to be able to use effective verbal communication in healthcare, the professional must be comprehensive, relevant and *perspicuous*, i.e., simple, clear and concise. Much attention must therefore be paid to specialised language, consisting of technicalities, which are expressions that do not exist in everyday language and are therefore not replaceable, at least not by a single word. Healthcare language also has many words in Latin and, especially in recent years, many in English. It can therefore be an obstacle to communication in non-English speaking countries. This is why it is *important to constantly check that the patient has understood, without ever taking anything for granted*. *Redundancy*, i.e., the repetition of the same information using different words, is also very useful. This is especially true for patients who do not know the language of the country that they are in, but not only. The *language barrier* is indeed one of the obstacles encountered in mammographic screening programs, especially in large cities (high immigration).

Knowing how to provide comprehensive and adequate information is important. In addition, it must be done in an appropriate, confident and professional manner. We play a fundamental role in regard to patients, about which very little is said, as far as radiographers are concerned. That is the *educational role, the* so-called **empowering.** It is defined by the World Health Organization

as that process through which patients are enabled to exercise greater control over their own health, thanks to the information they receive, so that they can participate more actively and consciously in their own care process.

The **non-verbal channel or non-verbal language is body language** [30].

It includes:

1. Facial expressions and gaze
2. Movements and posture
3. The position occupied in space and interpersonal distance
4. Body contact

It is not easy to control, and for this reason, it can allow meanings to filter through. It is simple, immediate and concise.

*What is perceived of a speech is greatly influenced by the non-verbal behaviour of the speaker.*

### 24.11.1 The Proxemics

It is part of non-verbal language and studies personal space, and the way we use and pass through it. It derives from the term proximity. It was introduced by the American anthropologist Hall in the 1960s and investigates the social significance of the distance that man interposes between himself and his neighbour. It takes on different meanings depending on the temperament of the person, her/his culture of origin and gender.

The space we have to consider is the diagnostic room where the mammograms are performed. It must be well known, so as to move around in it ergonomically and with confidence (see also Chap. 23). This gives the patient an idea of efficiency and therefore of the reliability of the operator and has a considerable relaxing impact. In addition, in order to be able to perform the examination, it is necessary to invade the so-called **intimate zone** of the patient (range from touching, up to 40 cm). It may not be particularly appreciated by patients, especially in certain cultures, such as the Northern European.

### 24.11.2   The Haptics

Even more important for breast radiographers is haptics, which concerns body contact. Mammography requires touching the patient in so-called *vulnerable areas*, usually only accessible to intimate people. The skin represents the largest organ that we have and the clearest boundary between us and the world.

However, that there can be difficulties even before touching the patient, especially if she: (a) is severely under or overweight; (b) does not live her body well and (c) has a dermatological disease or deformity. Even just asking her to undress, i.e., to deprive herself of the protection of her clothes, can be seen as a problem. One must act with extreme caution, strengthening one's position as a healthcare professional.

### 24.11.3   The Kinesics

Kinesics refers to the way human beings move their bodies in response to communication. *Gestures* are abbreviations of communication and encompass the communication of a wide range of mental states or ideas. Italians are very expressive in this sense, and this is known worldwide. There are in fact important cultural differences. For example, the Japanese, and to a lesser extent the British, place great value on not showing one's emotions; it what is called self-control. In some Neo-Latin cultures, as Mexican and Puerto Rican, averting one as Mexican and Puerto Rican, averting o-Latin culturmunication of a wide rang

Posture is then of particular interest to breast radiographers. Or rather, the **change in posture** is important, i.e., *the dynamism of the action is more significant than the action itself.* It must be taken into account in order to eventually modify our behaviour (see Sect. 24.19).

The **paraverbal channel** indicates that the way the voice is used to convey the message. It therefore concerns vocal aspects, such as *timbre*, *volume* and *rhythm of* the voice. Its judicious use can modify, emphasise or diminish the importance of words, and thus the relationship that is being established with the patient. For example, *tone* is a clear indicator of the intention and the meaning one wants to give to words. Also of interest is *volume*, i.e., the sound intensity. It must be clearly calibrated according to the distance of the patient. Just as important is modifying the rhythm of speech using pauses and slowing down the speed of communication (Sect. 24.19). We are talking about the *communication time.*

*We need to be able to capture the patient's feedback, in order to calibrate our behaviour appropriately.*

## 24.12   The Purpose of Strategic Communication in Mammography

What is desired is to put the patient at ease. Listening is the most effective communication technique: even if, given the tight schedule for each examination in the screening program, it has to be limited to a few minutes at most, it still requires vigilant attention and above all a considerable commitment. All this with the aim of obtaining the full cooperation of the patient, her **compliance**.

*A high degree of compliance sometimes incredibly improves the clinical quality of an examination, in terms of the appropriate extent and stretching of the acquired tissue. Also with respect to the degree of compression tolerance.*

The work of the breast radiographer is a complex amalgam of skills and knowledge, technical and communicative. *Each factor that describes the role of the mammographer has its own impact on the perception of the experience that the patient is having. Simultaneously, on the quality of the image that is being produced* [32–35].

## 24.13 Suggestions from Lived Experience, Step by Step, to Be Used in Performing a Mammography Examination

1. Accompanying the patient in the mammography room: if we can precede her, when she does not need our help, we must pay attention to our posture. Erect and decisive, to give ourselves authority, thus suggesting that we are competent and efficient.

2. Entering the room should mark a transition: the patient should be greeted with an open hand toward her, head reclined as a sign of welcome, in any case with signs of acceptance and openness. The message one wants to send is that the relationship becomes more intimate. The door closes and the patient can relax. The smile is important, and it is one of the most powerful means of communication.

3. One identifies oneself as the health professional who will perform the examination, the mammographer.

4. When collecting the patient's historical data (Chap. 16), there should be no physical barriers (computer, head always bent, eyes always elsewhere). While entering the data in the patient's personal file, one should therefore look up from time to time at the patient.

5. Answer the questions as best you can, following the criterion of flexibility and parsimony described above. This is why it is necessary to have answers ready, for the most frequent questions at least. This should be discussed in structured meetings between colleagues, because they must be based on guidelines, but also be contextualised.

6. We confirm the patient's first name and date of birth on the image acquisition workstation. Better to raise the volume of the voice doing it, the patient should never struggle to hear the operator.

7. We sanitise the detector when the patient is in front of it. This is a much appreciated gesture, especially, but not only, in times like the pandemic.

8. If the patient has a mammography for the first time, the procedure must be explained.

9. Generally, the patient at this point says that the examination is unbearable and that she does not understand how it is possible that in 2023, there are no other systems, that US sees more… the operator must understand, *the emotional states of the patient must be validated, even if they are not agreeable.* It is true, however, and I would say that it is undeniable, that mammography is "unpleasant", or even just "uncomfortable". As we know, pain is not the main problem. The advice is to create catchphrases and to use anecdotes and metaphors. This is a strategic expedient that can have a great impact: one speaks to the right hemisphere of the brain, which works with images, and it can be positive, creates a bond.

10. During the positioning, the suggestion is to lower the volume of the voice, lengthen the pauses, and make gentle movements, always warning and explaining. The idea is to suggest that there is no aggression, despite the invasion of the intimate area. A sort of self *deminutio (diminution) of the radiographer* should be made.

11. If one notices a change in the patient's posture, more precisely a stiffening, or a real withdrawal, the advice is to stop. It is something that comes unconsciously to the patient and could represent a **negative feedback.** The radiographer should physically step back, say something colloquial and then resume positioning. Sometimes, this is enough to make the patient relax.

12. It is crucial to observe, listen and modify our behaviour when necessary. This come from monitoring constantly, using the patient's feedback, throughout the patient's mammographic experience. It must be done, even if it is very demanding.

13. Even simple distraction through colloquial and joking conversation can be a method to be used in some cases. We have to be sure when and how much we can joke with the patient, and this is not easy to understand. It is a message to be deduced from the millions

of pieces of information that run over the practitioner, which are filtered in a completely automatic way. It could not be otherwise; the world is very complex. The filters, however, are connected to our defence systems that ignore or distort the patient's information that does not respond to our reference system. Communication has a rational component and an emotional one. It is essential to be able to decentralise from one's own reference system in order to understand that of another. It is a difficult process, and one learns by making mistakes and correcting oneself. The error should be seen as something that makes us better workers, if one is willing to *correct* oneself and makes a *revision of our behaviour*. In other words, one has to be *error friendly*.

14. At the end of the examination, it is necessary to make a summary of the important things using redundancy.
15. We thanks the patient and says goodbye. The suggestion is to include in the greeting the concept of returning, as in "see you next time." This is education on adherence to the screening program.

## 24.14   Communication in the Compression Procedure [36, 37]

Compression must be treated as a separate chapter, also for the communicative aspect. Compression's standardisation is as fundamental as for positioning. Even if there are no compression ranges expressly recommended in the European guidelines, there is a range in the section concerning technical quality, which is quite similar to those reported in the national guidelines of the various European and non-European countries (Chap. 11). In addition to the advantage of being able to better compare examinations performed by different radiographers, on the same patient, standardisation would have a further positive effect, that is, *making the patient's experience constant*, at least in terms of compression. The perception of how a woman who comes for a mammogram lives this experience certainly includes many aspects, among them: (a) the confidence in the professional practice shown by the radiographer; (b) her/his ability to establish an effective relationship with the patient, including the possibility to interact with her and (c) the ability that the operator has *to manage the patient's physical/emotional discomfort*. Motivating the patient, providing her with explanations as to why we need to compress, can become decisive for the production of quality images. Confirming ("validating") the pain sensation experienced by the patient is another aspect to point out. Besides, the pain reported is also in locations other than the breast, and this should not be overlooked.

*Patient's cooperation sometimes influences the quality of the examination more than physical factors.*

## 24.15   The Encounter Between Health Worker and Patient: Communication in Recalls

The American AIDET model [38] is one of the recommended approaches to modulate the encounter between health professionals and patients:

A: Acknowledge: acceptance
I: Introduction
D: Duration
E: Explanation
T: Thanks

What it is for: to introduce oneself, to start interacting and to de-escalate certain situations that might get out of hand. There should be no confrontation between health worker and patient (Sect. 24.10). In fact, when in the mammographic room, the patient may be under severe stress, this could be due to previous negative personal or family experiences. Her ability to communicate may be thus greatly reduced in both senses. Even an exaggerated expression of pain may convey a wrong message, that may be experienced as very disturbing by the radiographer, who is used to witnessing very serious situations, in polytraumatised or metastatic patients, working on other image modalities. However, it could be a system adopted by the patient to exorcise her stress; therefore, it is necessary to understand again.

It should then be added that the ***patient's perception of the radiographer's work may not be objective.*** People give more importance to some behaviour, to some words in an encounter and blur or even make everything else disappear from their memory. Everything, which does not confirm, does not align with their own convictions or previous knowledge. Generally, patients speak of the incorrect, cold, insensitive behaviour of the operator who gave her the mammogram the previous time, so different from the kindness and understanding shown by the one in front of her at that moment. The writer has referred to this behaviour as: *"The Stockholm syndrome in mammography": the radiographer who holds you "prisoner" in the present is always better and more understanding than the one who had you "prisoner" in the past* (Poggi, C.).

During the Level 2 or recall session (Chap. 13), patients are in the grip of an anxiety that is difficult to manage. For this reason, great care must be taken in one's communication.

To be noted:

1. Never say that she does not have to worry that everything will be all right. That is, do not make the typical mistake of entering the *caretaking phase.*
2. Ask why she is so upset: we know that ***out of 10 recalls, less than two are positive for lesions (average figure in Italy and Europe).*** The patient does not know this, but even if she did, she would think that she was among those with cancer. Moreover, her emotions should not be invalidated. That would be an example of ineffective communication.

Another important aspect to mention: patients often try, sometimes even becoming very manipulative, to get the radiographer to say something about the pathology eventually presents on the images. The advice is to distance oneself immediately: "I do another job, not the reporting, and mine is already very difficult," is the author's favourite.

## 24.16   The Gender of the Breast Radiographer

The gender of the radiographer performing mammography is internationally debated: mammography is still today a field of work dominated by female operators. In an interesting and recent review on the subject [39], the authors highlight various aspects that may deter male radiographers from choosing a job in Senology: (a) a lack of clinical experience during their studies (actually shared by female students), associated in some cases with (b) the outright denial of the male student's participation in the internship; this in addition to (c) the idea, still prevailing, that patients would not like or would even refuse the male operator (with or without chaperone). This is thought to lead to a worsening of the adherence to the screening program. In Italy, there is generally no discrimination in this respect; the male breast radiographer is accepted just as doctors of both genders are accepted. It is, however, true that sometimes satisfaction and relief are expressed at the sight of the female operator. In other countries, this is not accepted. It is not just a matter of religious motivations or cultural beliefs although they are certainly important. For example, in the United Arab Emirates until 2008 men were also working as mammographers. This was until the Abu Dhabi Health Authority intervened, imposing only the female gender to perform the examination. One-size-fits-all solutions for all countries can certainly not be indicated.

The chronic shortage of specialised personnel could indeed be solved, at least partially, by the entry of male colleagues in this field.

Another extremely interesting demographic study, conducted in the United States [40], clearly shows the situation in this respect. More than 96% of mammographers out of the total, even today, are women. From the point of view of training, there should be no restriction or discrimination according to the author. In fact, in many studies on this topic, it is emphasised that, regardless of the ethnicity of origin and the sociocultural and religious beliefs of the patients, what matters most is the professional competence and welcoming approach of the practitioner.

## 24.17 Human Error and Risk Management

When one speaks of planned actions, one must of necessity speak of failures to carry them out or errors in planning these actions. Error in healthcare can have serious repercussions and must be evaluated according to a *system approach.* That is to say, as a consequence rather than a cause, avoiding the "blame" idea. This applies to all types of error in healthcare, which in most cases do not result from a lack of skills and experience (*technical skills*), but from *non-technical* skills. These are related to cognitive, social and personal skills and are complementary to the technical ones. In other words, ***error must always be contextualised, precisely because it is often caused by intrinsic properties of the system and just as often stems from recurring patterns.*** The approach must therefore also be *proactive.* Risk management is based on this.

Medico-legal cases involving the branch of radiology see the highest percentage precisely in Senology (see last paragraph in Chap. 12). Establishing a good, trusting relationship with the patient, on the part of the radiographer and the radiologist, has been proven to be able to lower this percentage significantly. This also concerns effective communication between team members.

## 24.18 Communication Between Team Members [41–44]

According to Salas et al. [41], a group or team is a collection of two or more persons who: (a) interact dynamically, (b) influence each other; (c) aim to achieve common goals; (d) share rules of behaviour and (e) have been assigned specific roles and functions. The development of interaction is implicit in the definition of a group; it is the key to achieving greater safety and effectiveness in daily work. The exchange of communication, the coordination between the various figures, at all levels, the equal distribution of the workload and the monitoring of performance are important features of a group. Radiographers typically work as a team in all branches of diagnostic imaging although in different ways. In Senology patients perceive the quality of the overall service through interactions with all members, starting with the reception staff. Unfortunately, staff in healthcare are rarely trained for teamwork. In Italy, training focuses on technical skill and individual competence, what is referred to as **single-professional training.** This is the training which forms the technical basis of disciplinary knowledge, the **knowhow. Interdisciplinary training**, on the other hand, would allow an integration of one's own competence with that of others. This would mean acting collaboratively and interactively. However, it presupposes the creation and construction of a well-functioning group. A well-functioning group is composed of individuals who: (1) are individually competent; (2) communicate with each other clearly; (3) are motivated in the realisation of the group's task (*team self-awareness*) and (4) share the group's objectives.

*Leadership* is required to direct and coordinate in this sense: (1) encouraging individuals to work together; (2) evaluating performance; (3) developing the group's knowledge, skills and competences and (4) creating a positive atmosphere. Cooperation, mutual support and conflict resolution are the foundations for building good teamwork. And certainly, effective communication between the various team members influences not only the team itself, but also the professional satisfaction of the individual practitioners and the relationship with patients.

## 24.19 The Ethics of Data Management: The Privacy Act 101/2018 (EU 2016/679) and Artificial Intelligence (AI) [45–52]

In health care, privacy is specifically understood as the protection of personal data concerning her or his state of health and the way in which her or his pathology, current or former, may be treated. It is therefore a subject that also concerns the radiographer. The processing of data in its entirety must be carried out while guaranteeing confidentiality and respect for the rights and dignity of the person. A distinction is made between **personal** and **sensitive data.** The former concerns information on an individual's psycho-physical condition, including genetic data; hereditary traits, the photographs taken during a medical or surgical act, are included. The latter are such as to reveal ethnic origin, for example, or religious beliefs, possibly political opinions, state of health and sexual life. For all sensitive data, consent must be explicit (in accordance with GDPR General Data Protection Regulation 2016/679). Violation of privacy through unlawful processing of personal data is punishable with administrative fines and under the criminal code.

*Artificial intelligence (AI),* mentioned several times in this text, has extremely interesting applications precisely in the field of biomedical imaging. Its progress in recent years has been and still is overwhelming. The need to ensure that the data used, even during training and education of workers, are treated in a congruent and ethical manner has therefore become increasingly pressing.

Some definitions are provided first. Suggestion is to refer to dedicated texts for more information on such a complex but increasingly influential topic for those working in healthcare.

*AI: AI commonly refers to the set of methodologies and techniques that enable the design of hardware systems and software programs, through which it is possible to interpret a huge volume of data (big data), in a flexible manner (similar to the human approach). This is in order to achieve set goals.*

*Machine learning (ML): consists of the use and development of complex algorithms that are able to create models for analysing and drawing inferences from data. These data may be classified and unclassified (algorithms that are able-imilar to the human approach). This is in order to achi features in the data provided, automatically. One then speaks of **data mining,** especially when learning is unsupervised. Machine learning requires a large amount of data for training.*

*Deep learning (DL): this is an AI algorithm and is a sub-specialty of machine learning based on neural networks. Neural networks are adap-*
*tive, multi-layer, non-linear structures in which the data flowing through them are analysed according to their characteristics, from the simplest to the most complex. The aim is to provide an output that has an absolutely complex relationship with the input.*

The best known neural network model in the biomedical field is the ***convolutional neural network (CNN).*** It is mainly used in image analysis, and thus in ***radiomics*** and ***radiogenomics***, for the extraction of quantitative information from images, diagnostic or histological. This is done for the detection of tumour lesions, and to correlate them with their phenotypic characteristics. In general, for a classification useful for risk stratification and choice of therapies.

***Radiomics:*** *consists of extracting quantitative data from the image using AI algorithms, to provide information on patho-physiological phenomena of the lesion, which are not accessible to qualitative analysis (observation).*

***Radiogenomics:*** *correlates radiomics with the genomic characteristics of the lesion. This is generally only accessible through biopsy and histopathological analysis. The possibility of integrating different information, and its processing by platforms using AI algorithms makes it possible to identify similar patients who can benefit from specific treatments in advance.*

DL has been shown to be able to diagnose breast lesions up to 12 months earlier than conventional qualitative procedures are capable of doing, as some studies would have shown. Furthermore, it appears that the model combining deep learning and machine learning methods, known as the *hybrid algorithm*, gives the best results [46]. Very interesting the DL implementation of computational mammographic phenotypes [47] for automatic BI-RADS density classification (see Chaps. 1 and 3). There is a version based on large FFDM and 2D SM DBT (Chap. 20) images archives.

***The creation of relevant public databases (in terms of volume and classification) should be in fact regarded as a crucial necessity for the future.***

*European Society or Radiology (ESR) and European Institute for Biomedicine Imaging*

*Research (EIBIR)* have launched a project called *"chAImeleon,"* financed with European funds [48]. Its aim is to create an open-source cloud-based data-repository of images acquired by various methodologies, classified and labelled (i.e., equipped with the necessary information for their identification), of tumours, including BC. Eighteen organisations from all over Europe have joined, including three from Italy.

AI systems are technologies for processing data and information in general which can predict and help healthcare professional in the process of decision making [49, 50]. It is then understandable how important is that all actors in the process itself, whether virtual or physical, follow ethical rules aimed at protecting the patient. A Manual of Recommendations on the Ethics of AI has been drafted by UNESCO and made available on 23 November 2021 [51]. Fundamental concepts such as the respect, protection and promotion of human rights and the fundamental freedom and dignity of the individual are reiterated.

There has also been a multi-society statement on AI ethics in biomedical imaging since 2019, of which the *ESR* and *European Society of Medical Imaging Informatics (EUSoMII)* were part. *EFRS*, *ISRRT* and *Society and College of Radiographers (SCoR)* also produced a similar statement [52]. This parallelism between the two statements makes clear a fundamental aspect according to the author. That is, those who report and those who produce mammograms should aim at an increasingly important working collaboration and to share a common educational path, whenever possible.

## 24.20   The Breast Radiographer Profile in Italy and Common Frontiers

It is essential to predetermine the skills that operators, of whatever role, must possess in order to be part of the team, so as to standardise them. The specific training, what in the Anglo-Saxon world is called **job description**, has not yet been clearly outlined for what concerns the

mammographer in Italy. In the *Contratto Nazionale del Lavoro CNL (National Labor Contract)*, the figure of both the specialised and the expert breast radiographer is transposed, pursuant to Law No. 43 of 2006. Although master courses are also offered in Senology, *all master courses* (intended as specialisation courses, not to be confused with the master's degree), apart from the staffing management one, do not have a nationally recognised educational system in Italy. The title is awarded under the autonomous responsibility of the individual university (cit. Ministero dell'Istruzione MI, currently called MIM, dell'Istruzione e del Merito, and MUR, dell'Università e della Ricerca). This means that all master courses have no operational usability in Italy.

The courses for breast radiographers with expertise in Senology proposed to the Region of Tuscany in 2021 by *REte TEcnici SEnologi in ToscanA (RE.TE.SE.TA)* with *Centro di Riferimento Regionale Prevenzione Oncologica-ISPRO* of Florence and the working group of the Tuscany region have not yet started (interrupted by the pandemic).

***The difficulties in the profiling of the mammographer, not only in Italy*** [53, 54], ***also derive from the fact that she/he is a hybrid figure, including skills generally excluded from the general professional profile of the diagnostic radiographer*** (see also Chap. 26).

Below is a list of some specific traits:

1. Advanced anatomical and anatomo-radiographic knowledge, not only of the breast
2. Knowledge, skills and abilities relating to musculoskeletal and postural function, onere, including skilpatient
3. Knowledge of the organisation of clinical programmes and pathways and of the different mammographic examination, oncological follow-up, urgent by suspected lesion or by symptoms
4. Up-to-date knowledge of treatment and surgical procedures, so as to be able to collect patient data in a safe and professional manner

5. Knowledge expertise and skills in various areas of breast imaging, MRI, tomosynthesis, stereotactic biopsy... in addition to mammography, standard and recall
6. High communication competence, including both building a relationship with the patient, of trust. This is to achieve patient compliance, building a positive mammography experience. Also important is the communication with other staff members, both team members and outsiders
7. Ability to pass on the acquired theoretical and practical skills to the best of our own ability, to students and in general to those who want to learn this job

***Producing a Positive Mammography Experience Involves a Real Problem-Solving Process.*** One has to understand first what the problems will be, with the individual patient. Then, choose the most effective behavioural approach, thinking about and possibly trying at least two alternatives, selecting the best one. This also applies to the positioning technique, which must be adjusted for each patient. The aim is to finally produce the best possible examination, in terms of extension, stretching and acquisition geometry. That is to say, images with a high fidelity of reproduction of the actual anatomy of the individual patient. The result is monitored and its success or otherwise, evaluated. And all this within a matter of minutes. It is a ***process that takes years of work in a mammography department to be refined, and many, many mistakes***. Such hard-earned skills must be taught, that is, be part of the curriculum of that radiographer who wants to devote her/himself to Senology. This was the driving purpose behind the drafting of this text.

The professional qualification that enables the radiographer to practise provides the necessary minimum knowledge and competence, which among other things, have a short half-life [55]. Knowledge and competence must be kept up-to-date and developed, we should compulsorily speak of CPD, understood as that series of training activities by means of which one is able to maintain, but also develop, one's working abili-

ties. It must be strenuously pursued throughout one's working life.

Learning in an adult only occurs when he or she "feels" the need to know, and the most important motivation for the desire to learn is professional self-esteem. Unfortunately, the work routine is depersonalising and sometimes de-professionalising. Mammography is indeed a very difficult examination to teach and learn, daunting, especially at first. In addition, the acquired competence has to be refreshed often.

***All radiographers, as such, play a fundamental role in the overall quality of the diagnostic image. This is not sufficiently understood in Italy. Nevertheless, it implies a great responsibility toward the patients.*** This specific topic is dealt with by the Italian law known as Gelli, No. 24/2017. It highlights, among other things, the need to introduce control and performance evaluation mechanisms into professional practice.

In this regard, it is worth noting the previously mentioned EFSR White Paper [9], for the 2021–2031 decade. It clearly specifies how continuing education and acquisition of advanced qualifications are necessary to grow the profession, expanding and differentiating the role of the radiographer in response to the substantial change in healthcare.

As far as the AI approach is concerned, in an interesting work, Akudjedu et al. [56] investigated what radiographers' knowledge, perceptions and expectations of this topic are. The resulting benefits, for them to be truly enjoyed, will require training that is appropriate and contextualised to work practice. For example, benefits could be seen in the workflow, or in the assessment of clinical image quality. With regard to AI-based mammography quality assessment, it must be said that the quality criteria need to be refined, and based on EBP, so that these techniques can be implemented successfully [57].

In this perspective of comprehensive continuing education, the specific educational path for the breast radiographer should certainly be included. Also with a view to a revaluation of her/his role, which cannot be said often enough, is fundamental and irreplaceable in the pathway of breast cancer diagnosis.

# References

1. Il processo di Bologna e lo spazio europeo dell'istruzione superiore. https://education.ec.europa.eu/it/education-levels/higher-education/inclusive-and-connected-higher-education/bologna-process.
2. EHEA. https://ehea.info/page-full_members.
3. Description of the eight EQF levels. https://europa.eu/europass/en/description-eight-eqf-levels.
4. Prentakis AG, et al. Education, training and professional issues of radiographers in six European countries: a comparative review. J Eur CME. 2016;5(1):31092. https://doi.org/10.3402/jecme.v5.31092.
5. Couto JC, et al. An evaluation of the educational requirements to practice radiography in the European Union. Radiography. 2018;24:64–71. https://doi.org/10.1016/j.radi.2017.07.009.
6. Diagnostic radiographer. https://www.healthcareers.nhs.uk.
7. PGCERT breast imaging. https://www.lsbu.ac.uk/study/course-finder/breast-imaging. ultimo accesso 18 Dec 2022.
8. Challen V, Pronk-Larive D. A European perspective on the role of radiographers in imaging department, vol 11(3), 2011-Cover Story. https://healthmanagement.org/c/it/issuearticle/a-european-perspective-on-the-role-of-radiographers-in-imaging-departments.
9. EFRS white paper on the future of the profession radiographer education, research, and practice (RERP): 2021–2031. EFRS. https://api.efrs.eu/api/assets/posts/275.
10. ARRT education requirement for obtaining an maintaining certification and registration. American Registry of Radiologic Technologists; 2022.
11. How to become a mammographer—The complete Guide RadComm; 2020. https://radcomm.net/. Ultimo accesso 30 Jan 2023.
12. MTMI: MQSA requirements for mammography. https://www.mtmi.net/blog/. Ultimo accesso 25 Jan 2023.
13. Albus K. ACR, validation cycles: mammography. 2023. https://accreditationsupport.acr.org/support/solutions/articles/11000051607-validation-cycles-mammography-revised-02-22-2023.
14. ECM, Commissione Nazionale Formazione Continua. https://ape.agenas.it/ecm/ecm.aspx.
15. Hogg P, Holmes K. Rapid creation of a website to produce educational and clinical support resources for global use during and beyond the Covid-19. Radiography. 2022;28:S3. https://doi.org/10.1016/j.radi.2022.07.011.
16. Rainford L, et al. Education and training in radiation protection in Europe: an analysis from the EURAMED rocc-n-roll project. Insights Into Imaging. 2022;13:142. https://doi.org/10.1186/s13244-022-01271-y.
17. Comunicazione e performance professionale: metodi e strumenti. Ministero della Salute Direzione Generale della programmazione sanitaria, Ufficio III, I modulo Elementi teorici della comunicazione, Maggio 2015. https://www.salute.gov.it/imgs/C_17_pubblicazioni_2385_allegato.pdf.
18. European Qualifications Framework (EQF). Level 6 benchmarking document: radiographers, EFRS. https://api.efrs.eu/api/assets/posts/205.
19. GIMBE. https://www.gimbe.org/.
20. Grimm LJ, et al. Benefits and risks of mammography screening in women ages 40 to 49 years. J Prim Care Community Health. 13:21501327211058322. https://doi.org/10.1177/21501327211058322.
21. Whelehan P, et al. The effect o mammography pain on repeat participation in breast cancer screening: a systematic review. Breast. 2013;22:389–94. https://doi.org/10.1016/j.breast.2013.03.003.
22. Van Goethem M, et al. Influence of the radiographer on the pain felt during mammography. Eur Radiol. 2003;13:2384–9. https://doi.org/10.1007/s00330-002-1686-6.
23. Arthur L, et al. Effect of verbal communication on experiences of discomfort in women undergoing mammography examination. J Sci Multidiscip Res. 2013;5(1):42–53. issn:2277-0135.
24. Sterlingova T, Lundén M. Why do women refrain from mammography screening? Radiography. 2018;24:e19–24. https://doi.org/10.1016/j.radi.2017.07.006.
25. Arnold L. Patient care, communication, and safety in the mammography suite. Radiol Technol. 2016;88(1) SSRT CE directed Reading.
26. Impact of Communication in Healthcare. IHC. https://healthcarecomm.org/about-us/impact-of-communication-in-healthcare/.
27. Morreale SP, et al. Human communication motivation, knowledge, and skills. 2nd ed. Thomson Wadsworth; 2007. isbn:0-534-57024-0.
28. Debenedictis M, et al. Coming out of the dark: a curriculum for teaching and evaluation radiology residents' communication skills through simulation. ACR. 2017;14:87–91. https://doi.org/10.1016/j.jacr.2016.09.036.
29. Del Piccolo L. La comunicazione nonverbale. Dipartimento di Sanità Pubblica e Medicina di Comunità, Sezione di Psicologia Clinica, Università di Verona. https://www.dsu.univr.it/documenti/OccorrenzaIns/matdid/matdid775979.pdf.
30. Secci EM, Duo C. La comunicazione strategica nelle professioni sanitarie. Collana E-BOOK ECM seconda edizione elettronica; 2011. isbn:978-88-903376-2-8. http://www.aslcarbonia.it/documenti/7_189_20120328151144.pdf.
31. Metsala E, et al. European radiographers' challenges from mammography education and clinical practice-an integrative review. Insight Imaging. 2017;8:329–43. https://doi.org/10.1007/s13244-016-0542-1.

32. McCorry LK, Mason J. Communication skills for the healthcare professional. Wolters Kluwer/Lippincott Williams & Wilkins Health. isbn:978-1-58255-814-1.

33. Patel MM, Parikh JR. Patient diversity in breast imaging: barriers and potential solutions. J Breast Imaging. 2021;3:98–105. https://doi.org/10.1093/jbi/wbaa092.

34. Strøm B, et al. Challenges in mammography education and training today: the perspectives of radiography teachers/mentors and students in five European countries. Radiography. 2018;24:41–6. https://doi.org/10.1016/j.radi.2017.08.008.

35. Pal S, et al. Improving performance of mammographic breast positioning in an academic radiology practice. AJR. 2018;210:807–15. https://doi.org/10.2214/AJR.17.18212.

36. Mercer CE. Practictioner variation of applied breast compression force in mammography. PhD thesis. School of Health Science, University of Salford, UK. https://salford-repository.worktribe.com/preview/1496464/PhD_Thesis_Claire_Mercer_Practitioner_variation_of_applied_breast_compression_force_in_mammography.pdf.

37. Branderhorst H, et al. Mammography compression: a need for mechanical standardization. Eur J Radiol. 2015). https://pubmed.ncbi.nlm.nih.gov/25596915/.;84:596.

38. Valessa J. Incorporating Acknowledge, Introduce, Duration, Explanation, and Thank You (AIDET) framework and patient satisfaction in the primary case setting. Acta Sci Med Sci. 2020;4(1). issn:2582-0931. https://www.actascientific.com/ASMS/pdf/ASMS-04-0503.pdf.

39. Ashton J, Waren-Forward HM. Males in mammography—a narrative review of the literature. Radiography. 2019;25:392–9. https://doi.org/10.1016/j.radi.2019.05.001.

40. Mammography technicians demographics and statistics win the US ZIPPIA The Carrier Expert. https://www.zippia.com/mammography-technician-jobs/demographics/.

41. Salas E, et al. Does team training work? Principles for health care. Acad Emerg Med. 2008;15:1002–9. https://doi.org/10.1111/j.1553-2712.2008.00254.x.

42. Galli V. Valutazione e formazione Continua attraverso il Gruppo di Lavoro TSRM: L'esperienza della Regione Emilia-Romagna: un modello condivisibile? Verona convegno nazionale *GISMA* 25 Maggio. 2017.

43. Strudwick RM, Day J. Interprofessional working in diagnostic radiography. Radiography. 2014;20:235–40. https://www.sciencedirect.com/science/article/abs/pii/S1078817414000406.

44. Miller LC. What every mammography technologist would like their radiologist to know about: our patients/image quality/the role of the technologist. SBI; 2014. https://mammographyeducation.com/wp-content/uploads/2014/09/SBI-ARTICLE_MILLER-.pdf.

45. Lei Y-M, et al. Artificial intelligence in medical imaging of the breast. Front Oncol. 11:600557. https://doi.org/10.3389/fonc.2021.600557.

46. Nasser M, Yusof UK. Deep learning based methods for breast cancer diagnosis: a systematic review and future direction. Diagnostics (Basel). 2023;13:161. https://doi.org/10.3390/diagnostics13010161.

47. Gastounioti A, et al. Artificial intelligence in mammographic phenotyping of breast cancer risk: a narrative review. Breast Cancer Res. 2022;24:14. https://doi.org/10.1186/s13058-022-01509-z.

48. Chaimeleon. https://www.eibir.org/projects/chaimeleon.

49. Marino MA, et al. Lymph node imaging in patients with primary breast cancer: concurrent diagnostic tools. Oncologist. 2020;25:e231–42. https://doi.org/10.1634/theoncologist.2019-0427.

50. Ektefaie Y, et al. Integrative multiomics-hostopathology analysis for breast cancer classification. NPJ Breast Cancer. 2021;7:147. https://www.nci.nlm.nih.gov/pmc/articles/PMC8630188/pdf/41523_2021_Article_357.pdf.

51. Recommendation on the Ethics of Artificial Intelligence Corporate author UNESCO 66618, document code: SHS/BIO/PI/2021/1 https://www.unesco.org/en/artificial-intelligence/recommendation-ethics.

52. Walsh G, et al. Responsible AI practice and AI education are central to AI implementation: a rapid review for all medical imaging professional in Europe. BJR Open. 2023;5:20230033. https://doi.org/10.1259/bjro.20230033.

53. Albeshan S, et al. Evaluation of radiographers' experience in mammography: an explanatory study. Iran J Radiol. 2022;19(2):e121918. https://doi.org/10.5812/iranjradiol-121918.

54. Meystre NR, et al. Characterization of radiographers' mammography practice in five European countries: a pilot study. Insights Imaging. 2019;10:31. https://insightimaging.springer.com/articles/10.1186/s13244-019-0711-0.

55. Norman GR, Schmidt HG. The psychological basis of problem-based learning: a review ot the evidence. Acad Med. 1992;67(9):557–65. https://doi.org/10.1097/00001888-199209000-00002.

56. Akudjedu TN, et al. Knowledge, perceptions and expectations of artificial intelligence in radiography practice: a global radiography workforce survey. J Med Imaging Radiat Sci. 2023;54:104–16. https://pumed.ncbi.nih.gov/36535859/.

57. Waade GG, et al. Assessment of breast screening positioning criteria in mammographic screening: agreement between artificial intelligence software and radiographers. J Med Screen. 2021;28(4):448–55. https://doi.org/10.1177/0969141321998718. Sagepub.com/journals-permissions downloaded from Research Gate.

# Part VI

# The Poggi Method

# Radiographic Anatomy of the Breast: Subdivision by Zones, According to the Hands of the Clock and into Anatomical Parts

**25**

## 25.1 Breast Subdivision by Zones or Areas: CC Projection

The breast image can be subdivided into zones or areas, as shown in Fig. 25.1 (CC projection) and 2 (MLO projection).

**Fig. 25.1** Subdivision of the breast in zones on the mammographic image, in antero-posterior direction: retroareolar, anterior, central and posterior areas; in lateromedial direction: lateral, central and medial (or inner) areas, CC projection and left breast

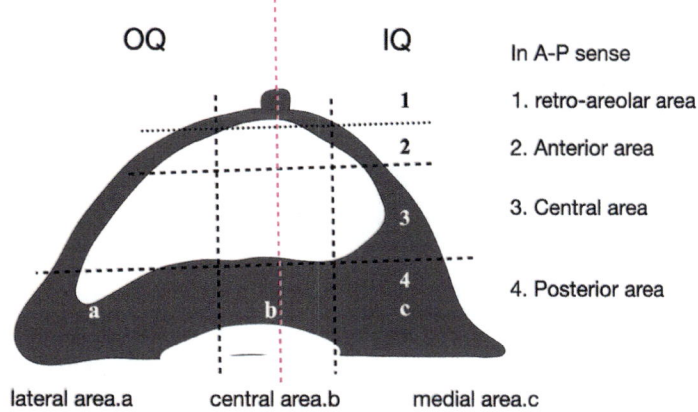

OQ     IQ     In A-P sense

1. retro-areolar area

2. Anterior area

3. Central area

4. Posterior area

lateral area.a     central area.b     medial area.c

In latero-medial sense: a. Lateral; b. Central; c. Medial

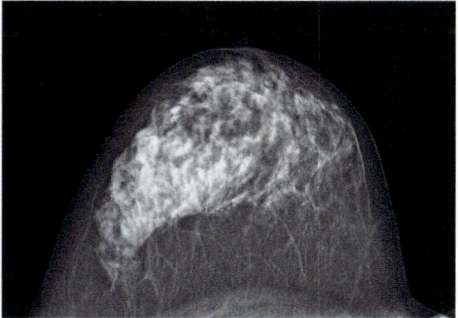

## 25.2    Breast Subdivision by Zones or Areas: MLO Projection (Fig. 25.2)

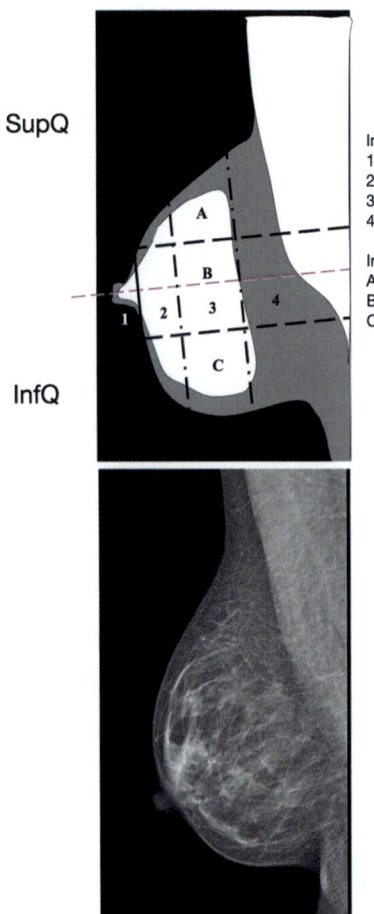

In A-P direction
1. Retroareolar area
2. Anterior area
3.Central area
4.Posterior area

In Sup-Inf direction
A. Superior
B. Central
C. Inferior

**Fig. 25.2** Subdivision of the breast in zones on the mammographic image in antero-posterior direction: retroareolar, anterior, central and posterior areas; in superoinferior direction, superior, central and inferior areas, MLO projection and right breast

## 25.3    Posterior Nipple Line (PNL) [1, 2]

PNL is a measurement that allows us to establish whether the mammogram has been correctly performed, from the point of view of the extension of the documented tissue in the antero-posterior sense, in the CC projection. It is called PNL, Fig. 25.3. It is the only objective parameter that can be used in assessing the clinical quality of the CC projection,

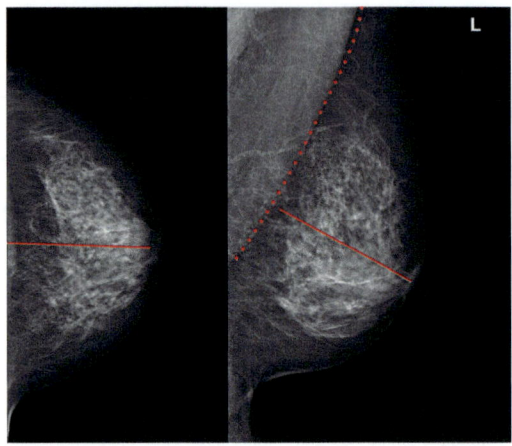

**Fig. 25.3** PNL: the CC projection includes the entire central retromammary space, as confirmed by the presence of the pectoralis muscle, and the length of the PNL. Identification with the midline in the CC projection and with the axial plane in the MLO

and it was introduced by the Americans. Unfortunately, it is not easy to use. It is measured on a successful MLO projection, which is subsequently transferred to the CC of the same side.

The deep (central) planes have been correctly documented in the CC projection if the PNL, measured from the nipple to the pectoral muscle if visible, or if not, to the posterior edge of the image (Fig. 25.3), is approximately equal to that of the MLO. At most, slightly shorter (see below). The PNL on the CC projection is always described perpendicular to the thoracic plane: in the case of a strongly eccentric nipple with respect to the median sagittal plane, however, the PNL would be much shorter than the breast AP-larger dimension. In this text, a different thesis is therefore advocated, identifying the PNL on the CC with the midline or rather with the *median sagittal plane*. The aim is the same to assess the correct documentation of the deep planes in CCs.

## 25.4    Other Lines and Areas to Be Considered in a Mammogram [3–10]

When looking at the mammography image produced, one can also consider various lines and the areas that these lines define and delimit. This allows one to:

1. compare the extent of tissue between the two sides
2. evaluate the centring of the organ in relation to the FOV
3. the left/right symmetry

**MIDLINE**: this is the line that divides the breast in mammography into two quadrants, ideally equal, called *inner* (or *medial*) *IQ* and *outer* (or *lateral*) OQ. It is traced from the nipple to the pectoral muscle, in the **CC projection**, generally perpendicular. When the breast is correctly positioned, and the quadrants mentioned are of equal size, the midline coincides with the *median sagittal plane*, which divides the breast into two parts (irrespective of the size of the quadrants themselves) and with the *central line* (see below). In this case, **the midline is the two-dimensional transposition of the median sagittal plane and is perpendicular to the thoracic plane.** However, if one of the two quadrants is larger than the other, the midline does not coincide with the sagittal plane, and it is no longer perpendicular to the thorax. If the midline is forced to coincide with the median sagittal plane, there will be a loss of part of the dominant quadrant (failure to meet the *second acquisition geometry parameter*, Chaps. 9, 26 and 27).

**PNL**: this is the line joining the front edge of the pectoralis major muscle to the nipple (or if the muscle is not visible, from the posterior edge of the image to the nipple), in the CC projection. It is transferred from the MLO, where it is obtained by drawing a line on the front edge of the pectoralis major muscle, from its super-anterior to the inferior–anterior angle, and then its perpendicular joining it to the nipple. They should be about the same length, shorter in the CC, but less than 1 cm.

The **PNL** divides the breast **in the MLO projection** into upper and lower quadrants. **Therefore is the two-dimensional transposition of the median axial plane**.

**Central line**: divides the mammographic image into two parts, in both projections, exactly in the centre of the image itself, in the typical layout. It identifies the perfect centring of the organ in relation to the available FOV. It coincides with the midline in the CC and with the median sagittal plane when inner and outer quadrants are the same size.

**Pectoralis major muscle**: it is the radio-opaque area that should appear, in the CC projection, lunette-shaped (semi-elliptical), central, convex anteriorly, more or less wide lateromedially, and more or less wide antero-posteriorly. It depends on the stretching operated by the radiographer and on the patient's anatomy. The size of the pectoral muscle demonstrable is influenced by many parameters, see Chaps. 9 and 11, and YouTube material on this link at the end of the book. In the MLO projection, it should appear as a wide fan, convex anteriorly, very wide at the axillary level and then decreasing, with a rounded tail (lower part), following its actual anatomy.

**Latissimus dorsi muscle**: this is part of the posterior wall of the axillary cavity, the only one visible, and not always, in the MLO projection alone. It presents itself as a more radio-opaque triangle than the pectoralis major and behind it. In reality, it is not only posterior, the two planes partially overlap. **Intermammary cleft**: this is the portion of deep medial tissue of the breast that looks toward the sternum. According to the method devised by the author (mentioned in Chap. 26), this is an anatomical area of high importance in assessing image quality for extension and proper stretching. Even better, when associated with a similar flaring on the opposite side (lateral end), the two flares make up the "tent sign" (see Chaps. 9 and 26), which identifies the attachment of the skin envelope containing the breast to the thorax.

**Retromammary space**: located at the front of the pectoralis muscle and, generally behind the glandular body, is of fundamental importance in mammography. It should be acquired at its best, both in extension and fidelity of representation, as it is a likely site of lesions, see also Chap. 17 on *forbidden zones* (Tabar).

**Inframammary fold (IMF)**: is the portion of the breast that identifies the inferior passage between the breast and the thorax, below the inferior margin of the pectoralis major muscle. It consists of the deep, inferior tissues of the breast and a portion of the thorax. A *fingernail IMF* is defined as one in which only the angle of connection of the breast to the thorax appears. The IMF position, in the up-down direction, associated with greater or lesser breast volume and degree of ptosis, is very interesting for the production of high-quality mammography; it has in fact a strong impact on that.

IMF documentation gives confidence that the *Posterior Inferior Quadrant POSTINFQ* has been included.

**Posteroinferior quadrant POSTINFQ**: this is a portion of posterior and inferior breast tissue, only visible if the MLO projection has been accurately performed. It must be documented, as it is not well visible on CCs. It is located above and somewhat anterior to the IMF.

**Axillary prolongation or lobe**: this is the portion that extends externally and superiorly to the UOQ. It can be documented in its entirety only in the MLO projection.

**Nipple areolar complex (NAC)**: is the portion of tissue comprising the nipple and areola, which can be studied in its entirety, including the retro-areolar area, only if the nipple is documented in profile.

By *nipple in profile,* we mean its projection outside the glandular tissue and outside the skin edge, i.e., when the X-ray beam is tangent to it. In the case of spontaneous retraction of the NAC to compression, a specific projection can be added. It is done with minimal compression, including only the anterior tissue, for its more effective documentation.

However, it must be said that the latest studies would show that this projection does not lead to an increase in the *detection rate* (see Chap. 6). Furthermore, in the PGMI system, it is considered sufficient that the nipple is in profile in at least one of the two projections on the same side.

[AN: *it should be added that the nipple should be in profile only if the quadrants are the same size, for the first acquisition geometry parameter. A rotation of a few degrees, in one of the two projections, may be acceptable. In the case that the upper and lower quadrants in the CC and/or medial and lateral quadrants in the MLO are not the same size, the nipple in profile condition should not be sought, as it leads to the loss of part of the dominant quadrant*]. See also Chap. 27.

## 25.5 Breast Subdivision According to the Clock

The breast can also be subdivided into portions, according to the clock, see Figs. 25.4, 25.5, 25.6, and 25.7. Figures 25.8, 25.9, and 25.10 show the same subdivision in the presentation layout for CC and MLO projections. In Fig. 25.11, an

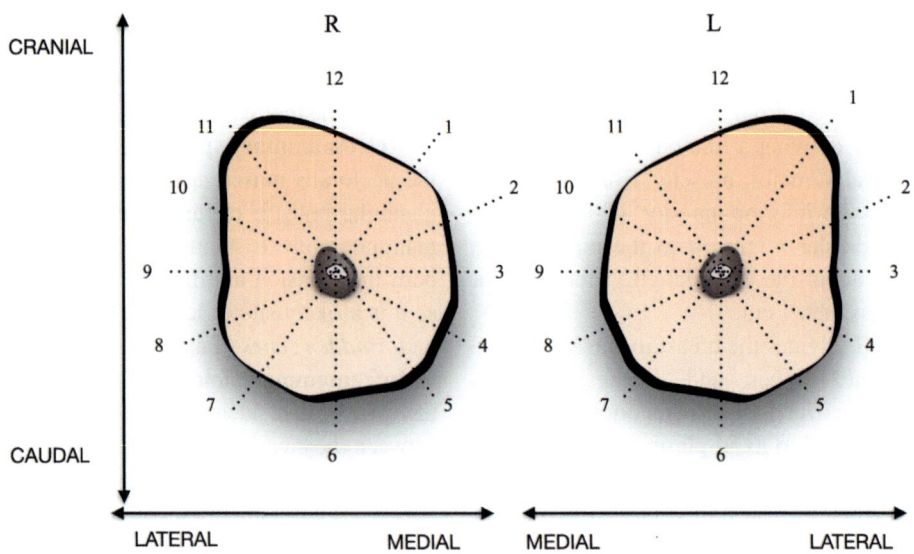

**Fig. 25.4** Breast subdivision, according to the clock. Right and left breast, on the coronal plane, which cannot be projected. It is necessary to acquire two projections in order to obtain all the information for the localisation of a lesion, CC and MLO projections in standard examinations

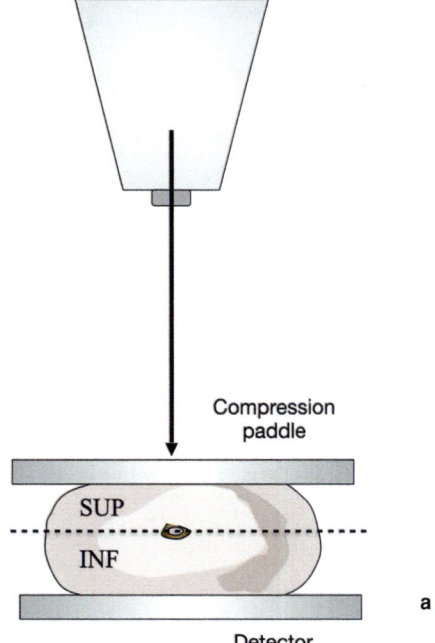

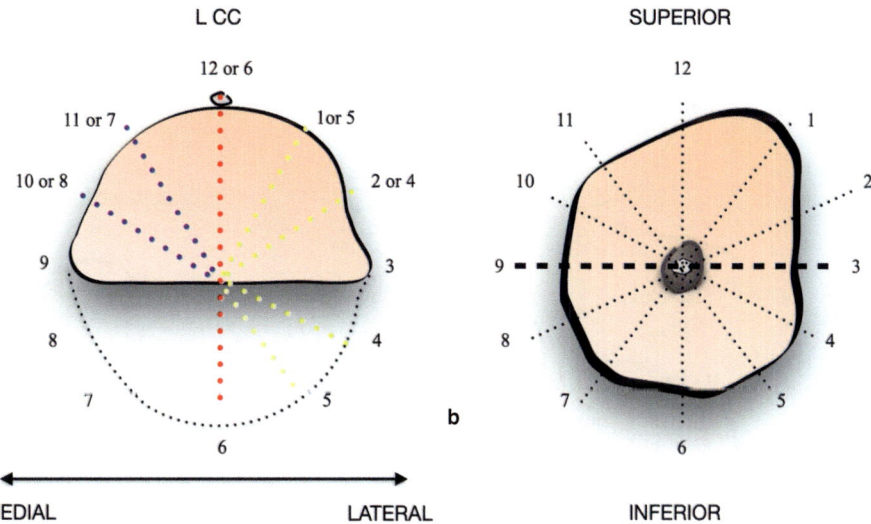

**Fig. 25.5** (**a**) Overlapping of upper and lower quadrants in the CC projection, along the beam direction. Subdivision according to the hands of the clock. (**b**) Overlap of the two portions shown in the CC layout, with nipple facing upward (anterior)

example of straight-line triangulation (Chap. 13) is correlated with this new information.

See Chap. 13 and material on You Tube @cristinapoggi7579 channel (2021):

1. First part: https://youtu.be/fHiX8YhMBe8
2. Second part: https://youtu.be/OnNpSSu-wmV8
3. Third part: https://youtu.be/mKtqr7LXoHk

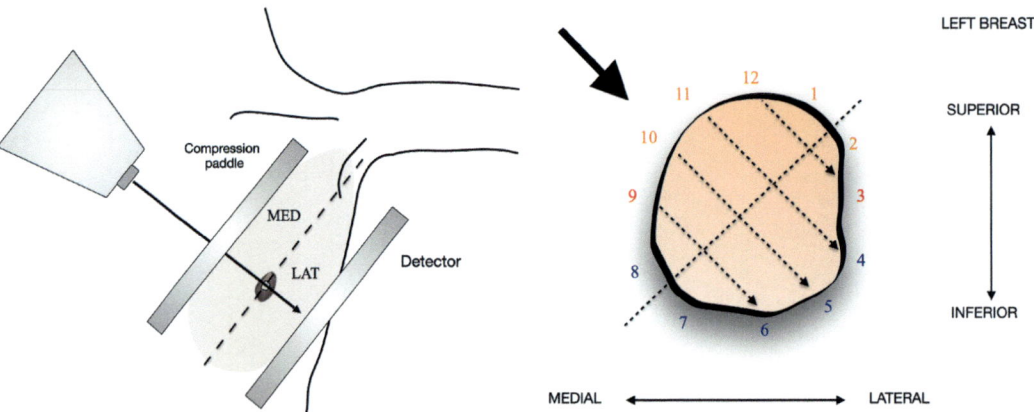

**Fig. 25.6** Overlapping of medial and lateral quadrants in the MLO projection. Due to the skew caused by the obliquity of the beam, the overlap is not exact, as is the case with the true lateral

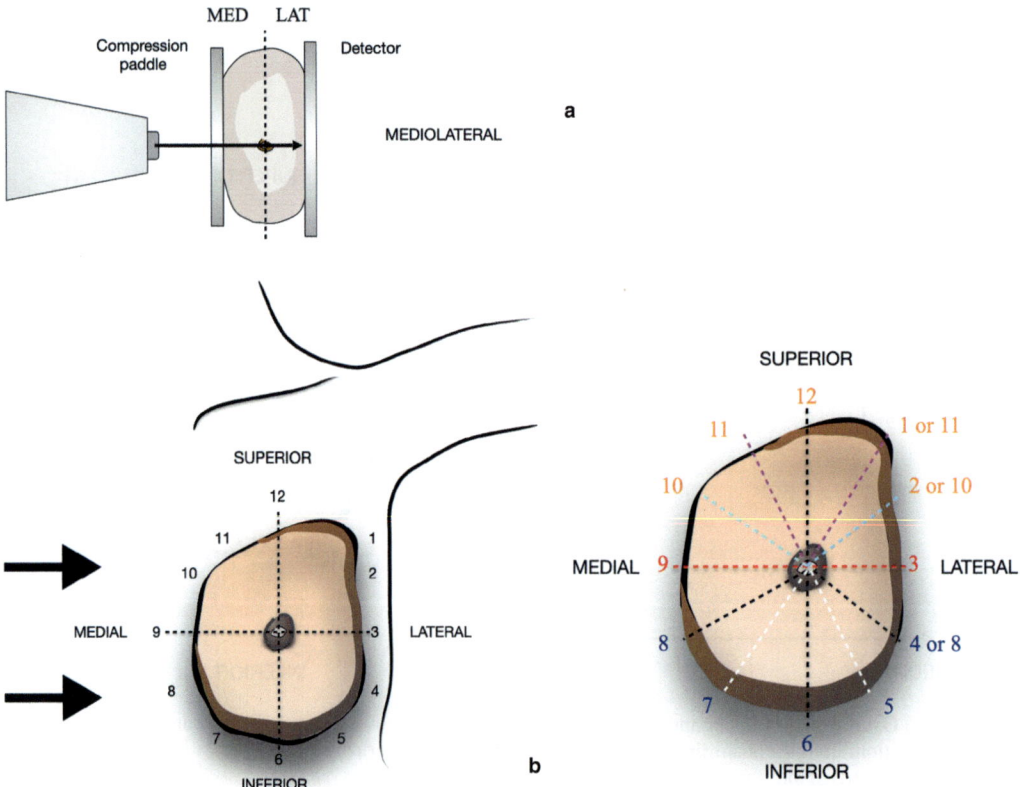

**Fig. 25.7** (**a** and **b**) Exact overlapping of medial quadrants over lateral quadrants in ML projection, between medial and lateral points, as shown in the drawing above, for left breast, ML projection

**Fig. 25.8** CC projection, left and right sides, in the presentation layout. The information that can be obtained about the position of a lesion is only in the lateromedial direction, as the upper and lower points are superimposed. Definitely lateral the points shown in purple, medial the points in yellow, central the white ones, both sides

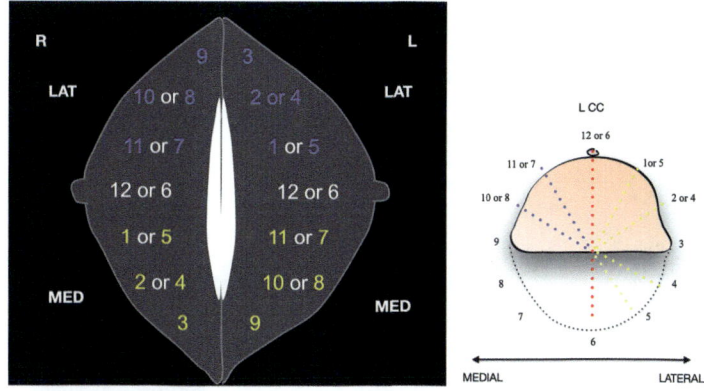

**Fig. 25.9** Inexact overlapping of medial and lateral portions in the two MLOs, due to beam obliquity, in the presentation layout. The information that can be obtained about the position of a lesion is in the superoinferior direction, but it is not exact. In orange the probably superior points, in blue the inferior, in red the central ones. This is evaluating only the oblique beam, thus considering a perfect positioning. To locate a lesion in the upper-lower direction, the true lateral is required

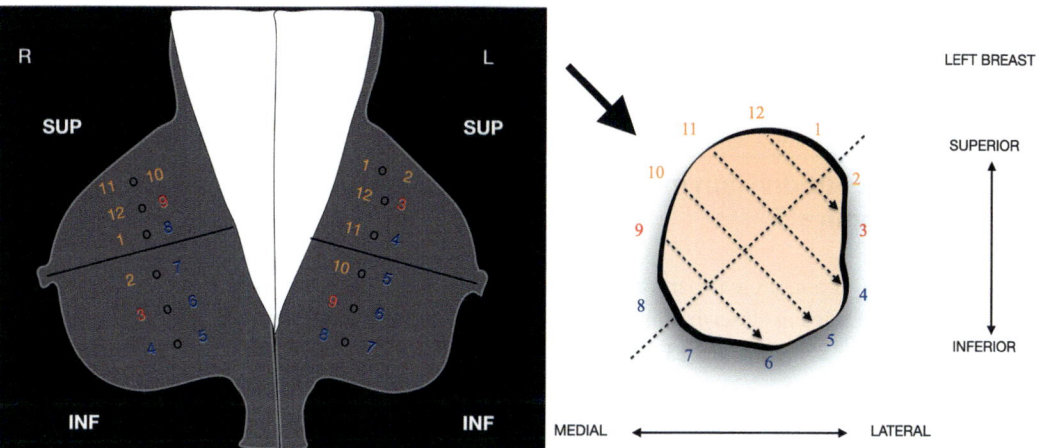

**Fig. 25.10** Exact superimposition of the medial and lateral portions in the two MLs, right and left. The information that can be obtained on the position of the lesion is in the superoinferior sense, and this time is real. In orange the definitely superior points, in red the central and in blue the inferior ones

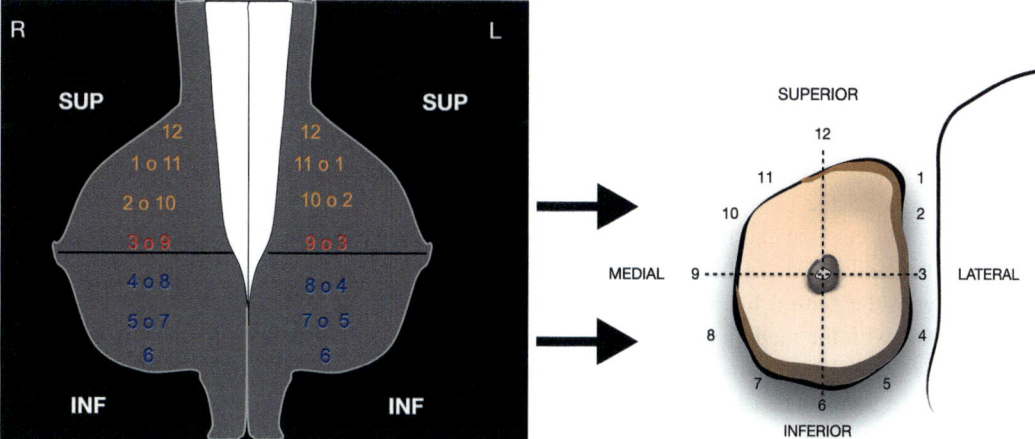

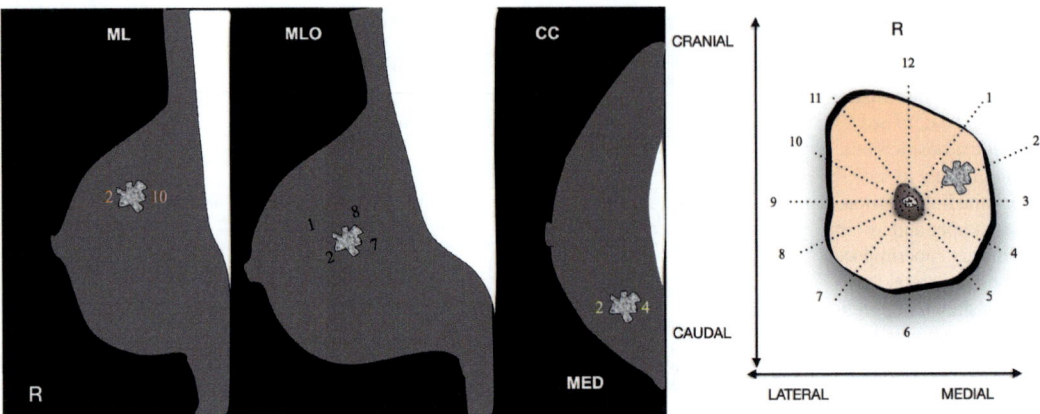

**Fig. 25.11** Lesion, which appeared central in MLO, appears in the upper quadrants in ML projection. It will therefore be identifiable (or 'triangulated') in the medial quadrant, in the case of the right breast, at 2 o'clock in the example shown. Compare with Fig. 13.7, topographic subdivision. Straight-line triangulation: the medial lesion 'rises' from MLO to ML (*MELE*, MEdiale saLE, cpoggimammoedu, MuffinRise)

## 25.6    Breast Subdivision into Anatomical Parts

The subdivision in anatomical parts is obtained using planes and lines as described in Sect. 25.4 and shown in Figs. 25.12 and 25.13.

1. Pectoralis major muscle: lunette-shaped and central, in well-executed CCs
2. Retromammary space
3. Glandular body
4. Intermammary cleft
5. Cooper's anterior ligaments or Duret' crests (or ridges)

Central line: divides the mammographic image up-down into two parts, in the typical layout, orange in Fig. 25.12. It can coincide with the midline in the CC, which divides the outer quadrant from the inner one, and with the median sagittal plane, which divides the breast into two parts. In the case shown, patient with breasts of different size and nipple position. On the right the midline (light blue line) does not coincide with the central line (orange). It coincides instead with the median sagittal plane. On the left the central line coincides neither with the median sagittal plane (green line), nor with the median line (the difference is however smaller than on the right).

1. Pectoralis major muscle: fan-shaped and convex, with wide documentation at the axillary level, in well-executed MLOs
2. Retromammary space
3. Glandular body
4. Creste del Duret
5. Posteroinferior quadrant (POSTINFQ), above and anterior with respect to IMF
6. Latissimus dorsi (its documentation depends on the patientti compliance, her anatomy and functionality of the upper limb: It represents the posterior wall of the axillary fossa)
7. Axillary lymph nodes.

High-quality mammography images provide very detailed anatomical information: in Fig. 25.14 are shown the crests of Duret, and the NAC, tending to retract on compression (Chap. 16). In Fig. 25.15, retracted and inverted nipples are shown. Section 25.4 indicates what to do if the patient shows this anatomical variant.

See also Chaps. 3, 9, 11, 17 and 27 for further information on radiographic anatomy, with a 360° view.

In the following pages, some mammographic examinations are presented, to sum up all the information given. In Fig. 25.16, a medium-sized breast: the anatomical parts described above are only fully visualised when considering both projections. It is thus possible to obtain a three-

**Fig. 25.12** Right and left CC projections

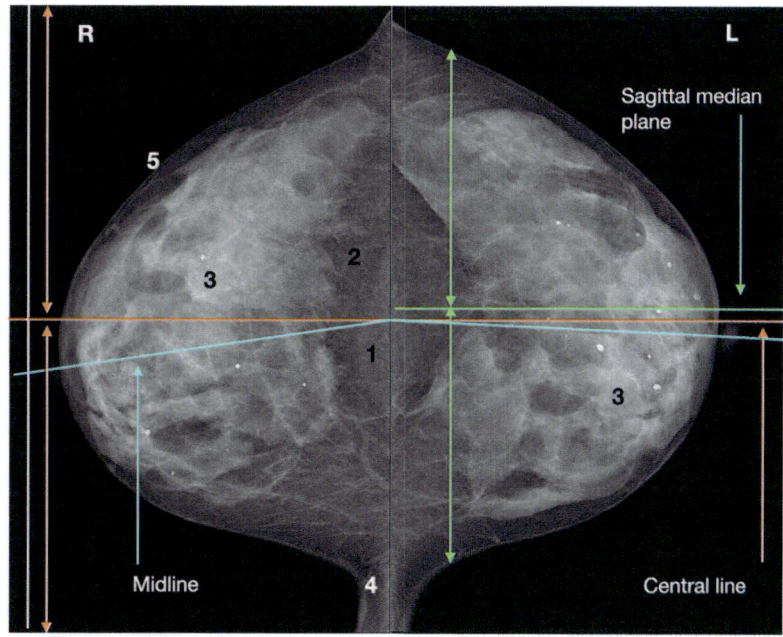

**Fig. 25.13** Right and left MLO projections

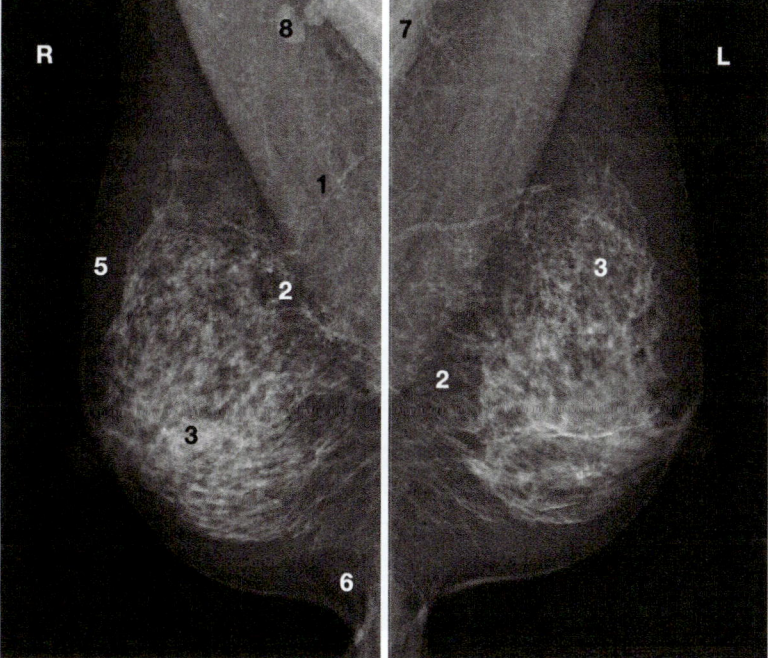

dimensional idea of the spatial distribution of the fibro-glandular tissue.

Figure 25.17 shows a very small breast; in most cases, due to the anatomy of the patient, it is very difficult to reach the deep tissue in the CC projection, even for a very experienced and competent radiographer

In Fig. 25.18, a breast of medium sized and consistency is shown. The two anatomical parameters, i.e. size and consistency, make it more difficult or easier to demonstrate all the tissue. In this example, the stretching manoeuvre and the process of compression appear optimal. Note the *hypodermis* (or subcutaneous fat), of similar

**Fig. 25.14** (**a**) Crests of Duret well demonstrated in dense breast (white arrow). (**b**) NAC tending to retract on compression

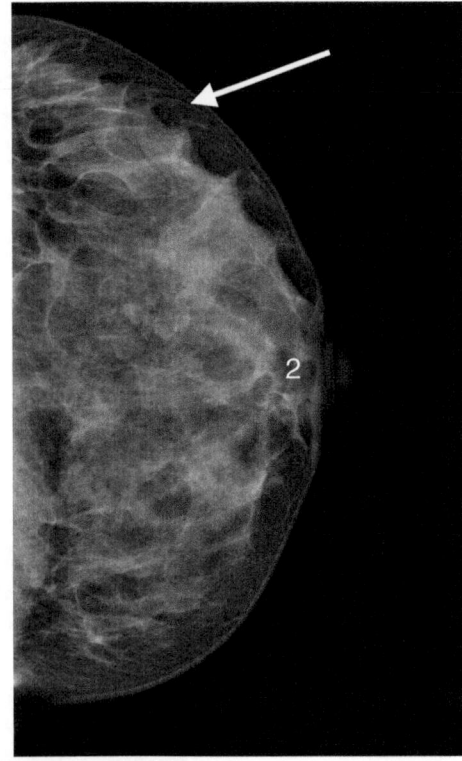

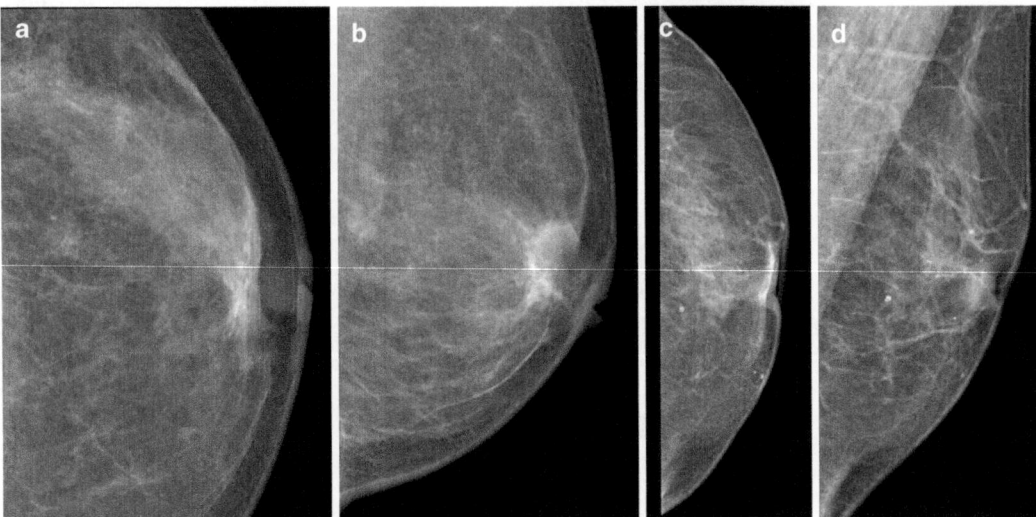

**Fig. 25.15** (**a, b**) Retracted nipple, in profile; (**c, d**) inverted nipple (or introflected), not in profile

thickness throughout, a factor associated with correct stretching and better reading of the mammary gland (Chaps. 3 and 9), as it is for the *tent sign,* Chap. 26, for both CCs. In spite of that, an important kinetic blurring can be seen at the axillary extension and the pectoralis major mus-

cle on the right side. The projection R-MLO must be repeated

The breasts on the two sides can be very different in size and consistency in the same woman. This anatomical factor complicates the work of the breast radiographer. The iconographic results

**Fig. 25.16** Medium-sized breast: OQ visible in its entirety only in the MLO projection, in CCs that do not fully document the deep planes (the fibroglandular tissue in the UOQ in the left MLO appears to extend deeper than in the right)

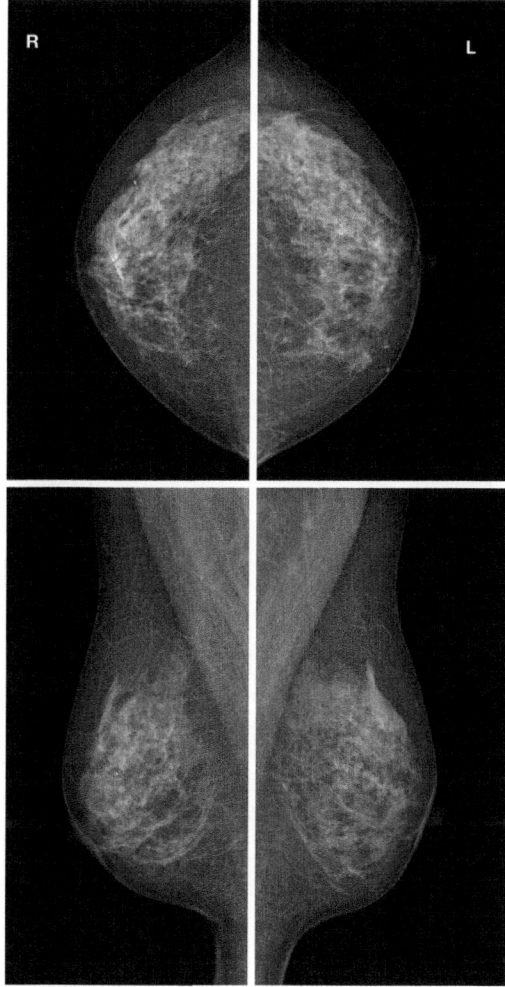

can therefore be very different, this time complicating the reader size and consistency in thdicated radiographer must adjust her/his technique for each individual breast (Fig. 25.19). Features are clearly seen in this example: (1) the transition between supQ and axillary prolongation (orange arrow); (2) the nipples, naturally pointing laterally and (3) the fingernail IMF (Sect. 25.4), see also Chaps. 26 and 27

As repeatedly reported, documentation of the IMF is considered to be one of the most difficult quality criteria to meet. Again, this should be closely related to the anatomy of the patient, especially for breast consistency. Despite the anatomical differences (see Fig. 25.20 for some of them, IMF level), the posterior–inferior quadrant (POSTINFQ) should always be included, see also Sect, 25.4, Chaps. 9, 11, 17 and 27.

**Fig. 25.17** Very small breast: difficulty in documenting the retromammary space in the CC projection, particularly the left side

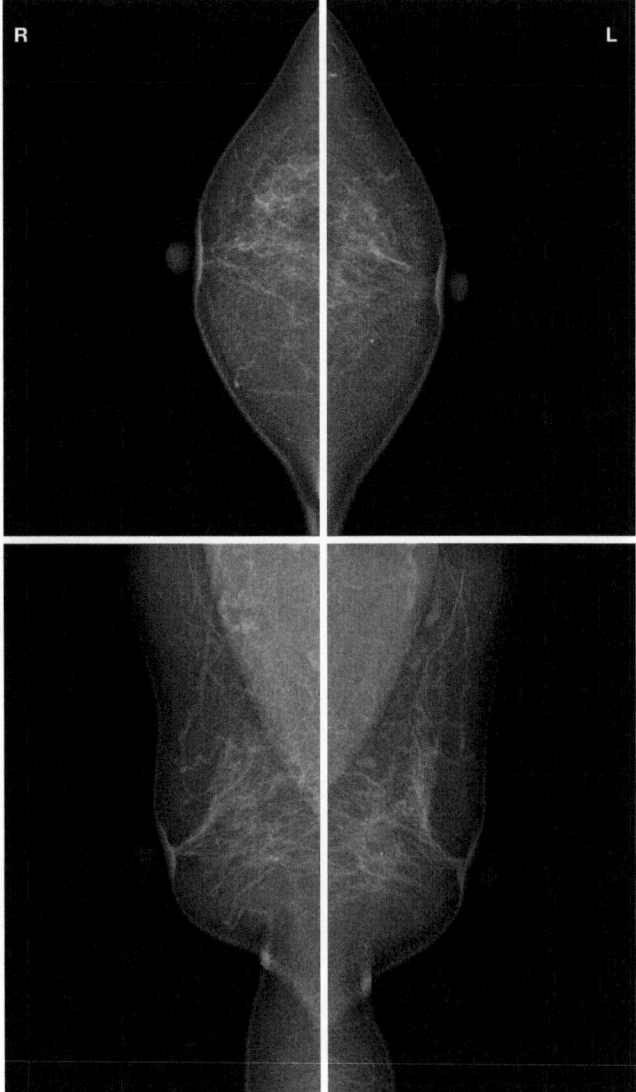

**Fig. 25.18** Breast of medium size and consistency. Excellent examination for positioning. Note the hypodermis, of almost similar thickness throughout. *Tent sign* for both CCs. Severe kinetic blurring at the axillary extension and the pectoralis major muscle on the right

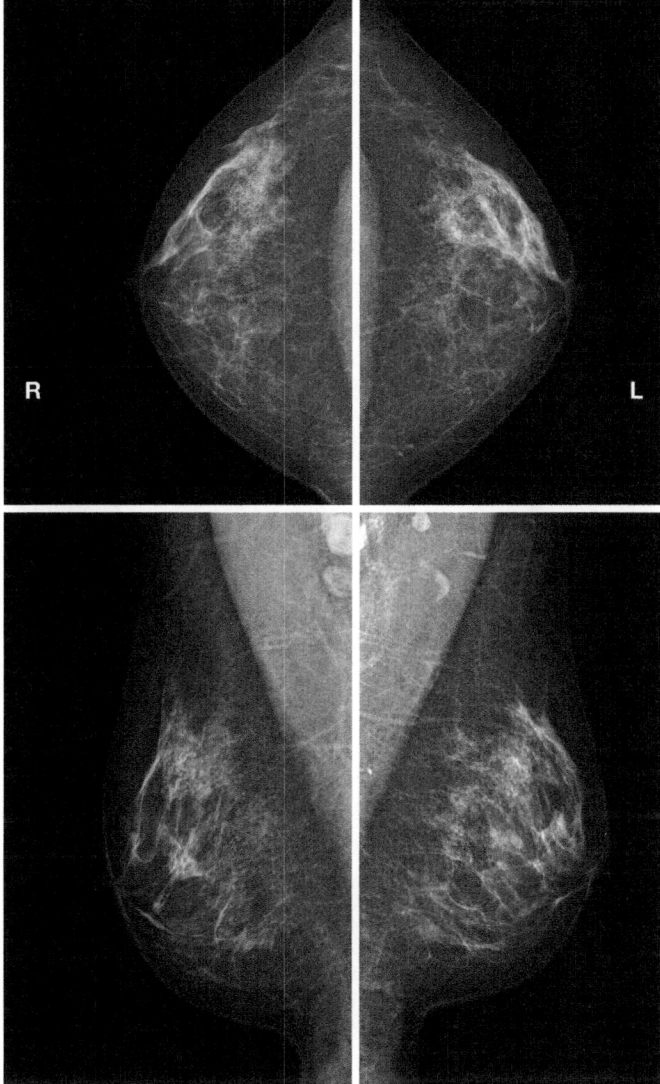

**Fig. 25.19** Breasts very different in size, natural direction of the nipple outward. Fingernail IMF. Clearly visible the transition between supQ and axillary prolongation (orange arrow)

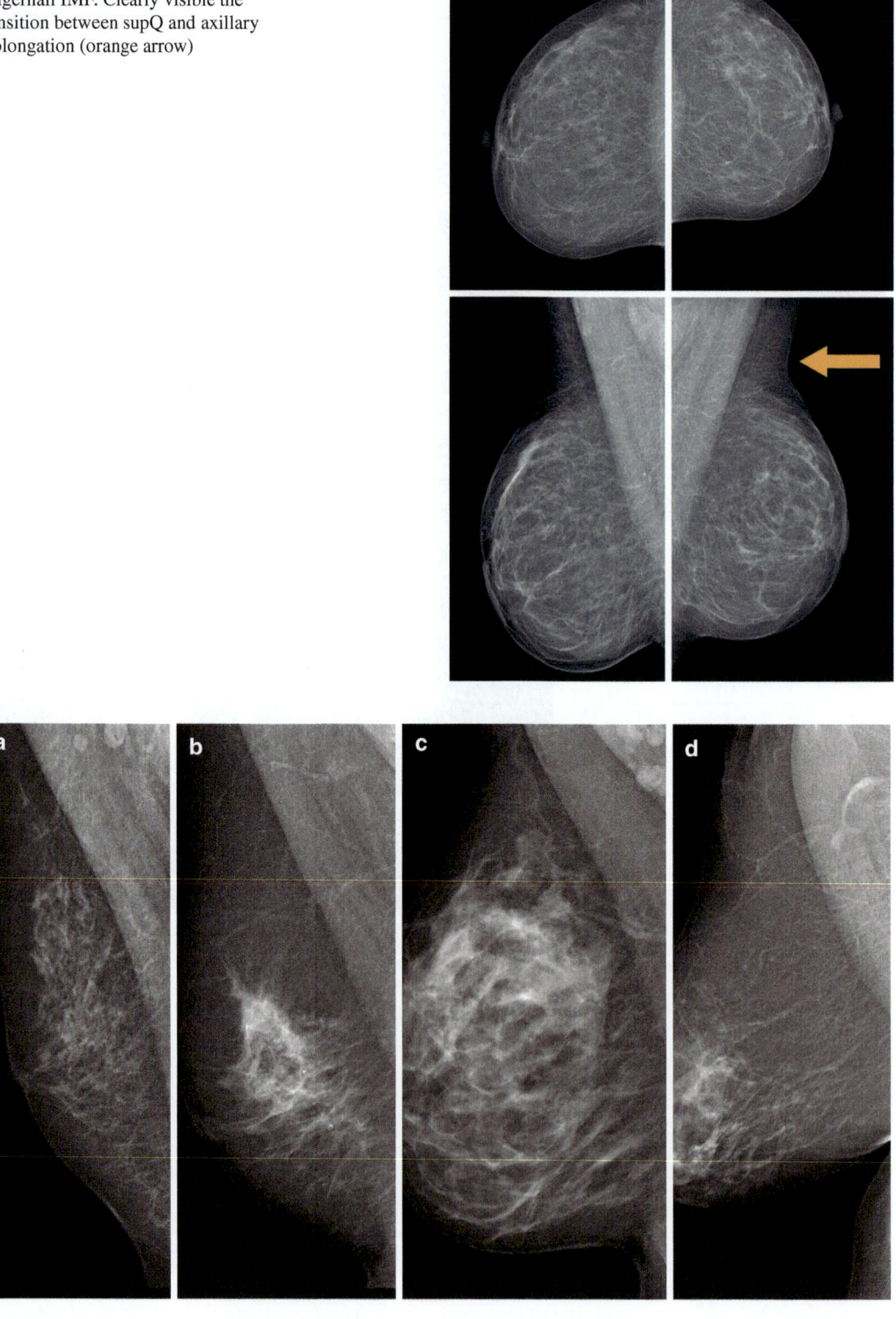

**Fig. 25.20** Different documentation of the IMF, right breast, by presentation high and ease of documentation. (**a**) Seamless with the chest, in small, medium-sized breast; (**b**) coming in low in medium-sized breast; (**c**) standard; (**d**) IMF very high in tuberous-like breast: POSTINFQ non fully shown

# References

1. Galli V, et al. Il Protocollo di valutazione della qualità tecnica dellcesame mammografico. Contributi 95 Regione Emilia Romagna RER; 2017.
2. Spurr K, et al. Mammography image quality: model for predicting compliance with posterior nipple line criterion. EJR. 2011;80:713–8. https://doi.org/10.1016/j.ejrad.2010.06.026.
3. Bentley K, et al. Mammography image quality: analysis of evaluation criteria using pectoral muscle presentation. Radiography. 2008;14:189–94. https://doi.org/10.1016/j.radi.2007.02.002.
4. Borrelli C, et al. NHS Breast Screening Programme *NHSBSP* publication number 49, 4th ed. 2016, PHE publications gateway number 2016426.
5. Breastscreen Australia National Accreditation Standards October (2015) BreastScreen Australia Accreditation Review Committee April (2017).
6. ACR clinical image testing: mammography (Revised 3-3-2023). https://accreditationsupport.acr.org/support/solutions/articles/11000065937-clinical-image-testing-mammography-revised-3-3-2023.
7. Perry N, et al. European guidelines for quality assurance in breast cancer screening and diagnosis. European Communities, 2006. isbn:92-79-01258-4.
8. Spurr K, et al. Mammography image quality and evidence based practice: analysis of the demonstration of the inframammary angle in the digital setting. EJR. 2018;100:76–84.
9. Spurr K, Poulos A. Evaluation of the pectoral muscle in mammography images: the Australian experience. EJR. 2009;1:12–21. https://doi.org/10.1016/j.ejradi.2008.11.003.
10. Gullien R, et al. Identifying the most common deviations in mediolateral-oblique (MLO) mammograms classified as framammary angle in the digital setting: POSTINFQ non fully shown. DeECR. 2010. https://doi.org/10.1594/ecr2010/B.059.

# Further Reading

Andolina V, Lille SL. Mammographic imaging: a practical guide, 3rd ed. Wolters Kluwer Lippincott Williams & Wilkins; 2011. isbn:978-60547-031-3.

Bassett WL, et al. Diagnosis of diseases of the breast. W.B. Saunders Company; 1997. isbn:0-7216-3796-5.

Fisher U, et al. Mammografia Capire, Applicare, Ottimizzare. Verduci Editore; 2005. isbn:88-7620-707-7.

Hogg P, et al. Digital mammography: a holistic approach. Springer; 2015. isbn:978-3-319-04830-7, 978-3-319-04831-4 (e-book). https://doi.org/10.1007/978-3-319-04831-4.

Pacifici S. Lo standard di qualità nella mammografia di screening. MB Edizioni; 2015. isbn:978-8894085303.

Tabar L, Dean PB. Teaching atlas of mammography, 4h ed. Thieme; 2012. isbn:978-3-13-640804-9.

Tabar L, et al. Breast cancer—The art and science of early detection with mammography. Thieme; 2005. isbn:3-13-135371-6 (GTV).

Tabar L, et al. Understanding the breast in health and disease in 3D, vol. 1. C & C Offset Printing; 2012.

Van Landsveld-Verhoeven, C. The right focus manual on mammography positioning technique. LRCB; 2013. isbn/ean:978-90-821079-1-3.

# The Poggi Method: A New Approach to the Production of High-Quality Mammography

# 26

## 26.1 Training the Breast Radiographer

The first thing to point up when talking about the radiographer working in Senology is that she/he is a hybrid figure, which is difficult to describe. By "hybrid", we mean that advanced skills are required in fields generally not included in the diagnostic radiographer profile. They are briefly and incompletely summarised in Table 26.1, see also Chap. 24 on *job description*.

The process by which a mammography examination is performed is extremely complex. In the author's opinion, it must be dealt with a ***problem-solving*** approach. It involves a series of decisions to be made, and steps to be taken, in order to meet the quality criteria in terms of extension and proper stretching of the acquired tissue and acquisition geometry. Often, the steps are to be also taken in the exact sequence because otherwise the result may vary greatly. This includes the appropriate choice of compression value. The process is presented, simplifying enormously, in Table 26.2.

It is a process that requires years of work in a Senology division to hone and many mistakes. Skills acquired so painstakingly must be absolutely taught and thus form part of a specialised course that concretely and effectively trains the breast radiographer.

**Table 26.1** Competences of the mammographer

| | |
|---|---|
| 1 | Advanced anatomical and anatomical–radiographic knowledge (not only of the breast), including musculoskeletal/postural function |
| 2 | Of an organisational nature on screening programmes, and the various clinical-diagnostic pathways |
| 3 | Always up-to-date on treatment therapies and technical-surgical procedures for appropriate hystorical data collection |
| 4 | In various areas of biomedical breast imaging, in addition to mammography: magnetic resonance imaging, tomosynthesis, stereotaxis, CESM, etc. |
| 5 | For dose monitoring and overall patient safety |
| 6 | For the overall management of the patient from an anatomical-functional point of view, but also from a relational point of view, to achieve patient compliance |
| 7 | In building a shared role with the other professionals in the team |

**Table 26.2** Procedure for performing the mammographic examination

| | |
|---|---|
| 1 | The problems to be addressed with the individual patient, of a behavioural nature, and of adapting the positioning technique to produce quality mammograms, must be identified |
| 2 | Solutions to the problems encountered must be implemented, thinking of possible alternatives, and selecting the best ones, carrying out our mental process |
| 3 | The result should be monitored, so that it can be used again under similar conditions, depending on its success |
| 4 | All this within a few minutes |

**Table 26.3** The three steps for categorizing patients into the three groups, Poggi method

| | |
|---|---|
| Step 1 | Visual evaluation of the anatomy and volume of the breast to be studied: "**Mammography as photography©**". For this, it is absolutely essential that the patient is made to undress up to the waist. The posture of the patient should also be considered |
| Step 2 | Visual evaluation of the width of the attachment base of the breast to the thorax and the AP base/volume relationship. This indicates the degree of ease with which it is assumed that the breast will be detachable from the thorax, and thus, how easy it will be to document deep planes. This is referred to in the Poggi method as: "**Theory of anatomical relationships©**" |
| Step 3 | Touch evaluation of the consistency of the breast, including the skin envelope, and its thickness. It allows the selection of the appropriate compression value. It is described in the Poggi method as the "**Evaluation of the compression and stretching resistance index©**" |

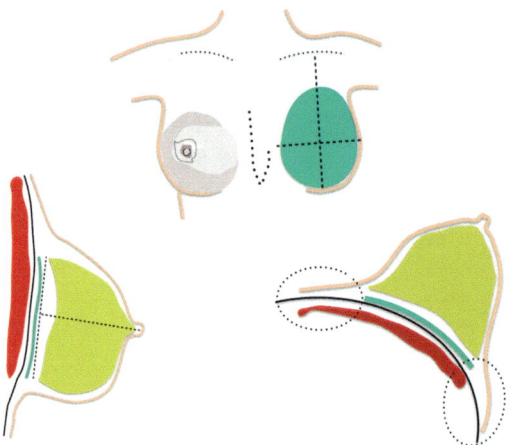

**Fig. 26.1** Breast attachment base or footprint in green; conus or volume in yellow and skin envelope in pink. Indicated the relationships between volume in AP and footprint with dashed line and connections of the breast to the thorax with dotted ovals

## 26.2 Categorisation of Patients into Three Groups: The Three Steps

In the first instance, the standardisation of positioning and compression must be pursued, despite the incredible anatomical and cooperation variability of patients. In the Poggi method, this is simplified by categorising patients into three groups. The idea is to be able to manage patients with any physicality, foreseeing the macro problems that may arise in each group. This can be done knowing the specific adjustments to do in order to improve the final result. The division into the three groups takes place in three steps (Table 26.3).

## 26.3 Anatomo-radiographic Parameters: Breast Attachment Base on the Thorax, Volume or Conus and Skin Envelope

These are parameters derived from the reconstructive surgical school of Dr. Blondeel, P.N., MD, an internationally renowned plastic surgeon

[1]. This was learned from a series of articles written by doctor Blondeel, from 2009 and later. Subsequently declined, adapted and modified for the radiographic study of the breast to form the basis of the Poggi method. The method was then implemented, progressively refining it, in the following years of activity.

**Breast attachment base:** *this is the area where the breast is attached to the chest wall* (Fig. 26.1). It is a parameter that strongly impacts the mammographic product. In general, the more extensive the base of attachment, the less easy it is to document the deep planes of the breast. It should be assessed in the superoinferior and laterolateral directions. Also known as *footprint.*

**Breast volume:** *this is its projection outward* (Fig. 26.1). It is an anatomical parameter that breast radiographers are used to assess immediately, having to choose the size of the compression paddle appropriate for each patient (Chap. 16). However, not only the antero-posterior dimension must be considered, but also the laterolateral, in some cases very important, even in the presence of a medium-sized breast. The height of the patient, and therefore the actual size proportion of the breast volume in relation to the detector, must also be considered.

**Skin envelope:** *this is the anatomical part that surrounds the breast and anchors it to the chest, consisting of skin and subcutaneous fat* (Chap. 3 and Fig. 26.1). The lateral and medial anchor points are important, as they give information on the documentation of the relative deep planes (dotted ovals in Fig. 26.1).

## 26.4    Notes on the Method Poggi (Dealt with Extensively in the Text: *Performing the Mammography Examinations: The Poggi Method*, Poggi, C., Not Published)

The Poggi method aims to demonstrate the breast as extensively as possible and as faithfully as possible. Hence, the method's first dogma, "*mammography as photography*". To achieve this, *it is necessary to acquire a solid theoretical basis on anatomy and radiographic anatomy*. It enables one to relate *the images produced (2D) to reality (3D) and thus to know how to correlate them exactly.*

The patient must therefore be made to undress up to the waist, completely. This is the only way to observe how the breast develops, in all its directions, in that specific patient. Also to actually hypothesise what its boundaries are with the bony and muscular parts. For example, there are women in whom the base of attachment of the breast to the chest extends far toward the axilla. In such cases, attention should be paid to complete documentation (as far as possible) of the OQ. This is to be obtained without rotating the breast. The frontal visual assessment of the patient can be misleading, as the nipple may appear very lateral as in dominant inner quadrant-breast, but in reality, part of the outer quadrant could be hidden in the axilla (see below).

The extension of the breast must also be considered globally in the anterior–posterior direction from the nipple to the base of attachment. There are congenital malformations of the thorax that must be known, Chap. 10. This in order to improve the documentation of the breast as far as

possible, always adopting the right manoeuvres to protect the protruding bony parts. Reducing the patient's discomfort for the passage of the compression paddle, or for the simple leaning on the detector, is important. The breast radiographer needs to know the exact boundaries of the breast with the *pectoralis major muscle*, and how this extends in all directions, so as to be able to document it and to assess on the image its correct shape, width and length. She/he has to know how much can and should be obtained of it for each individual patient. Adopting the three-group system is assumed to simplify this step. Equally, it is necessary to know how the shape of the muscle and breast change when the patient lifts her arm, to perform the oblique projection. What the position and anatomy of the latissimus dorsi is, and how to document it, when possible. And of course, to do so without artefacts. All the other anatomical portions apart from the breast that must be part of the mammographic images are also to be considered. That is to say, everything that surrounds the breast itself, in all directions.

It must also be known how to manage the *skin envelope, which is to be understood as the first great variable in the production of quality mammograms*, and this is despite the fact that it is not usually mentioned in mammography textbooks. There are in fact considerable differences in thickness and consistency between one person and another, and more generalised differences between one area and another, in the same breast. For example, the connective fibres are denser toward the sternum. This influences: (1) the positioning technique; (2) the results that can be obtained for each individual patient; (3) the compression and (4) the stretching action, for the lesser or greater ease of producing skin folds, but also for the extent of tissue that can be demonstrated (Fig. 26.2). see also Chaps. 9 and 17.

The **acquisition geometry is** very important (first parameter: *parallelism between superior and inferior planes in the CC and medial and lateral in the MLO*. Second parameter: *perpendicularity between the thoracic wall and median axial and median sagittal planes,* Chap. 9), Fig. 26.3.

The **documentation of the connections to the thorax, internal and external** could be

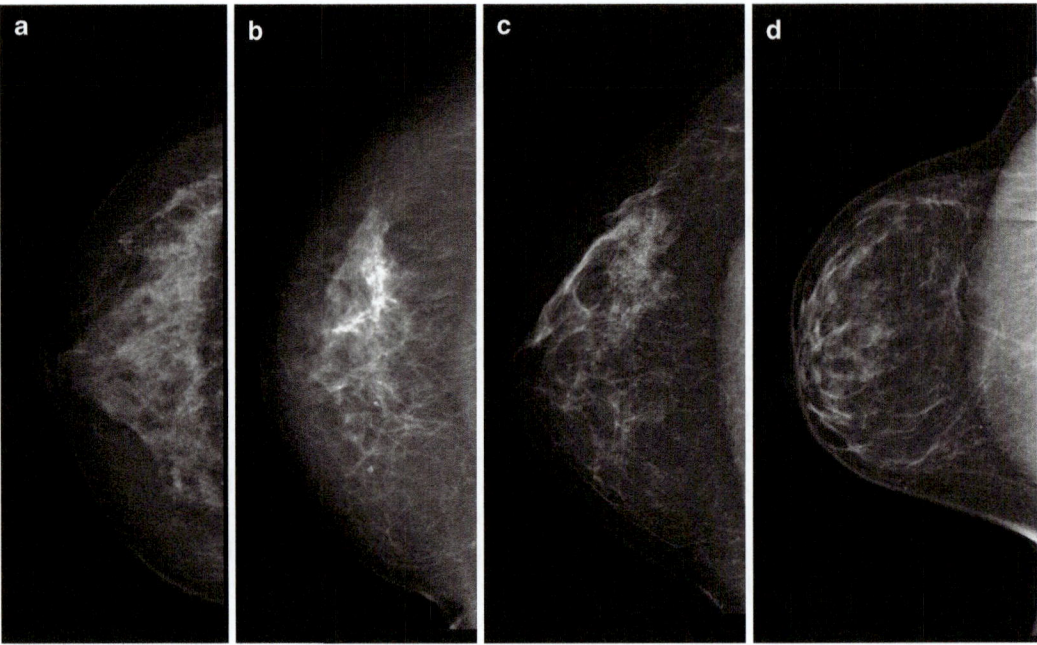

**Fig. 26.2** Different degree of breast consistency or texture and detachability from the thorax. Going from a to d decreases the consistency, i.e. increases the detachability from the thorax and ease of stretching. Note how these two parameters affect the documentation of the deep planes, both central (pectoral muscle), external and internal (connections to the thorax)

**Fig. 26.3** Acquisition geometry parallelism between the upper and lower planes in the CC projection and perpendicularity between the chest wall and the median axial and median sagittal planes of the single side (1 and 2 parameter)

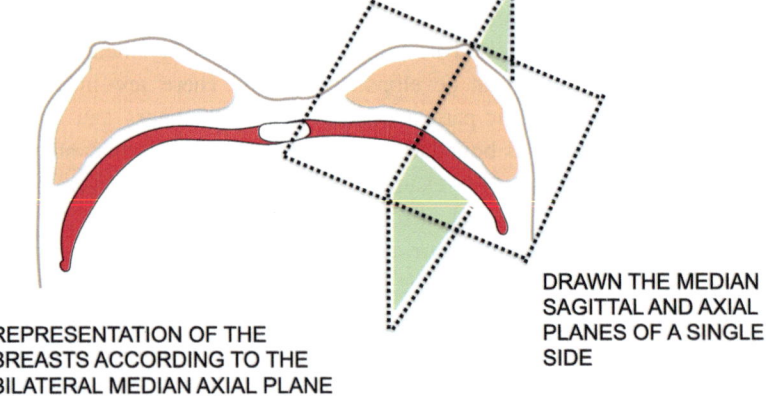

REPRESENTATION OF THE
BREASTS ACCORDING TO THE
BILATERAL MEDIAN AXIAL PLANE

DRAWN THE MEDIAN
SAGITTAL AND AXIAL
PLANES OF A SINGLE
SIDE

added, in the author's opinion, as a new quality criterion for the documentation of the deep planes, in addition to the pectoral muscle. The muscle in fact only concerns the central part and showing it on the CC projection does not necessarily imply that the connections have also been documented. The connections give information about the extent of the acquired tissue and give the correct acquisition geometry.

One aspect that is very little considered overall in mammography is the patient's **posture**, which is part of the three-step assessment as proposed in this method (see below).

## 26.5 Describing the Three Groups A, B and C

The rationale behind this categorisation is that standardising positioning and compression is a very complex process. It is therefore proposed to make it simpler by individuating group-specific errors, which can thus be prevented, or at least minimised. The results of the retrospective qualitative multicentre project **CATER** (Poggi, C.) **CATegorisation of Error by anatomy and posture** (unpublished) would appear to tend, as hypothesised, in that direction. This is in spite of the many confounding factors determined in large part by the insufficient preparation from which almost all operators in the field suffer. Mammography is not considered to be a difficult modality as MRI, for example, and therefore would not require lengthy training. It seems that there are indeed specific and characteristic errors in each group, for which ad hoc solutions are proposed. Below are the tables with the parameters of the individual groups, called A, B and C, simply, Tables 26.4, 26.5 and 26.6.

See Fig. 26.4, for example, of group A, Fig. 26.5 for group B and Fig. 26.6 for group C.

**Table 26.4** Parameters group A: visual and tactile assessment of the patient

| | |
|---|---|
| Footprint | Very extensive, always in the superoinferior direction, often also in the laterolateral direction |
| Volume | Small/medium; footprint/AP volume > 2 |
| Skin envelope | Hard to the touch |
| Consistency | Very high (poor elasticity). High stretching resistance index, especially in CC projection. High, medium/high compression resistance index, for both CC and MLO projections |
| Degree of ease of detachability of the breast from the chest | Poor. Connections to the thorax difficult to document; also very difficult to show IMF |

**Table 26.5** Group B parameters: visual and tactile assessment of the patient

| | |
|---|---|
| Footprint | Small to medium |
| Volume | Medium to large (but there is also a small volume group); footprint/AP volume = 1 |
| Skin envelope | Mobile, soft |
| Consistency | Medium stretching resistance index, intermediate compression resistance index |
| Degree of ease of detachability of the breast from the chest | Good. Generally well demonstrable chest connections, both medial and lateral. IMF also generally well documented |

**Table 26.6** Parameters group C: visual and tactile assessment of the patient

| | |
|---|---|
| Footprint | Small to medium |
| Volume | Large to very large. The smallest dimension is in the superoinferior direction, the largest dimension in the AP direction; footprint/AP volume < 1 |
| Skin envelope | From mobile to too mobile |
| Consistency | Low, very low stretching resistance index. No resistance to compression. Skin envelope tends to be loose, ease of creating skin folds high |
| Degree of ease of detachability of the breast from the chest | Very well detachable from the chest. Degree of ptosis sometimes severe, connections generally well documented. If one can block the breast effectively, and avoid artifacts from a prominent abdomen, IMF generally well documented |

**Fig. 26.4** Example group A, footprint in green and volume in AP in yellow. See text

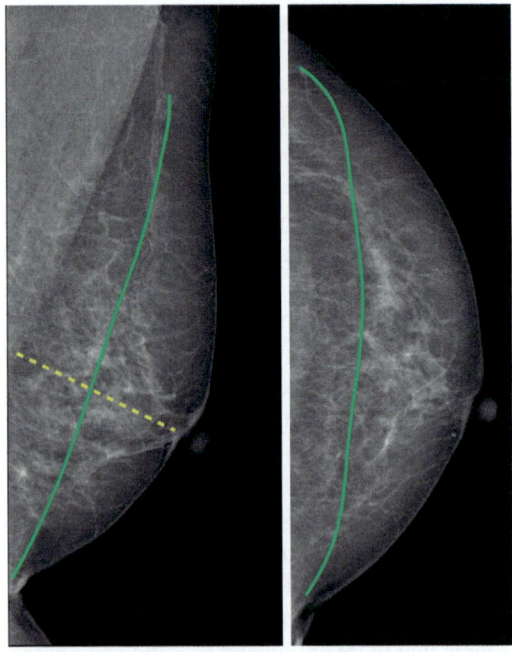

**Fig. 26.5** Example of group B

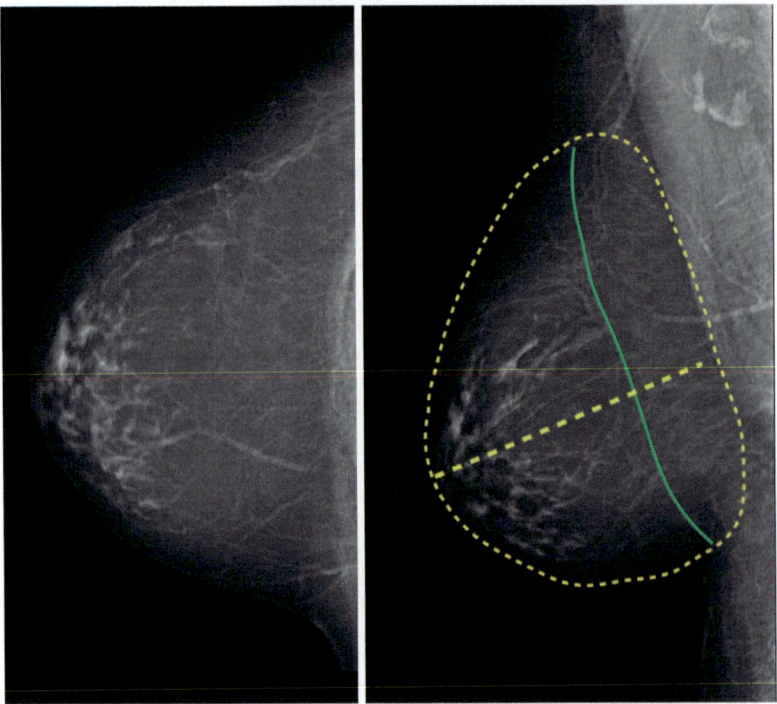

**Fig. 26.6** Example of group C

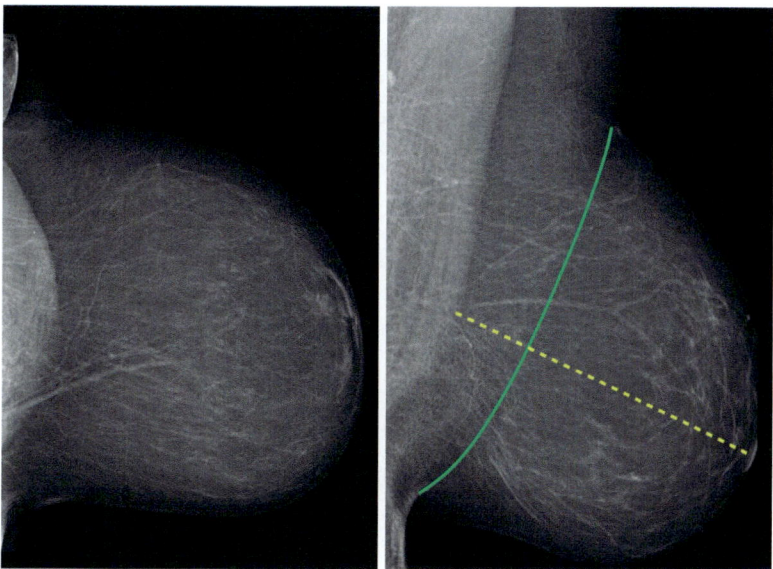

## 26.6    On Captured Images, Categorisation

In Fig. 26.4, example of group A: the ratio of the footprint (in green) to the volume in the anteroposterior direction (yellow line) is greater than two. Footprint also very large in the laterolateral direction. In Fig. 26.5, example of group B: footprint represented in green and the volume in the AP direction with the yellow dotted line. The ratio between them is approximately 1. Both medial and lateral chest connections are more easily documented. Generally well-shown the IMF. In Fig. 26.6 example of group C: the volume in AP direction is very important, the footprint is medium, sometimes small, if compared to volume.

## 26.7    The Correct Acquisition Geometry

Perpendicularity of mid-sagittal plane to the thoracic wall, as stated by the second geometry parameter, is fundamental to include deep places correctly without rotations. Forcing the midline coincides with the median sagittal plane, in breasts with different IQ and OQ in size, leads to tissue loss (Fig. 26.7a). In Fig. 26.7b, the geometrically correct acquisition. The two images

were taken on the same patient, see also Chaps. 9 and 17.

In Fig. 26.8a, the tent sign is shown (orange lines): indicates having documented lateral and medial connection in the CC projection, and so how the skin envelope that wraps the breast anchors it to the chest. It appears as a tent with the vertex on the nipple. In Fig. 26.8b, complete documentation of the deep planes, tent sign present, in a case of a patient with OQ very developed toward the axilla (much bigger than the IQ).

In Fig. 26.9, right and left side MLOs are compared, in the case of equal-sized medial and lateral quadrants. In the left side, it could be seen: (1) the nipple is not in profile, obliterating the retroareolar area; (2) the upper anterior outline of the gland is "crowded" (large red oval) and not readable and (3) the pectoralis major muscle is more extensively documented than the right. This last feature could be considered positive; however, it is at the expense of deep tissues in the direction of rotation. There is certainly a rotation, since if the medial and lateral quadrants are of equal size, being placed correctly parallel to each other, the nipple as a result appears naturally in profile. Assuming that it is a laterally directed rotation, lateral deep tissue will be missing to a greater or lesser degree depending on the extent of rotation.

**Fig. 26.7** Perpendicularity of mid-sagittal plane to the thoracic wall (second parameter) and documentation of deep planes. In image **a**, laterally directed rotation to make the midline coincide with the median sagittal plane, in breasts with unequal IQ and OQ. Note the difference in extension of the acquired tissue between the two images **a** and **b**, taken on the same patient

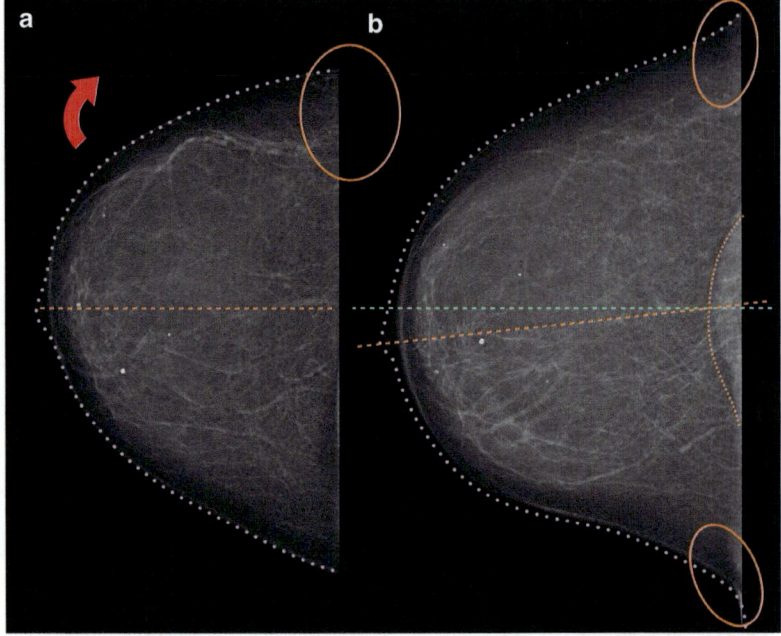

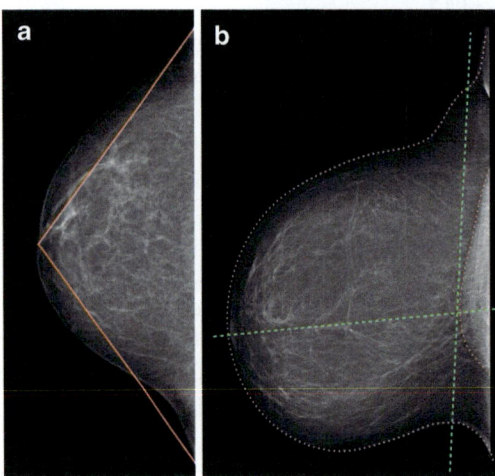

**Fig. 26.8** Tent sign (Poggi, C.©): it appears as a tent with the vertex on the nipple (image **a**). (**b**) Complete (external, internal and central) deep plane documentation in the CC projection, in the case of a patient with significant development of the OQ toward the axilla

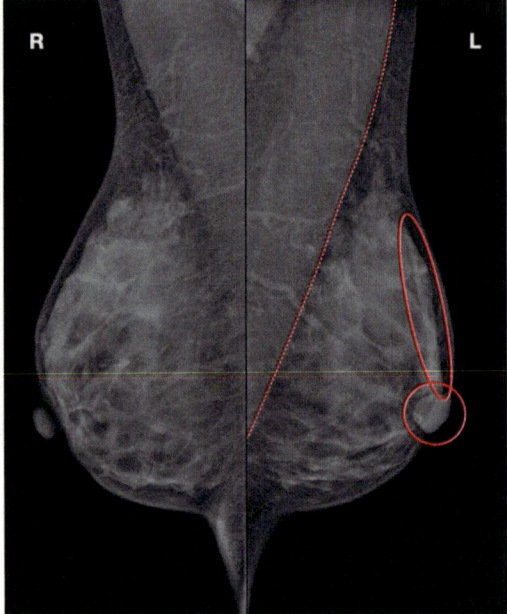

**Fig. 26.9** Parallelism between medial and lateral planes in MLO projection (first parameter) with equal-sized medial and lateral quadrants: left and right compared. The left breast presents: (1) The nipple not in profile; (2) The upper anterior outline of the gland is 'crowded' (large red oval); (3) The pectoralis major muscle is more extensively documented than the right. However, it is at the expense of deep tissues in the direction of rotation. Incorrect

**Fig. 26.10** (**a** and **b**)
Same patient: woman in
whom the OQ extends
toward the axilla. The
failure to implement the
manoeuvre for
later-extended OQ,
image **a**, resulted in the
loss of the deep planes
demonstrated in image **b**

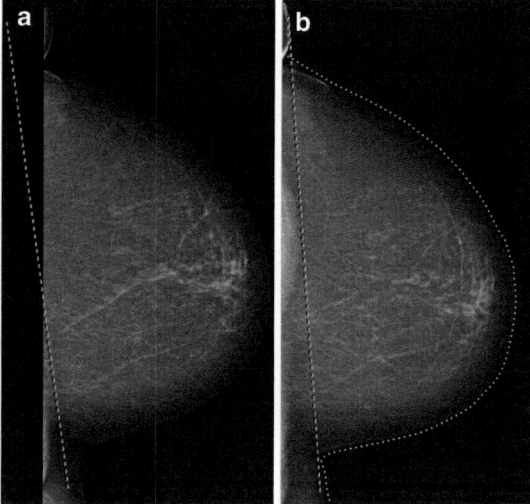

In Fig. 26.10a, b, a CC projection of the same patient is compared. It is the case of a woman in whom the outer quadrant extends toward the axilla. Failure to consider this anatomical feature in Fig. 26.10a has led to a loss of the deep planes, demonstrated instead in Fig. 26.10b. It is although a not perfect satisfaction of the second acquisition parameter, but better than that achieved in image 1 (compare the angle of the red dotted lines: that line should be perpendicular to the mid sagittal plane).

In Figs. 26.7, 26.8, 26.9, and 26.10 could be noted that the extent of the tissue acquired is greater when the two acquisition geometry parameters are met, and how this allows a more faithful demonstration of the organ studied.

## 26.8 Manoeuvre for Documentation of OQ that Develops Toward the Axilla

There are women who have an OQ that develops very much toward the axilla, especially in group C, and which can escape, as already indicated above, from an initial frontal assessment. It is easier to see when the patient is on her side.

Once the breast has been brought onto the detector, the OQ must be pulled further forward, taking care that the repeatedly mentioned geom-etry conditions are met, especially the perpendicularity with respect to the median sagittal plane, see Chap. 9 and Fig. 26.10.

## 26.9 Assessing at a Glance the Satisfaction of the Correct Acquisition Geometry and Stretching: The "Arc Sign"

In order to quickly assess the appropriateness of acquisition geometry and stretching in the CC projection are important:

1. Both the shape and position of the pectoralis muscle
2. The presence of the two connections of the skin envelope to the thorax (tent sign)
3. The thickness of the hypodermis layer, which must remain the same all around

One could mention a further sign, which is not always possible to observe, because it depends on multiple anatomical factors, named by the author *"arch sign (with the arrow stuck)"*. It is assessed looking how the anterior profile of the FGT is "drawn" in the CC projection. In general, it is arranged in both quadrants, in women of child-bearing age, to form a kind of arch (Fig. 26.11a). Even in menopausal women, the FGT tends to

**Fig. 26.11** (**a**) Arc sign with the arrow stuck (which corresponds to the median sagittal plane, Chap. 25); (**b**) CC for OQ in which the second parameter is obviously not satisfied, first parameter is (*positive arc sign*); (**c**) First and second parameter sufficiently satisfied, but due to incorrect stretching the convexity is partly lost, with flattening of the glandular profile (*negative arc signs*)

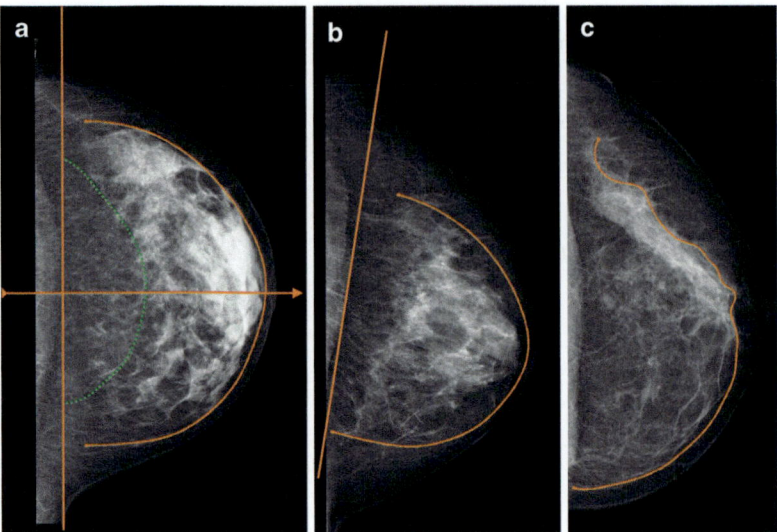

maintain this characteristic anterior convexity, even as it is gradually lost with advancing age. A second, more internal convexity, which is the anterior wall of the retromammary space, is sometimes well visible (green in Fig. 26.11a).

The deformation of this natural convexity of the FGT (*negative arc sign*) is sometimes produced by the radiographer with an incorrect rotation or stretching, but in some cases, it can also be due to an ongoing pathological process. Once again, therefore, the extreme importance of the quality of the radiographer's work is to be highlighted.

## 26.10 The Patient's Posture in Mammography

Various aspects are taken into account in the Poggi method:

1. The angle of approach of the patient's thorax to the detector
2. The posture of her hips
3. Shoulder and neck position
4. Relative thorax–hips position

See also Chap. 9 and the material on YouTube on the pectoral muscle (links at the back of the book).

## 26.11 In the Case of Patients with Lordosis or Hyperlordosis

They present an anterior tilt of the pelvis, leading to a posterior angle, and a consequent accentuation of the curvature of the lumbar spine. The posterior angle of the pelvis is counterbalanced by an identical angle of the thorax. This means that it will be more likely in these cases to lose the upper deep tissues, in the CC projection, as can be seen from the drawing in Fig. 26.12. This is because the upper and lower quadrants have to be parallel to each other.

### 26.11.1 Posture Correction in Lordotic Patients

CC projection: it is necessary to re-balance thorax and pelvis, bringing them on the same line. In this way the condition of geometry of parallelism mentioned above is fulfilled. Furthermore, it will be possible to choose the right height of the detector, a step in conducting the examination that is fundamental precisely for reaching and documenting deep tissues.

MLO projection: equally important is the alignment of thorax and pelvis. The anterior tilt of the pelvis can result in a receding POSTINFQ

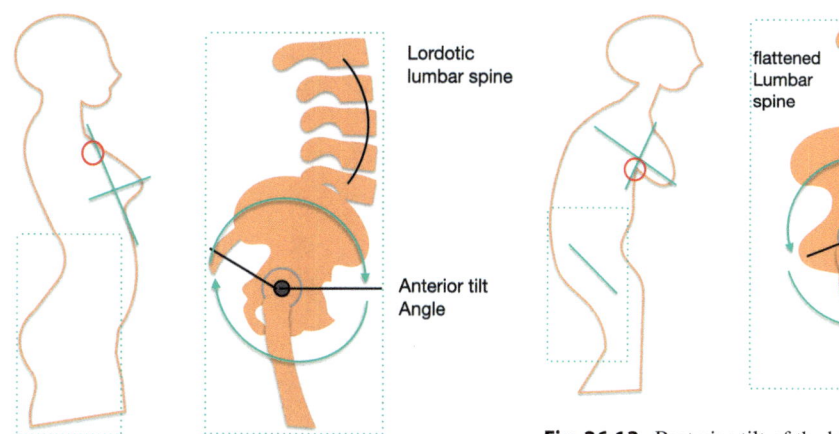

**Fig. 26.12** Anterior tilt of the hips inducing an accentuation of the lumbar curvature. Lordosis or hyperlordosis; associated posterior thoracic angle. Probable loss of upper deep breast tissue in the CC projection. In MLO projection: probable loss of the lower deep tissues (poor IMF), and sometimes poor documentation in width of the pectoralis major muscle (for stiffening)

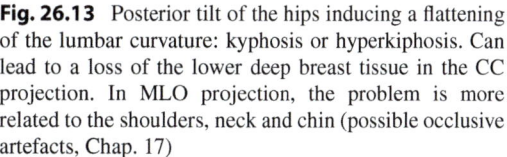

**Fig. 26.13** Posterior tilt of the hips inducing a flattening of the lumbar curvature: kyphosis or hyperkiphosis. Can lead to a loss of the lower deep breast tissue in the CC projection. In MLO projection, the problem is more related to the shoulders, neck and chin (possible occlusive artefacts, Chap. 17)

and IMF. This posture is common in patients belonging to group A. Usually, the IMF is of small size and the breast is of high consistency. The two features make the documentation of the inferior posterior area not easy.

## 26.12   In the Case of Patients with Kyphosis

Kyphotic patients, but more accurately they should be called hyper-kyphotic, are patients for whom the production of quality mammograms is even more complex than usual. The shoulders and neck are forward, and for this reason, the neck muscles may be constricted and stiffened. There may be an anterior shift or angulation of the hips, associated with a flattening of the lumbar curvature, as well as pathological accentuation of the thoracic curvature.

For these patients, again, the main problem is determined by the difficulty of documenting the lower deep tissues in CC projection, and moving the neck and shoulders away from the FOV.

**Correction of posture in (hyper)kyphotic patients**: as far as the thorax and pelvis are concerned, it is necessary to bring them back to the same line, as far as possible. That is to say, bringing the hips back a little for CC projection and straightening the shoulders. It is especially difficult to move the neck backward and medially (Chap. 9) because of the stiffening of the muscles in the area. The shoulders are also often blocked with anterior rotation of the humeral head, leading to a loss of lateral deep tissue and associated occluding artefact (see Chap. 17), Fig. 26.13.

These general considerations on patient's posture in mammography should also include assessments of her *physical phenotype,* or *somatotype,* which are based on anthropometric measurements (Parnell, Heath-Carter system). This include stature, weight, diameters and circumferences, with a classification using a scale of 1–7. Although it has been widely used in sports, and the results are certainly interesting, it is a system that has not yet been sufficiently studied in the field of diagnostic imaging. Moreover, to my knowledge, it has never been applied for mammography studies, for which a simplification related to the timing of the examination would in any case be necessary.

The influence of the relative angle between the patient's thorax and hips on the extent of the acquired tissue could be noted in Fig. 26.14. In Fig. 26.14a, the image presented denotes excellent arm and shoulder positioning and therefore

**Fig. 26.14** Influence of the relative angle between the patient's thorax and hips on the extent of the acquired tissues. (**a**) Very good positioning of shoulder and arm, but no documentation of the IMF. (**b**) Central and inferior deep tissues (red oval 2) are missing. (**c**) POSTINFQ (red oval 3) and the IMF are missing. Sagging breast

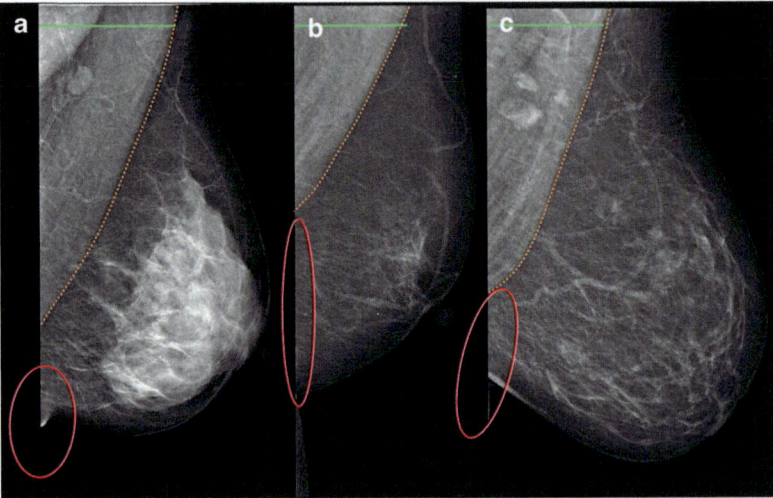

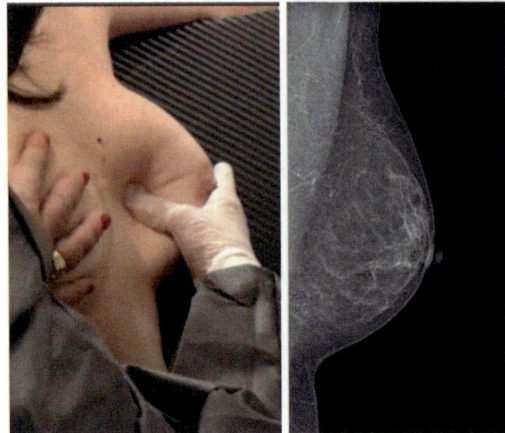

**Fig. 26.15** Thorax and hips on the same line, after lateral rotation and advancement (if any) of the hips, for documentation of the IMF. Screen shot from video. Arm and shoulder not positioned

a large documentation of the axillary fossa. The hips back, however, did not allow documentation of the IMF. In Fig. 26.14b sufficiently correct positioning of arm and shoulder, but the patient bowed at the waist, with straight hips. This resulted in the loss of deep central and inferior tissue (red oval 2). IMF just behind the FOV. In Fig. 26.14c, there is an optimal documentation of the pectoralis major, but the posterior–inferior quadrant and IMF (red oval 3) are missing. The probable cause of this sagging breast is inadequate compression, rather than positioning.

In Fig. 26.15 shown the relationship between thorax and hips required for a correct mammography; they must be on the same line.

## 26.13 Posture in the Three Groups, A, B and C

Posture has a substantial impact in mammography positioning technique. In particular, patients with lordosis/hyperlordosis and hyperkhyphosis are found in group A. In group B, posture of the hips forward in relation to the chest is common, as in group C. In the latter, in some cases, it is associated with a prominent abdomen.

These aspects must be taken into account in the positioning in order to achieve a high-quality result (see examples Cases 1 and 2 shown below).

## 26.14 CATER Project Results

The CATER project was interrupted by the SARS-CoV-2 pandemic (unpublished). Considering the data resulting from it, it would appear that the patients in group A and group C are the most difficult. In fact, the number of *inadequate* images (Chaps. 11 and 12) is higher in A and C groups, although group B is by far the most represented. Furthermore, the most frequent errors are significantly different in each of the three groups. Proposing therefore an "adjusted" technique for each group, as depicted in the Poggi method, by posture anatomy and breast consistency, could actually be a winning strategy.

*The mammography positioning technique must absolutely be standardised, despite, or rather because of its extreme complexity. However, multiple aspects, such as those mentioned above, must be taken into account. This is in order to know in advance what difficulties are most likely to be encountered in that individual patient, depending on her belonging to one of the three groups, and what are the best solutions to deal with them successfully.*

## 26.14.1  Future Investigations in the Field of Mammography

It would be interesting to extend the study of the **patient's somatotype,** to see what impact it might have on the quality of the examination produced in mammography, beyond what the author evaluated. It would also be interesting to study what **potential** could be **exploited in individual mammographers, according to their somatotype.** Again, the aim is to make performing mammography easier and more ergonomic, so to

produce images richer in diagnostic information, in extension of the tissue captured, and in accuracy of representation (fidelity of reproduction). And above all, make it in a standardised manner, for an increasingly earlier diagnosis of breast cancer.

Below are two examples of group B women. The photographs presented are of patients who have granted their permission according to the law on privacy protection EU2016/679 and transposition in Italy D.Lgs 101/2018.

### Case 1. Poggi Method Compared to Standard Method
#### Step 1: Visual Assessment of the Anatomy and Volume to Be Documented, Patient Posture

*"Mammography as photography"*

It can be seen in Fig. 26.16 that the volume is medium. The nipples are medial to the sagittal plane, and pointing decisively downward. An extension of the OQ toward the axilla can be seen, evidenced by the bulging indicated by the red arrow in the frontal view photograph. It is especially seen under the arm in the lateral view photograph (short arrow). The two breasts are different in size, but this is due to the surgery performed on the right. The shape is oblong, ptotic.

With regard to posture, one notices a slight unevenness of the shoulders and hips, and a sway

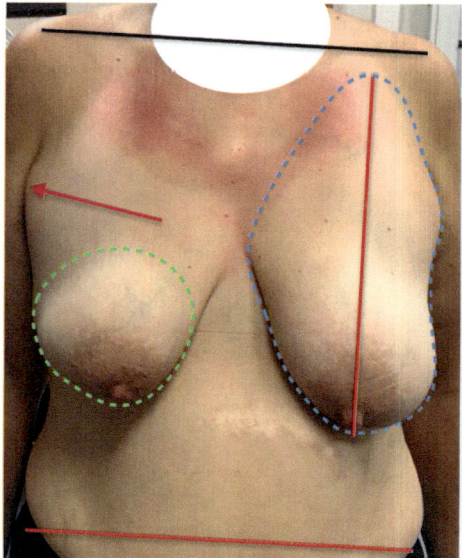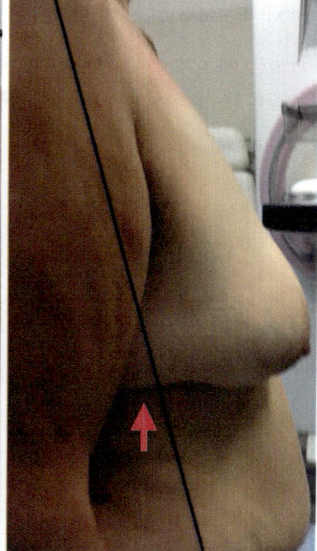

**Fig. 26.16** Patient in menopausal age. She underwent surgery on the right. Scar in the IMF, not visible, in ptosis breasts. First step Poggi method

posture, with the hips forward (black lines, Fig. 26.16).

**Step 2: Visual Assessment of the Extension of the Base of Attachment to the Thorax and the Base/Volume Ratio in AP**

*"Theory of Anatomical Relationships"*

The base of attachment (green in Fig. 26.17) is not large; the volume (pink dotted line) is also medium. The ratio of volume to base would therefore place the patient in group B. The breasts have a low consistency, intermediate thickness and loose skin envelope. It is expected that both breast connections to the thorax, as well as the deep central tissues (i.e. the pectoralis muscle) are easily documented. Thus, the stretching out action would not require great physical effort on the part of the radiographer (see Chap. 23), and relatively low compression values should be chosen. The nipples are naturally medial, so the midline is not coincident with the median sagittal plane (see also Chaps. 25 and 27).

**Step 3: Tactile Assessment of Breast Consistency, Including Skin Envelope and Thickness**

*"Evaluation of the compression and stretching resistance index".*

The tactile assessment apparently confirms the hypothesis put forward in Step 2.

**Discussion of Case 1, evaluation at the acquisition monitor and correlation between the image produced and the patient**: it is a good mammography (Fig. 26.18), in particular

the MLOs. However, the breasts are depicted with roundish shape in CCs that is not real. In fact, only the ptosis part is roundish. The right breast would seem bigger, but it is not known if it was like that before the operation. The deep planes are missing in the left CC. The nipple is not perfectly in profile, but this was not a parameter that could be expected to be fulfilled, given the severe degree of ptosis. Quite the contrary: being bigger the superior quadrant than the inferior one, the nipple must *not be* in profile in CCs (Chaps. 9 and 25).

There is no overall sense of what the breast really looks like. The nipples are positioned medially in the CC and very inferiorly in the MLOs, and this is real. The shape of the right pectoralis muscle, which is oval and tends to narrow superiorly (see Chap. 17), could be due to a functional impotence of the ipsilateral shoulder.

**Same patient, after surgery, performed with the POGGI method, CCs:**

In the right CC, Fig. 26.19, there is a medially directed rotation, as shown by:

1. The nipple is more medial than the left.
2. The width of the pectoralis muscle is greater in AP direction on the lateral than on the medial portion (thick orange strokes).
3. There is a slight deformation of the shape of the breast itself (ogive-shaped tip, indicated by the thin red arrow, see Chaps. 9 and 17). Above all, by the flattening of the medial

**Fig. 26.17** Second step

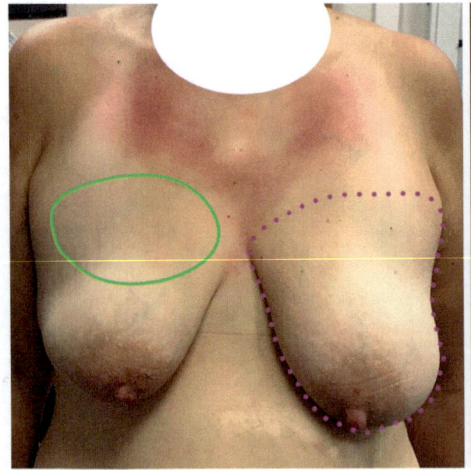
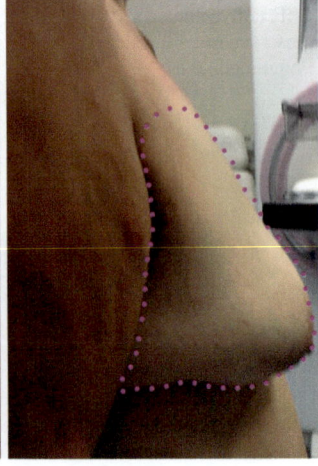

**Fig. 26.18** Mammography performed before surgery, case 1, performed by standard method

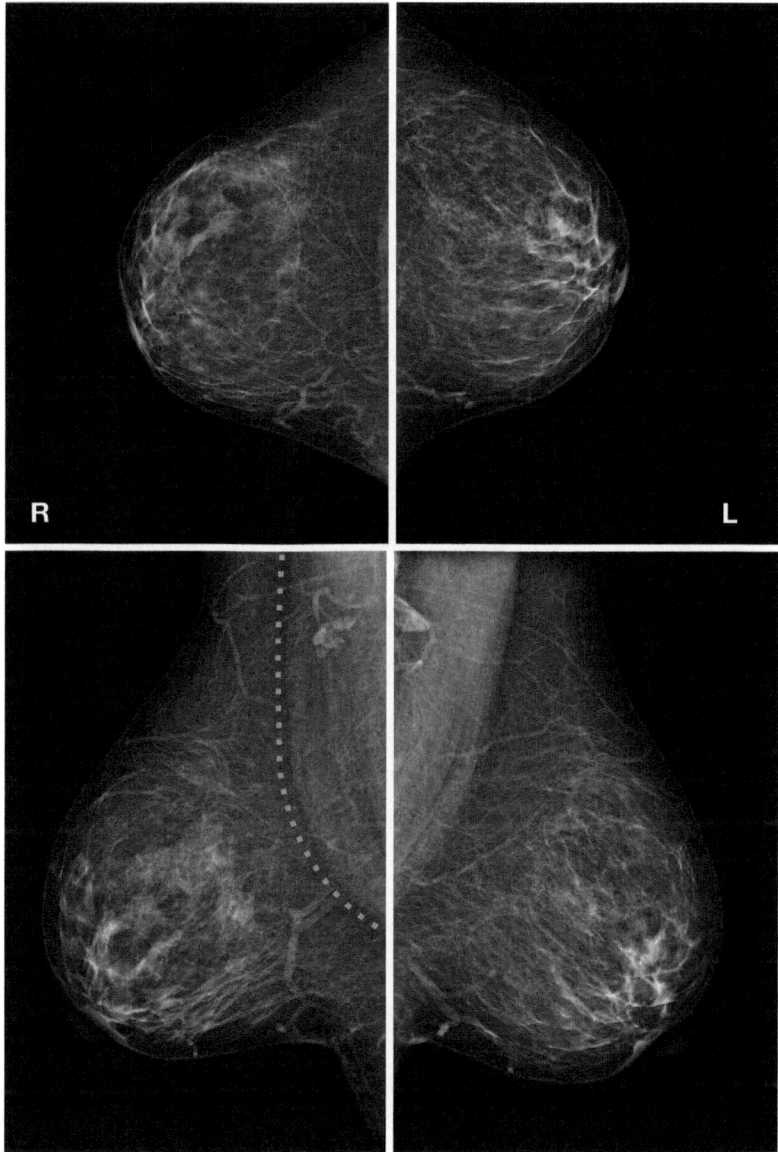

attachment to the thorax (short white arrows), to the right in relation to the left.

It can be assumed that too strong a stretching was applied for the type of breast (very mobile and of low consistency), and not neutral. More exactly, the stretching is medially directed (Fig. 26.19, red arrow). The positioning of the chest wall is also incorrect; there is a slight rotation of the right hemithorax, again directed medially. That is, the second acquisition geometry parameter was not exactly met. It can also be deduced from the shape of the pectoral muscle, which is wider laterally than medially. Regarding the nipple completely present in the retroareolar area, this must be accepted. The breast is ptotic, and more, a scar is present in the lower quadrants with a retraction effect. However, the deep planes are well documented, including the lateral and medial connections (better on the left side than on the right). The right projection is, however, more than adequate. The shape of the breast all in all reflects the anatomical reality, much more so than in the previous mammogram (Fig. 26.18).

**Fig. 26.19** Mammography exam, case 1, CC projections, performed by the Poggi method

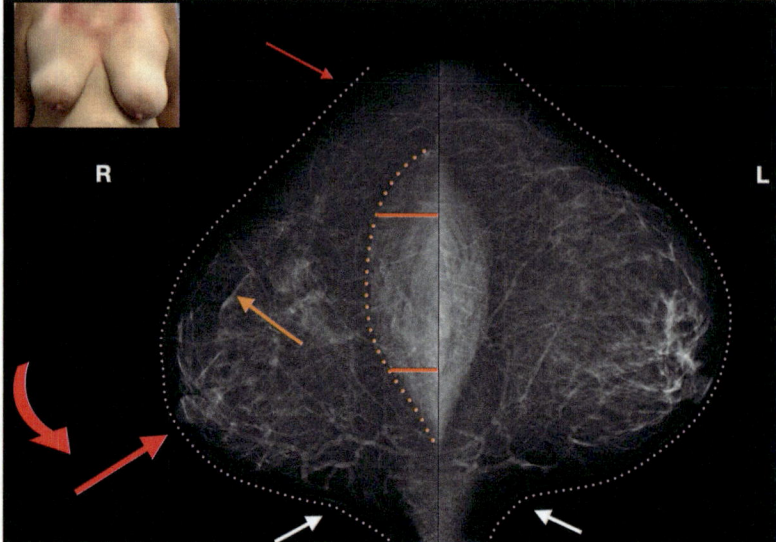

**Fig. 26.20** Mammography exam, case 1, MLO projections, performed by the Poggi method

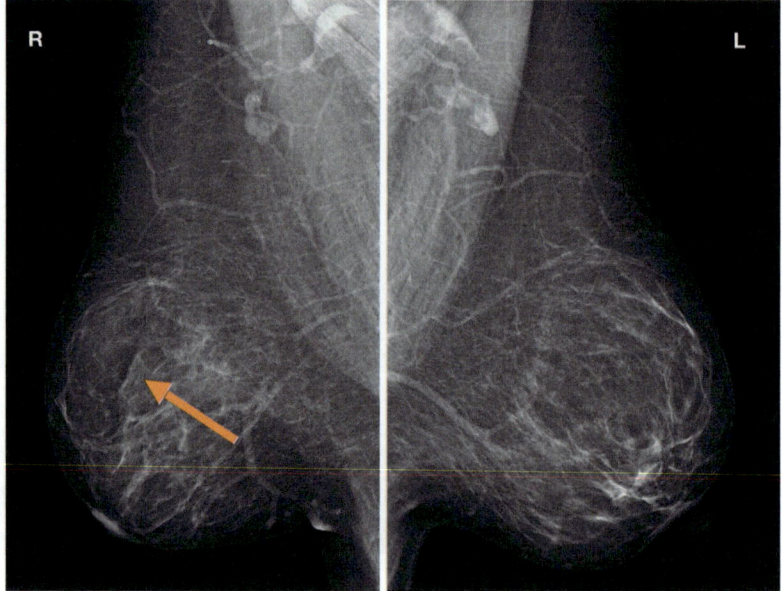

**Same patient after surgery, performed with Poggi method, MLOs:** MLO projections very good (Fig. 26.20), all quality criteria for tissue extension and acquisition geometry are met. The IMF shows some minimal artefacts to be expected given the laxity of the skin envelope.

The optimal shape of the pectoralis muscle, both right and left, compared with that of the previous mammogram, may be due to a resolution of the previous joint pathology. It could also be to the positioning technique alone. Optimal stretching action, also of the scar area, indicated with light green arrow.

The founding axiom of the method is fully respected: mammography as photography.

**Case 2. Poggi Method Compared to Standard Method**

**Step 1: Visual assessment of the anatomy and volume to be documented, patient posture**

*"Mammography as photography"*

It can be seen in Fig. 26.21 that the breasts have a lesser degree of ptosis than in Example 1. The nipples appear to be directed laterally, but the OQ extends toward the axilla. Looking at the breast more closely in its entirety, one notices that in reality the nipples are in the median sagittal plane of the breast. That is to say, the OQ is partially hidden and thus falsely 'translates' the nipple to a lateral position. The shape is approximately triangular. Slight lordosis, perhaps also determined by the photographic 'pose'.

The presence of protruding abdomen, not only in size, but also in the slight accentuation of the lumbar curvature.

**Step 2: Visual assessment of the extension of the base of attachment to the thorax and the base/volume ratio in AP**

*"Theory of anatomical relationships"*

Medium base of attachment to the thorax, in relation to breast volume: this is probably again a group B patient (the most common).

It is expected to have to exert a fairly firm force for stretching, but to be able to document easily the two connections and the pectoralis muscle in the CC projection. Also the IMF in MLO projection should be easily shown (see Chap. 9). The nipples should be documented on the midline that coincides with the midsagittal plane. This is to be obtained making sure that the part of OQ hidden toward the axilla is brought onto the detector.

**Step 3: Tactile assessment of breast consistency, including skin envelope and thickness**

*"Evaluation of the compression and stretching resistance index".*

Intermediate consistency, medium thickness; typical features of group B. Skin envelope sufficiently mobile, but not loose (Fig. 26.21).

**Discussion of Example 2, monitor evaluation and correlation with patient,** Fig. 26.22: CCs are good, even if artefacts are observed in the deep IQ (see Chap. 17). The midline coincides with the median sagittal plane, rightly so. The connections to the thorax on the left side are not shown. This contradict the hypothesis: both connections should be easily shown in patient belonging to group B. The pectoralis muscle can only be glimpsed on both sides. The MLOs are good as they allow a good reading by the reporter. The pectoralis muscle shows optimal length, but a somewhat oval shape, suggesting stiffening on the part of the patient (see Chap. 17) and/or suboptimal arm–shoulder positioning. The IMF are "fingernail-like" Fig. 26.22), contrary to what was assumed in Step 2. It was supposed to be it fairly easy to obtain a wide one, as belonging to group B. The correlation anatomy–radiographic anatomy is of intermediate grade.

**Same patient, next round, performed with the POGGI method**

CCs (Fig. 26.23): the CCs also show artefacts in the deep inner quadrant as in Fig. 26.22, although reduced compared to the previous images. This could indicate an intermammary cleft which is not easy to document, despite the fact that from the photograph it appears open,

**Fig. 26.21** Patient of menopausal age participating in the mammography screening program, first and second steps

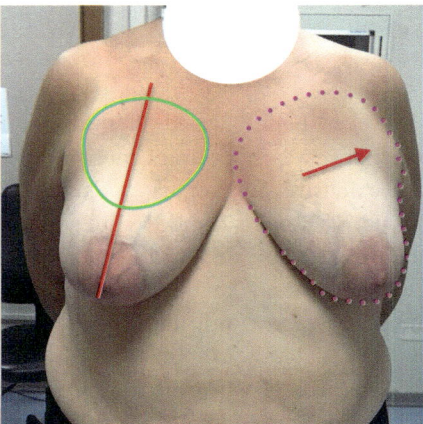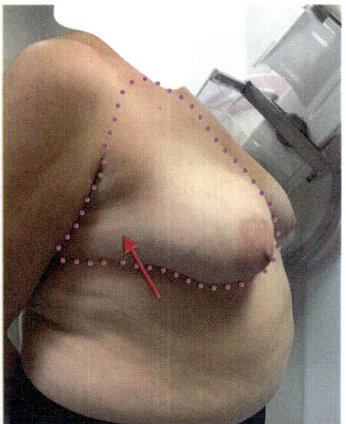

**Fig. 26.22** Mammography performed by standard method

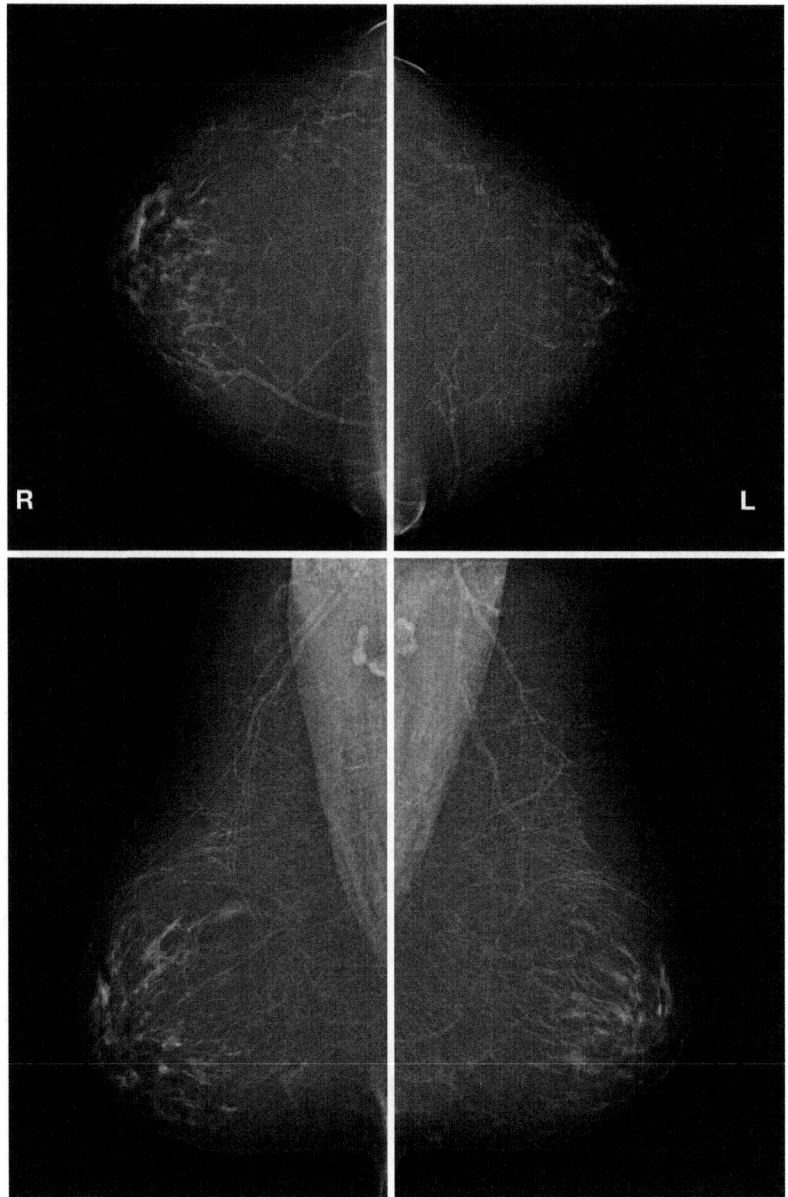

with the breasts well separated. However, both medial and lateral connections to the thorax were depicted. The deep planes were more extensively documented than in the previous round. There is a slight difference in the shape of the breasts, effectively associated with reality, which was less perceptible in the previous mammogram (especially in MLOs).

**MLOs**: (Fig. 26.24): the slight difference in shape and size between the sides is also con-firmed in the obliques projections. Optimum pectoral muscles are obtained in width length and shape. The latissimus dorsi is also present. The IMFs are perfectly represented and without major artefacts. The compression is also optimal, for tissue stretching and spatial resolution, in the two projections of the standard examination.

Correlation between anatomy and radiographic anatomy of the examination: high grade.

**Fig. 26.23** Mammography case 2, CC, performed by the Poggi method

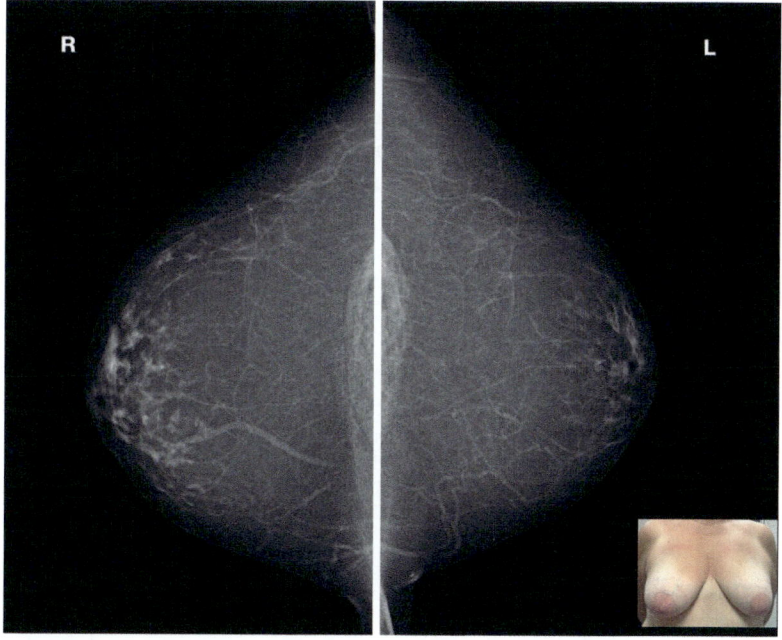

**Fig. 26.24** Case 2 mammography exam, MLOs, performed by the Poggi method

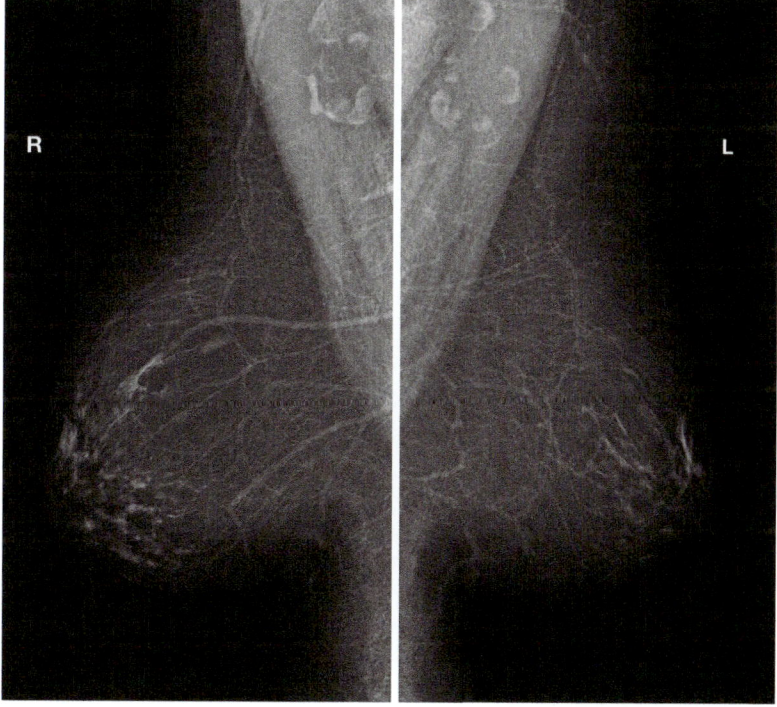

That is, the examination is more faithful to the original object, and all the hypotheses of Step 2 seem to be confirmed.

The Poggi method is dealt with extensively in the text 'Performing the mammography examination: the Poggi method', Poggi, C., (as of today unpublished).

See also Chap. 27.

## References

1. Blondeel PN, et al. Shaping the breast in aesthetic and reconstructive breast surgery: an easy three step principle. Plast Reconstr Surg. 2009;123(2):455–62. https://doi.org/10.2097/PRS.0b013e3181954cc1.

## Further Reading

Andolina V, Lille SL. Mammographic imaging: a practical guide, 3rd ed. Wolters Kluwer Lippincott Williams& Wilkins; 2011. isbn: 978-60547-031-3.

Bassett WL, et al. Diagnosis of diseases of the breast. W.B. Saunders Company; 1997. isbn:0-7216-3796-5.

Fisher U, et al. Mammografia Capire, Applicare, Ottimizzare. Verduci Editore; 2005. isbn:88-7620-707-7.

Hogg P, et al. Digital mammography: a holistic approach. Springer; 2015. isbn:978-3-319-04830-7, 978-3-319-04831-4 (e-book). https://doi.org/10.1007/978-3-319-04831-4.

Pacifici S. Lo standard di qualità nella mammografia di screening. MB Edizioni; 2015. isbn:978-88940853.

Pacifici S. La relazione Tecnico di radiologia-Paziente nel percorso enologico: alla ricerca di un approccio olistico. MB Edizioni; 2017. isbn:978-8894085358.

Tabar L, Dean PB. Teaching atlas of mammography, 4th ed. Thieme; 2012. isbn:978-3-13-640804-9.

Tabar L, et al. Breast cancer—the art and science of early detection with mammography. Thieme; 2005. isbn:3-13-135371-6 (GTV).

Tabar L, et al. Understanding the breast in health and disease in 3D, vol 1. C & C Offset Printing; 2012.

Van Landsveld-Verhoeven C. The right focus manual on mammography positioning technique. LRCB; 2013. isbn/ean:978-90-821079-1-3.

# Evaluation of the Mammographic Image Produced, According to the Point System

**27**

## 27.1 Assessing the Clinical Quality of the Image Produced in Mammography: POINT Scoring System

The thesis strongly advocated in this text is that the overall evaluation of the image is to be done correlating it with the patient's anatomy as faithfully as possible (Chaps. 25 and 26). Nevertheless, it must be added that *having a series of descriptors that can help in the first learning phase, indicating how much and in which way the quality criteria have been missed, can be of help* [1–9], see Chap. 11 and Annex 1. The assessment system that is proposed is intended to be as objective as possible; therefore, more reproducible than the PGMI system from which it derives. More exactly from the POBMI, used in Italy

(Chaps. 11 and 12). It was proposed and used in the sphere of two Tuscan projects on the performance of the breast radiographer. It is called **POint, POBMI and Integrated POGGI** and was elaborated by the writer. In this system, the deviation from the international quality criteria is evaluated in a differentiated way with penalties of three degrees, "slight", "fair" and "important". However, the images are still divided into the five POBMI classes. *Overall quality is represented by the three sets of POINT descriptor parameters.* The penalties are correlated with these parameters by means of a specific table (Table 27.1). This is intended as a tool to learn how to assess the quality of the image produced.

*In the case of intermediate assessment between classes, the exam should be weighted according to the average of the operator and the centre in*

**Table 27.1** POBMI classification with the point system

| N | Classes | Description | Penalisation |
|---|---------|-------------|--------------|
| 1 | Perfect | All criteria, both general and those associated with positioning, (Chap. 11) are met | 0 |
| 2 | Optimal | Almost all criteria are met, there are some minor penalties | Up to 1.5 in the total of the 4 projections |
| 3 | Good | Almost all criteria are met, there are some slight penalties+1 discrete penalty, in each pair of projections (R CC and L; R MLO and L, or R and L side) | Between 2 and 5 in total |
| 4 | Mediocre | At least two discrete penalties, plus several slight penalties. The examination is nevertheless sufficient for diagnostic purposes | Between 5.5 and 8.5 in total |
| 5 | Inadequate | Important penalties are present, the examination is non-diagnostic and must be repeated (1 or more projections) | ≥9 |

*which she/he works.* The system provides for the gradual training of operators, up to complete independence in the evaluation of the image produce. The aim pursued is the acquisition of full awareness of how a high-quality image should appear for diagnostic purposes. The POINT described below is a simplification of the first one created in 2017 by the writer and is called POINT.2.

## 27.2   First Set of Descriptors POINT.2

It evaluates descriptors of less impact on overall image quality. They are penalised with two different values: −0.25 for minor deviation and −0.5 for the upper one. The failure to meet these deviations from the quality criterion in this list makes the mammogram not perfectly readable, but still with sufficient diagnostic information.

**A: Asymmetry**, both for CC and MLO projections, with respect to the central line of the image and with respect to the contralateral breast (see Annex 1). Given the possibility of alignment present in all the reporting workstations, it is by now of little importance from the point of view of the reader. It is still very useful to the breast radiographer to evaluate if she/he has documented all the tissue on both sides, right and left. It is measured by assessing how far the *midline* (which divides the breast in two) and is from the *central line*. The latter identifies the centre of the mammographic image, see Fig. 25.12 in Chap. 25.

- A penalty of −0.25 is given for a deviation from the central line of between 5 and 10 mm.
- A penalty of 0.5 is given for a deviation >10 mm.

This parameter is related to: (a) the centring of the two breasts in relation to each other and (b) of the organ examined in relation to the available FOV.

**OQ**: **Non-full documentation of the outer quadrant** (OQ) in CCs. The OQ must be documented as extensively as possible (see Chaps. 9 and 11). The OQ parameter is assessed by considering the two halves of the breast, produced by drawing a line through the nipple, the midline. It must coincide with the mid sagittal plane if the quadrants are of equal size. The outward deflection of the nipple is quantified by evaluating the distance between the midline and the mid-sagittal plane. This is done continuing both lines toward the front edge of the image, just outside the skin edge. To be noted: the direction of nipple deflection indicates the direction of the missing tissue.

- It is decided not to penalise deviations of less than 0.5 cm;
- A deviation greater than 0.5 cm is penalised with −0.5.

However, if the inner quadrant is dominant (larger), the nipple will naturally shift outward. In this case, it should not be penalised. In order to understand whether the nipple is truly lateral in anatomical reality, these two conditions must be fulfilled: (1) there is no tissue missing in the direction of the supposed rotation and (2) the pectoralis muscle is central and lunette-shaped (semi-elliptical).

**A&F S: Small artefacts and folds**: the term "small" indicates: (a) the size; (b) the radio-lucency or poor radio-opacity and (c) the location. Small artefacts are always outside the fibro-glandular tissue FGT. For both CC and MLO projections, the decision is made not to penalise: (a) small folds of low radio-opacity: the tissue over-underneath can be seen and (b) radio-transparent folds, unless they are wide fan-shaped (see Chap. 17);

- Small folds of medium-to-high radio-opacity are penalised with −0.5;

In those are included: (1) Saturn ring artefacts, if short; (2) thin radio-transparent folds that may form in the retromammary space (RS) and in IMF or (3) in the axillary extension.

**S: Not correct shape of the pectoralis major muscle**, only for MLO projection.

The decision is made not to penalise rectilinear-shaped muscle or muscle of the same width all along the superoinferior direction if the width of the muscle is sufficient for the study of deep planes (see Chap. 17).

- We penalise the concave muscle with −0.5.

It should be emphasised that the correct shape of the pectoralis muscle cannot be documented in patients with acute or chronic functional impotence of the shoulder or in cases of pathological kyphosis or in congenital thoracic cage malformations. These data must be noted.

## 27.3   Second Set of POINT.2 Descriptors

In this list, there are descriptors whose non-satisfaction may render the mammography poorly readable, with medium-to-low diagnostic information. Minor penalty −1 and high penalty −1.5.

**R: Nipple rotation:** both superoinferior (or vice versa) in CCs and lateromedial (or vice versa) in MLOs. This is only in the case of superior/inferior quadrants, and lateral/medial quadrants equal in size. The R descriptor indicates the *satisfaction of the condition of the nipple in profile,* in this text called the *first parameter of acquisition geometry,* see on the matter Chaps. 9 and 25. The first parameter must always be satisfied if the quadrants mentioned are of equal size. If they are not, forcing the nipple in profile will lead to tissue loss in the direction of rotation.

- It is penalised with −1 when the nipple touches the edge of the skin. That is to say, is "transected" or partially protuding. The rotation is thus minimal and consequently the tissue lost is minimal. At most 2–3 mm;
- It is penalised with −1.5 when the nipple is all contained in the FGT. It is, therefore, a major rotation, or in any case more than 3–4 mm.

The measurement is taken from the posterior to the anterior margin of the nipple not in profile, contained within, along its largest diameter.

The information of the diversity of the medial and lateral quadrants size can be inferred by:

1. Carefully observing the patient; beware of the 'hidden' OQ in the axilla, see Chap. 26;
2. From the MLOs, on which this information is sometimes easier than in vivo in the case of a major ptosis.

**IQ: Not complete documentation of the inner quadrant,** for CC. The IQ must be documented in its entirety in the CC projection. This descriptor is assessed by considering the two halves of the breast. This is obtained drawing the midline and the mid-sagittal plane, which, in the case of inner and OQ of the same size, must coincide. If the nipple instead points medially, the distance between the two lines identifies the amount of tissue lost. The measurement is made by continuing both lines to the front edge of the image.

- A deviation of less than 0.5 cm is penalised with −1;
- A deviation greater than 0.5 but less than 1 cm is penalised with −1.5.

*If the lateromedial rotation is even greater, the image is to be considered inadequate (−9 penalty). It needs to be retaken.*

The presence of the intermammary cleft gives certainty that the deepest part of the IQ has been documented and is recommended in this text. When the OQ is actually dominant, the resulting medial nipple on the image will be natural and should not be penalised.

In order to understand whether the nipple is truly medial in anatomical reality two aspects must be satisfied: (1) there is no tissue missing in the direction of the supposed rotation and (2) the pectoralis muscle is central and lunette-shaped (see Chap. 17).

**IMF: Insufficient documentation of the IMF and part of the POSTINFQ** (Appendix 1), only for MLOs. This descriptor is related to several incorrect acquisition geometries, as: (1) the *drooping breast*; (2) insufficient documentation of the pectoral muscle and (3) exaggerated documentation of the latissimus dorsi (Chap. 17).

It is decided not to penalise the non-documentation of the IMF, or its obliteration with major folds, as long as they do not extend above it. This is only when the POSTINFQ has been fully documented:

- We penalise with −1.5 the absence of the IMF, or its obliteration with important folds, in case there is an even very small lack of POSTINFQ.

It is helpful to observe the lower edge of the breast depicted; it should be parallel to the lower edge of the image. A more or less important obliquity of the breast directed superiorly in AP direction identifies a consequential loss of POSTINFQ.

**WAP: Insufficient width (in AP sense) of the pectoral muscle,** at axillary level, only for MLOs. A width of at least 3 cm is suggested. The presence of the latissimus dorsi is decisive in this respect.

- A width of less than 2.5 cm is penalised with −1.
- A width of less than 2 cm is penalised with −1.5.

It should be noted again that any pathologies of the patient's shoulder or congenital malformations should be carefully noted, as they do not allow a documentation of the proper width of the pectoral muscle.

**A&F L: Large artefacts and folds:** (1) the term "large" indicates: 1) folds which only marginally involve the FGT; (2) are radio-opaque; (3) are *pocket or* 3D *folds*, i.e. they contain tissue, but only if they are in the pectoral muscle and (4) they are such that the mammogram is still readable.

- They are penalised with −1 long (>1 cm), but thin radio-opaque folds. They are typically: (a) in the IMF or in the pectoralis muscle; (b) in the axillary tail, e.g. as extended Saturn's rings-like and (c) at the extreme edges in the CCs, but only if contained;
- They are penalised with −1.5 radio-opaque folds ≥3 mm thick, even if they are of poor radio-opacity. Fan-shaped folds in the OQ are included. See Chap. 17.

**STR: Insufficient and/or wrong FGT stretching and spreading,** for both CCS and MLOS. The term *stretching* refers to the operation performed by the radiographer's hand, which moves anteriorly ("neutral" direction, see Chaps. 9 and 17), as the compression paddle descends. The force applied must be important and effective; insufficient stretching may result in a more

difficult image reading. This is due to the consequent bundling of the dense linear structures and Cooper's ligaments, resulting in an ineffective resolution of the summation artefact. Furthermore, the insufficient stretching leads to the production of a series of minute but disturbing folds, especially in the case of a loose skin envelope, see Chaps. 3, 9, 17 and 26. Insufficient stretching may also result in ineffective documentation of the deep planes, particularly the RS (Chap. 17).

- It is penalised with −1.

In addition, imparting a direction to the stretching operation ("non-neutral") can lead to flattening or alteration of the glandular anterior profile. This is physiologically defined with an anteriorly directed convexity (see *arch sign* in Chap. 26). Not only, it can lead to an incorrect acquisition geometry and to the bundling of the dense linear structures and Cooper's ligaments, until their distortion, see Fig. 26.9 in Chap. 26.

Wrong or "non neutral" stretching:

- It is penalised with −1.5.

It can be identified in some cases in the CCs, by measuring the *hypodermis layer* (Chap. 3). It should be the same throughout the breast. Interesting in this respect also the *sign of the negative arch* (Chap. 26).

**COMP: Inadequate compression,** both for CCs and MLOs. In this text, 8 daN has been indicated as the minimum value.

- They are penalised with −1 compressions of less than 7 daN
- They are penalised with −1.5 compressions of less than 6 daN

The appropriate compression force depends on many factors, see Chaps. 8, 9, 17 and 26. It should be chosen considering each individual patient characteristics. The calibration of the individual mammographic machine's pressure system also matters. However, as a first approach in the radiographer learning phase, it is important to have a minimum compression value to aim for.

It should be considered that inadequate compression can result in:

(a) Gland depiction alteration
(b) Increased geometric unsharpness
(c) The possibility of kinetic blurring
(d) The production of false positives and sagging breasts (camel nose)

## 27.4   Third Set of POINT.2 Descriptors

In this series, the descriptors included show significant deviation from the quality criteria. Thus, the degradation of the clinical quality of the mammography image is important. It may lead to the downgrading of the examination to MEDIOCRE or directly to INADEQUATE, i.e. with insufficient diagnostic information.

**RS: Insufficient documentation of** retromammary space: in CC and MLOs. This descriptor considers the PNL, see Chaps. 11 and 25. RS leads to a:

- Penalty of −3.5 in case the lack of deep planes is very limited. The RS is represented in the other projection at its best;
- Penalty of −6 in case of important lack of the deep planes.

**INFQ: Insufficient documentation of the posteroinferior quadrant (POSTINFQ).** For MLO projections.

- It is penalised with a single value, −6;

It is associated with an absence of the IMF and a drooping breast. The lower breast profile is oblique superiorly in the AP direction with respect to the lower edge of the image. There may also be an absence of documentation of the central deep tissues, see also Chaps. 17 and 26.

**AD: Insufficient documentation of the axillary extension and FOSSA,** only for MLOs. It is calculated by measuring the distance in an up-down direction between the upper edge of the image and the transition between the axillary extension and the upper quadrant (Fig. 25.19). This angle may be more or less pronounced but is generally clearly visible.

The distance between the lower edge of the breast and the lower edge of the image is then measured. It should be less than that measured at the top. That is to say, the ratio should be in favour of the upper part, and it is valid in a large percentage of cases out of the total.

- It is penalised with a single value of −3.5;

The documentation of the axillary cavity is important. The descriptor is related to:

1. The wrong choice of detector height, when the detector is too low, or patient too high.
2. The wrong centring of the breast in the available FOV.
3. The wrong choice of the dimension of the compression paddle (Chap. 16).

**PML: Pectoral muscle incomplete in length:** only for MLOs. The adjective "incomplete" refers to the failure to achieve the PNL (Chap. 25). The retromammary space will not be complete, the posterior wall of the same being represented precisely by the pectoral muscle.

- We penalise with −3.5 a distance between the lower edge of the muscle and the PNL less than 0.5 cm;
- A distance greater than 1 cm is penalised with −5.

**KB**: **Kinetic blurring,** both for CC and MLO;

- It is penalised with a single value: −9;

**MD: Pectoralis muscle deficiency,** only in MLOs;

- It is penalised with a single value: −6.

A summary of POINT.2 descriptors is presented in Table 27.2.

Congenital developmental abnormalities or severe functional impotence in the shoulder or

**Table 27.2** Summary table of POINT.2 descriptors, list

| A | ASYMMETRY between sides and with respect to FOV |
|---|---|
| OQ | Incomplete documentation of the OQ |
| A&F S | Small artefacts and folds |
| S | Wrong shape of the pectoral muscle (but sufficient width) |
| R | Nipple rotation sup-inf (or vice versa) in CCs and mid-lat (or vice versa) in MLOs, in breasts with similar sized quadrants |
| IQ | Incomplete documentation of the inner quadrant |
| IMF | Insufficient documentation of the IMF and a small part of the POSTINFQ |
| WAP | Insufficient documentation in width (AP) of the pectoralis muscle |
| A&F L | Large artefacts and folds |
| STR | Insufficient or incorrect FGT stretching and distribution |
| COMP | Inadequate COMPRESSION |
| RS | Insufficient documentation of the RS |
| INFQ | Insufficient documentation of POSTINFQ |
| AD | Insufficient documentation of axillary extension and cavity (measured in sup.inf. sense) |
| PML | Pectoralis muscle incomplete in length |
| KB | Kinetic blurring |
| MD | Pectoralis muscle deficiency |

arm should be indicated in the notes for the reader and not penalised. If there are several deviations from the quality criteria in the same anatomical site, it is proposed to enter only the highest penalty, even if it is less than the sum of the penalties present. A borderline final score is to be discussed taking into account the performance of the centre in which the operator in question works (*contextualisation and collective improvement*).

The POint system was implemented in the *VMM Evaluation Improvement and Monitoring of the performance of the breast radiographer project*, in the Central Tuscany Area from 2017 to 2019. It was discontinued by the pandemic. It was thought as complete system, with the purpose of:

1. Evaluating the knowledge, skills and competence necessary to produce mammograms of sufficient quality, to be easily read.
2. Identify the systematic error and therefore the training need of the individual operator. This was by far the most important aim of the project. The prospect was in fact offering customised training to all the operators involved. The project was incorporated, modified and improved, into the Tuscan regional project "288" (ISPRO)

A summary of penalties related to the POINT.2 descriptors is offered in Table 27.3.

*The use of the POint requires training, since it is a qualitative evaluation system.* The POint evaluator must be accompanied by an expert until understanding and uniformity of judgement. At the first assessment made independently, the data deduced must be compared with the expert operator. She/he must also be available for clarification even afterward.

This book was conceived for its use in the workplace to improve performance through the acquisition of theoretical–practical skills. However, an interesting note should be made on this topic: the evaluation of the quality of the image produced by the radiographer is a decision-making process that is a mixture between two types. The first, intuitive and fast, and the second, systematic, analytical, more difficult and certainly slower. This complex approach requires a lot of training and expertise. Even if we can say that the first type tends to prevail over time, it still relies on a very large amount of data. A system such as the Points speeds up, in the author's opinion, the acquisition of data on which to base an informed decision.

Below are some of the tools proposed:

**Table 27.3** Summary table of POINT.2 descriptors, penalties

| Descriptors CC | Penalty. Minor | Penalty. Major | Descriptors MLO | Penalty Minor | Penalty |
|---|---|---|---|---|---|
| IQ | −1 | 1.5 −9 | AD | −3.5 | |
| OQ | N.P | 0.5 | PML | −3,5 | −6 |
| A | N.P | 0.5 | IMF + INFQ | −1 | −6 |
| R | −1 | 1.5 | WAP | −1 | −1.5 |
| | | | S | N.P. | −0.5 |
| | | | MD | | −6 |
| RS | −3,5 | −6 | A | −0,25 | −0.5 |
| KB | −9 | | R | −1 | −1.5 |
| STR | −1 | −1.5 | KB | −9 | |
| A&F | | | A&F | | |
| S | N.P | −0.5 | S | N.P | −0.5 |
| L | −1 | −1.5 | L | −1 | −1.5 |
| COM | −1 | −1.5 | COM | −1 | −1.5 |
| | | | STR | −0.75 | −1 |

POINT DESCRIPTORS TABLE rad name._____PERIOD_____CENTRE_____

| N | CC | IQ | OQ | A | R | RS | K B | STR | A&F S+L | Com | MLO | AD | PML | IMF+ infQ | WAP/ S/MD | A | R | KB | STR | A&F S+L | Com | Score Class |
|---|---|---|---|---|---|---|---|---|---|---|---|---|---|---|---|---|---|---|---|---|---|---|
| 1 | R | | | | | | | | | | R | | | | | | | | | | | |
| | L | | | | | | | | | | L | | | | | | | | | | | |
| 2 | R | | | | | | | | | | R | | | | | | | | | | | |
| | L | | | | | | | | | | L | | | | | | | | | | | |
| 3 | R | | | | | | | | | | R | | | | | | | | | | | |
| | L | | | | | | | | | | L | | | | | | | | | | | |
| 4 | R | | | | | | | | | | R | | | | | | | | | | | |
| | L | | | | | | | | | | L | | | | | | | | | | | |
| 5 | R | | | | | | | | | | R | | | | | | | | | | | |
| | L | | | | | | | | | | L | | | | | | | | | | | |
| 6 | R | | | | | | | | | | R | | | | | | | | | | | |
| | L | | | | | | | | | | L | | | | | | | | | | | |
| 7 | R | | | | | | | | | | R | | | | | | | | | | | |
| | L | | | | | | | | | | L | | | | | | | | | | | |
| 8 | R | | | | | | | | | | R | | | | | | | | | | | |
| | L | | | | | | | | | | L | | | | | | | | | | | |
| 9 | R | | | | | | | | | | R | | | | | | | | | | | |
| | L | | | | | | | | | | L | | | | | | | | | | | |
| 10 | R | | | | | | | | | | R | | | | | | | | | | | |
| | L | | | | | | | | | | L | | | | | | | | | | | |

**Fig. 27.1** Point descriptors form

1. POINT descriptors form, for ten exams (Fig. 27.1).
2. Percentage sheet according to POBMI (see Chap. 11), per single operator, for at least ten exams; percentage achieved by the individual operator per each descriptor. POINT. The tool is designed to bring to light the greatest difficulties encountered by the operator, on her/his average and in the average of the facility in which the monitoring is implemented (Fig. 27.2).

## SHEET 2: CLASS PERCENTAGES ACCORDING TO POBMI (PGMI+OPTIMUM)

Rad name_____Period_____centre_____

| P | % | O | % | B | % | M | % | I | % |
|---|---|---|---|---|---|---|---|---|---|
|   |   |   |   |   |   |   |   |   |   |

| Results for Radiographer: | | Recommended GL percentages | Divarication from GL |
|---|---|---|---|
| N | % | | |
| P+O+B= | | >85% | - |
| M | | <12% | + |
| P+O+B+M | | >97% | - |
| I | | <3% | + |

Mark with X (UPPER CASE) the parameters in which the radiographer has the greatest difficulties, according to the her/his average, with x (lower case) compared to the centre's average

| CC | IQ | OQ | A | R | RS | KB | STR | A&F | COM | |
|---|---|---|---|---|---|---|---|---|---|---|
| MLO | AD | PML | IMF+ INFQ | WAP/S/ MD | A | R | KB | STR | A&F | COM |

**Fig. 27.2**  Percentage sheet according to POBMI (PGMI + Optimum) and descriptors percentages per single operator

| Comp (N) | No. Projections | R CC | L CC | No. Projections | R MLO | L MLO | Global No. same value |
|---|---|---|---|---|---|---|---|
| <60 | | | | | | | |
| <70 | | | | | | | |
| 80 | | | | | | | |
| 90 | | | | | | | |
| 95 | | | | | | | |
| 100 | | | | | | | |
| 105 | | | | | | | |
| 110 | | | | | | | |
| 115 | | | | | | | |
| 120 | | | | | | | |
| 125 | | | | | | | |
| 130 | | | | | | | |
| 135 | | | | | | | |
| 140 | | | | | | | |
| 145 | | | | | | | |
| 150 | | | | | | | |
| 155 | | | | | | | |
| 160 | | | | | | | |
| 165 | | | | | | | |
| 170 | | | | | | | |
| 175 | | | | | | | |
| 180≥ | | | | | | | |

## SHEET 6: COMPRESSION VALUES PER SINGLE PROJECTION AND GLOBAL EVALUATION

RAD_____PERIOD_____CENTRE_____

**Fig. 27.3**  Compression value sheet, per single operator. The term "global" is referred to the number of projections with the same compression value, out of the total of examinations evaluated

3. Compression value sheet, per single operator. The analysis is made on at least ten exams, considering the number of projections with the same compression value in relation to the total number of projections acquired (Fig. 27.3);

**SHEET 7: TECHNICAL RECALL TC to be audited**

| DESCRIPTORS | PROJECTION | | DESCRIPTORS | PROJECTION | |
|---|---|---|---|---|---|
| | R CC | L CC | | R MLO | L MLO |
| insufficient IQ | | | Insufficient axillary lobe documentation | | |
| Insufficient OQ | | | Pectoralis muscle not up to PNL, shape and width non correct | | |
| Insufficient retromammary space RS | | | Insufficient documentation of IMF and POSTIINFQ | | |
| Rotation (nipple not in profile) R | | | Rotation (nipple not in profile) R | | |
| Insufficient or incorrect stretching/distribution FGT | | | Insufficient or incorrect stretching/distribution FGT | | |
| Artifacts and/or folds | | | Artifacts and/or folds | | |
| Kinetic blurring | | | Kinetic blurring | | |
| More | | | More | | |
| | | | | | |
| Exam STD date | | | Recall date | COD ID | |
| Patient full name | | | | Birth date | |
| Exam STD radiographer name | | | recall radiographer name | | |
| RADIOLOGISTS/REPORTERS names | | | | | |
| Quadrant studied | | | NOTES: | | |

**Fig. 27.4** Recall sheet to be used in audit, per single case

4. Recall sheet, to be used in audit, for single case (Fig. 27.4).

Four examples of evaluation are also presented:

1. Example 1 of quality evaluation using POINT (Fig. 27.5), in which some of the penalties shown involved asymmetry (A), with respect to the central line, and insufficient documentation of RS, for CCs; PML, and lack of IMF + INFQ for MLO projections. Score class is identified.
2. Example 2 of quality evaluation using POINT (Fig. 27.6), in which the only penalties relate to the documentation of the RS and nipple rotation (R) for CCs that had to be retaken. Score class is identified.

3. Example 3 of quality evaluation using POINT (Fig. 27.7), in which, besides RS, also a not full documentation of the OQ is revealed to be noted in fact the non-central muscle on both CCs.
4. Example 4 of quality evaluation using POINT (Fig. 27.8), in which a slight asymmetry and a small artefact (A&P S) can be observed; the lateral rotation is contained and therefore not penalised. The MLOs show mainly a wrong FGT stretching and spreading (STR), especially on the left side. Also on the left side, not only the IMF, but also the posterior inferior quadrant is missing (IMF + infQ). Score class is identified.

Finally, the subdivision generally used, and chosen in this text, of the image displayed on the monitor is shown in Fig. 27.9.

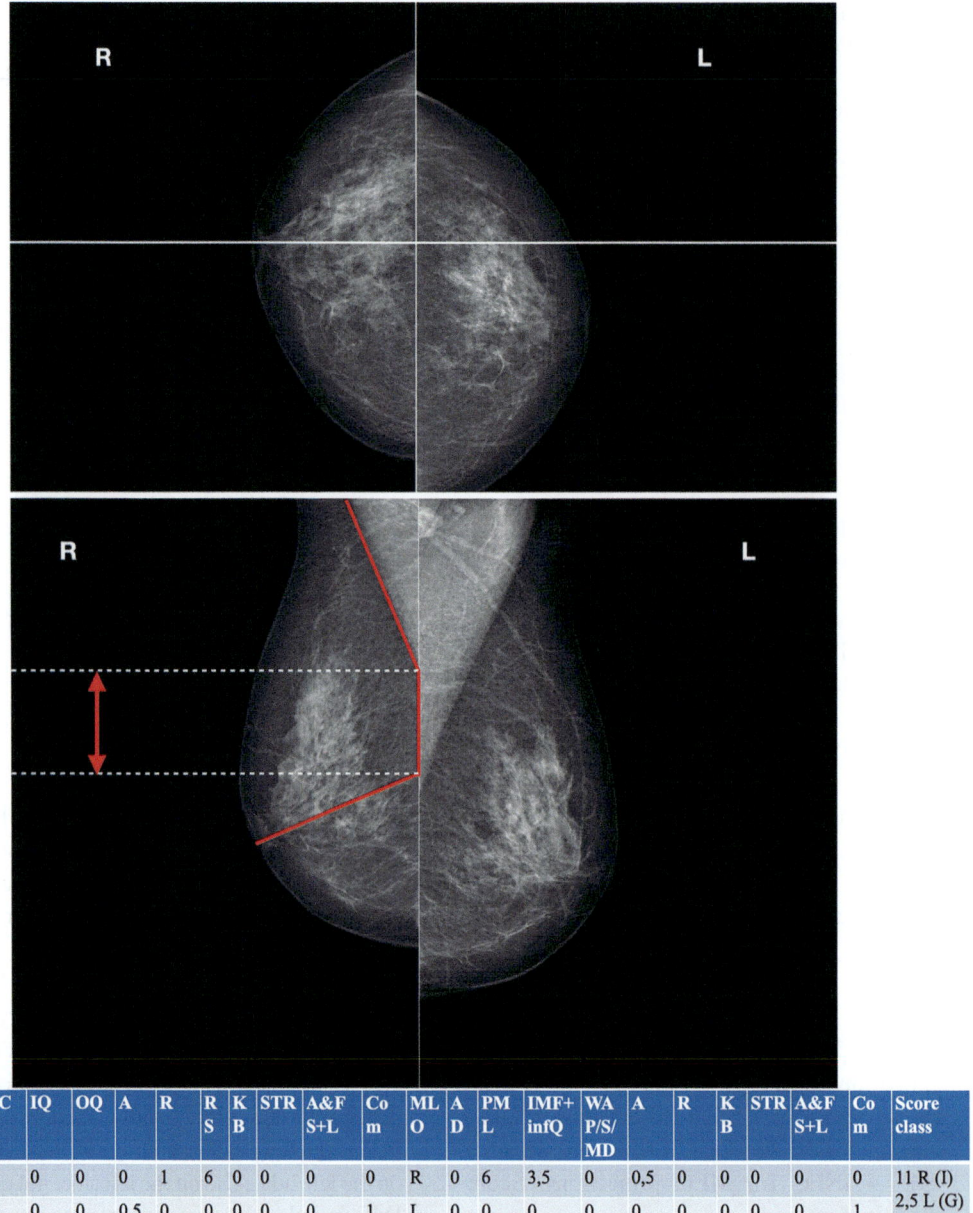

| No | CC | IQ | OQ | A | R | R S | K B | STR | A&F S+L | Co m | ML O | A D | PM L | IMF+ infQ | WA P/S/ MD | A | R | K B | STR | A&F S+L | Co m | Score class |
|----|----|----|----|----|----|-----|-----|-----|---------|------|------|-----|------|-----------|-----------|---|---|-----|-----|---------|------|------------|
| | R | 0 | 0 | 0 | 1 | 6 | 0 | 0 | 0 | | 0 | R | 0 | 6 | 3,5 | 0 | 0,5 | 0 | 0 | 0 | 0 | 0 | 11 R (I) |
| | L | 0 | 0 | 0,5 | 0 | 0 | 0 | 0 | 0 | | 1 | L | 0 | 0 | 0 | 0 | 0 | 0 | 0 | 0 | 0 | 1 | 2,5 L (G) |

**Fig. 27.5** Example of quality evaluation using POint, from the Manual. In this case, evaluation considered the two projections of one side. Penalties are to be summed separately CC and MLO right side, and CC and MLO left side. Right side: inadequate. Left side: good

**Fig. 27.6** Example from the POint Manual. To be noted MLO projections are practically perfect, while CCs are both to be retaken. In this case, therefore evaluation must be done for CCs and for MLOs in a separate way. CC are Inadequate I (13.5 penalty score). MLOs perfect P (0 penalty)

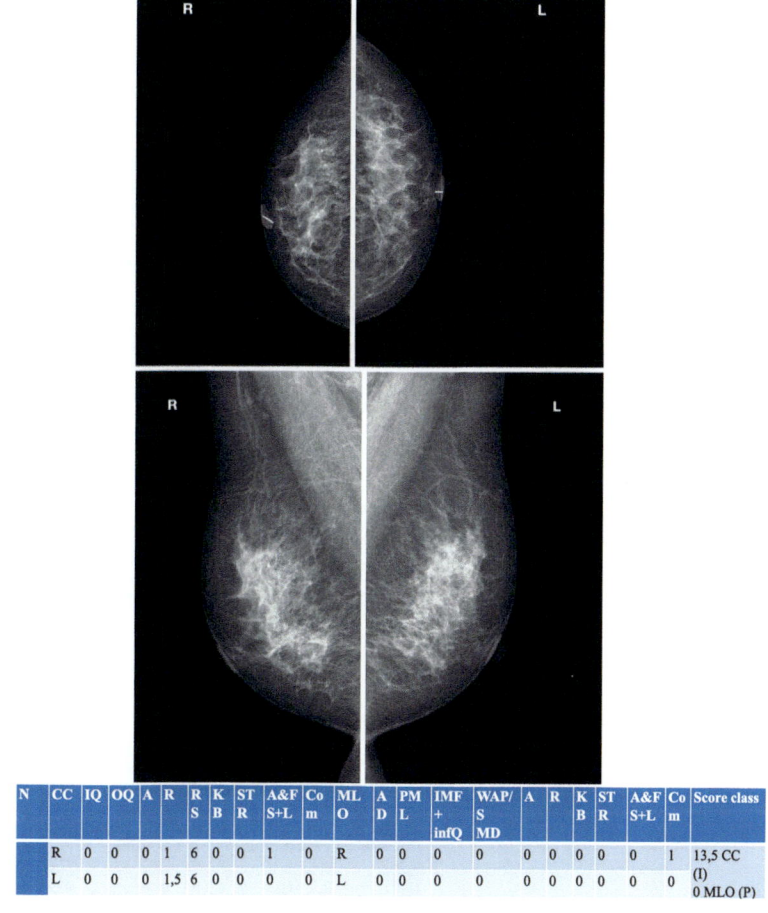

| N | CC | IQ | OQ | A | R | RS B | KB | STR | A&F S+L | Com | MLO | AD | PML | IMF+ infQ | WAP/S MD | A | R | KB | STR | A&F S+L | Com | Score class |
|---|----|----|----|---|---|------|----|-----|---------|-----|-----|----|-----|-----------|----------|---|---|----|-----|---------|-----|-------------|
|   | R  | 0  | 0  | 0 | 1 | 6    | 0  | 0   | 1       | 0   | R   | 0  | 0   | 0         | 0        | 0 | 0 | 0  | 0   | 0       | 1   | 13,5 CC (I) |
|   | L  | 0  | 0  | 0 | 1,5 | 6  | 0  | 0   | 0       | 0   | L   | 0  | 0   | 0         | 0        | 0 | 0 | 0  | 0   | 0       | 0   | 0 MLO (P)   |

**Fig. 27.7** Example of quality evaluation with POint, Good exam. Evaluation can be done on all the four projections together. The midline was forced to coincide with the median sagittal plane, in patient with an OQ larger than the IQ: to note the pectoralis muscle position in CCs. Fingernail IMFs

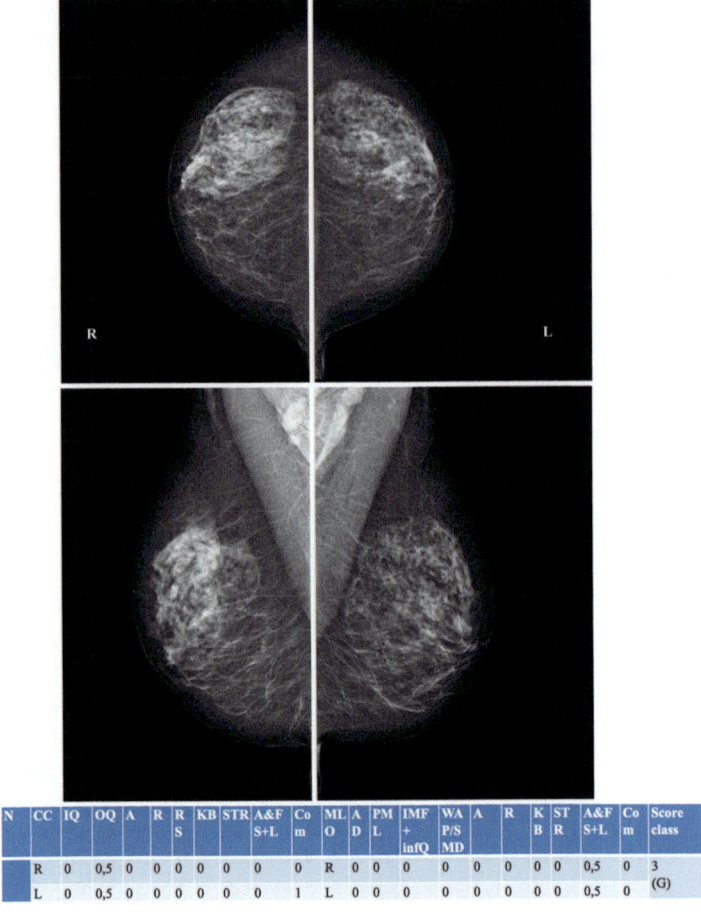

| N | CC | IQ | OQ | A | R | R S | KB | STR | A&F S+L | Co m | ML O | A D | PM L | IMF + infQ | WA P/S MD | A | R | K B | ST R | A&F S+L | Co m | Score class |
|---|----|----|-----|---|---|-----|----|-----|---------|------|------|-----|------|-----------|----------|---|---|-----|------|---------|------|-------------|
| | R | 0 | 0,5 | 0 | 0 | 0 | 0 | 0 | 0 | | R | 0 | 0 | 0 | 0 | 0 | 0 | 0 | 0 | 0,5 | 0 | 3 |
| | L | 0 | 0,5 | 0 | 0 | 0 | 0 | 0 | 1 | | L | 0 | 0 | 0 | 0 | 0 | 0 | 0 | 0 | 0,5 | 0 | (G) |

**Fig. 27.8** Evaluation done for pairs of projections places CCs in Good category. The lateral deviation of LCC is contained, and for this is not penalised. MLOs in Mediocre category, especially for insufficient and wrong stretching (STR). Also for the partial lack of POSTINFQ, left side

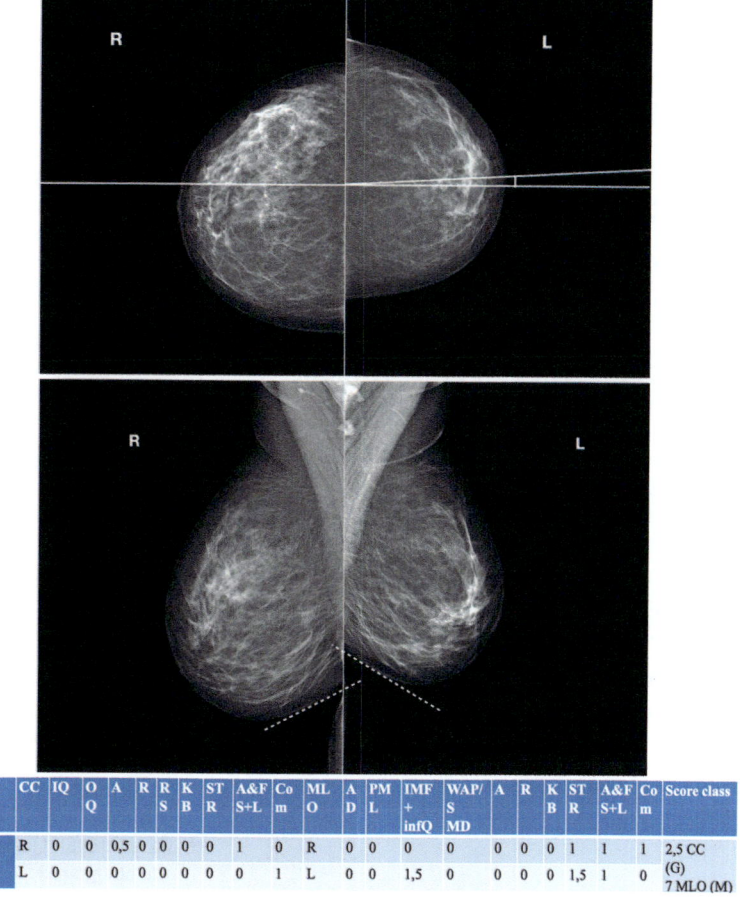

| N | CC | IQ | O Q | A | R | R S B | K B R | ST R | A&F S+L | Co m | ML O | A D | PM L | IMF + infQ | WAP/ S MD | A | R | K B R | ST R | A&F S+L | Co m | Score class |
|---|----|----|-----|---|---|-------|-------|------|---------|------|------|-----|------|------------|-----------|---|---|-------|------|---------|------|------------|
|   | R | 0 | 0 | 0,5 | 0 | 0 | 0 | 0 | 1 | 0 | R | 0 | 0 | 0 | 0 | 0 | 0 | 0 | 1 | 1 | 1 | 2,5 CC (G) |
|   | L | 0 | 0 | 0 | 0 | 0 | 0 | 0 | 0 | 1 | L | 0 | 0 | 1,5 | 0 | 0 | 0 | 0 | 1,5 | 1 | 0 | 7 MLO (M) |

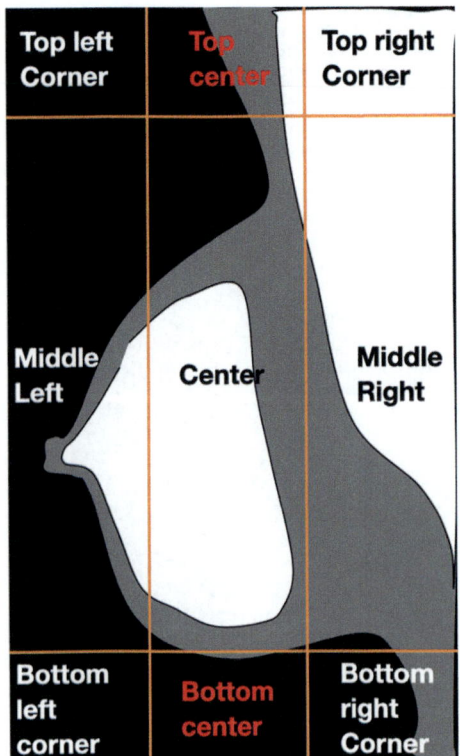

**Fig. 27.9** Image subdivision on the acquisition computer display

## References

1. Taylor K, et al. Mammographic image quality in relation to positioning of the breast: a multicentre international evaluation of the assessment systems currently used, to provide an evidence base for establishing a standardized methods of assessment. Radiography. 2017;23:343–9. https://doi.org/10.1016/j.radi.2017.03.004.
2. Boyce M, et al. Comparing the use and interpretation of PGMI scoring to assess the technical quality of screening mammograms in the UK and Norway. Radiography. 2015;21(4):342–7.
3. Gullien R, et al. Identifying the most common deviations in mediolateral-oblique (MLO) mammograms classified as "moderate" before and after implementation of improvement initiatives. EPOS ™ ECR. 2010. https://doi.org/10.1594/ecr2010/B-059.
4. Spurr K, et al. Mammography image quality: model for predicting compliance with posterior nipple line criterion. EJR. 2011;80:713–8. https://doi.org/10.1016/j.ejrad.2010.06.026.
5. Whelehan P, et al. Observer variability in accept/reject classification of clinical image quality in mammography. EPOS ™ ECR. 2015. https://doi.org/10.1594/ecr2015/C-2432.
6. Vee B, et al. Chapter 5. Directions for radiographers in the quality assurance manual of the Norwegian Breast Cancer Screening Program (NBCSP), Oslo; 2011. pp. 10. https://www.kreftregisteret.no/globalassets/mammografiprogrammet/arkiv/publikasjoner-og-brosjyrer/kval-man-radiograf_v1.0_innholdsfortegnelse.pdf.
7. Blancks R, et al. NHS Breast Screening Programme Guidance on collecting, monitoring and reporting technical recall and repeat examinations. 2017; Public Health England PHE publication gateway number: 2017608.
8. Reis C, et al. Quality assurance and quality control in mammography: a review of available guidance worldwide. Insight Into Imaging. 2013;4:539–53. https://doi.org/10.1007/s13244-013-0269-1.
9. Hendersson LM, et al. The influence of mammography technologists on radiologist's available guidance worldwide, all and repeat examinations. Acad Radiol. 2015;22(3):278–89. https://doi.org/10.1016/j.acra.2014.09.013.

# Annex 1

## Iconographic Quality Criteria in Mammography

### Quality Criteria for Cranio-Caudal (CC) Projection

Listed in Fig. A.1.

1. The medial aspect or inner quadrant IQ must be fully visualised (particularly in depth).
2. As much as possible of the lateral side or outer quadrant OQ.
3. The PNL, a transposition of that measured on a successful MLO projection of the same side (see Chap. 25), must be approximately similar to it, at most slightly shorter (less than 1 cm).
4. Nipple in profile, and on the midline when appropriate (i.e. when the outer and inner quadrants are about the same size).
5. If possible, the pectoralis muscle should be documented, central and lunette-shaped (semi-elliptical).
6. Symmetry between the two sides, left and right.

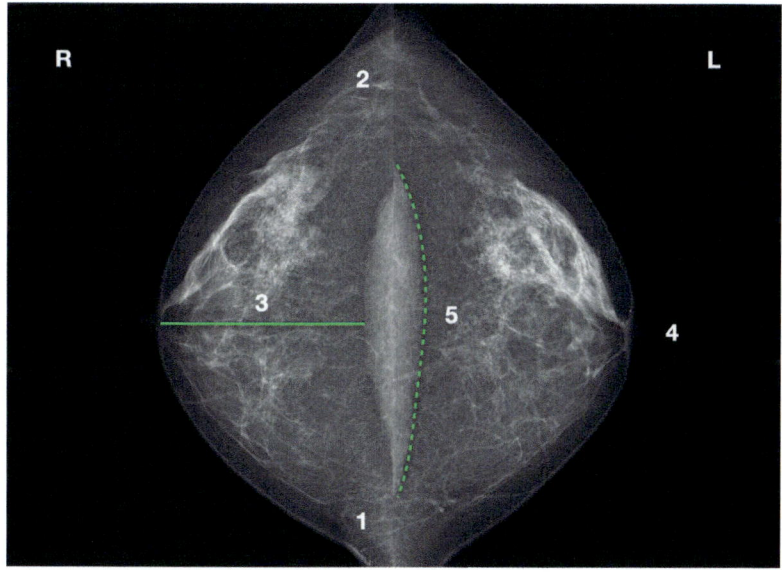

**Fig. A.1** Quality criteria for CC projection

**Fig. A.2** Quality
criteria for MLO
projection

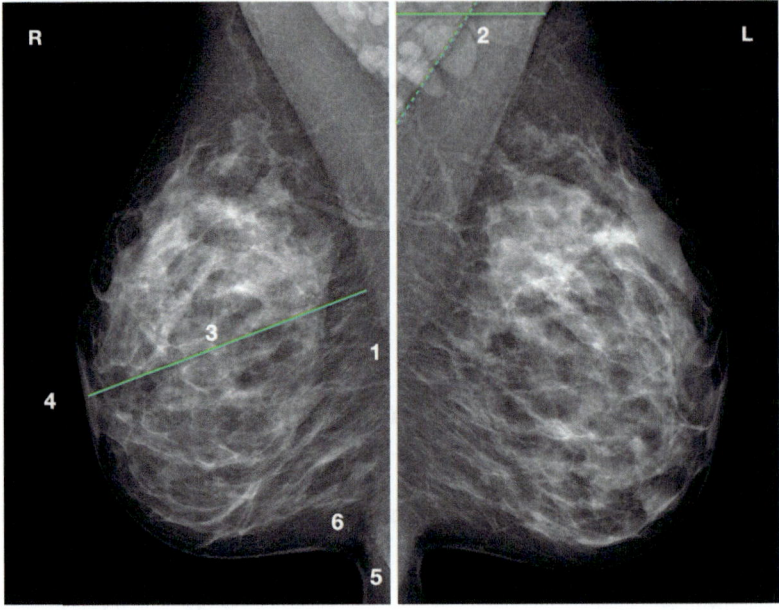

## Quality Criteria for Medio-Lateral Oblique (MLO) Projection

Listed in Fig. A.2.

1. The pectoralis muscle must reach in length at least the PNL (maximum documentation of the retromammary space).
2. Have a large axillary portion (plus possible documentation of the latissimus dorsi), with a convex or at most rectilinear shape.
3. The PNL must generally be greater than that which is subsequently measured on the CC of the corresponding side.
4. The nipple in profile.
5. The IMF must be present, and free of artefacts.
6. The posteroinferior quadrant POSTINFQ (above and somewhat anterior to IMF) must be present.
7. Symmetry between the two sides, left and right.

# Annex 2

## Radiographic Geometric Factors in Mammography

### Radiographic Geometric Factors

There are four main radiographic geometric factors to consider:

    1. Magnification.

    2. Distortion.

    3. The intrinsic characteristics of the mammographic unit.

    4. The characteristics of the X-beam.

### 1. **Magnification**

*All biomedical images produced by radio-diagnostic imaging represent objects that are larger than they are in reality.*

Magnification is determined by the ratio of the source-image distance SID to the object-image distance OID. Magnification could be used as it done in mammography, to study small findings Fig. B.1.

This means that to achieve the desired magnification (see Chap. 13), the source-object distance must be reduced and the object-image distance increased.

### 2. **Distortion**

*If the object to be studied is large enough, the magnification due to its radiographic reproduction will not be the same for the entire object.* This leads to *distortion,* to which the size and shape of the object contributes. Also important is its position in relation to the beam. In mammography, it is difficult to find very

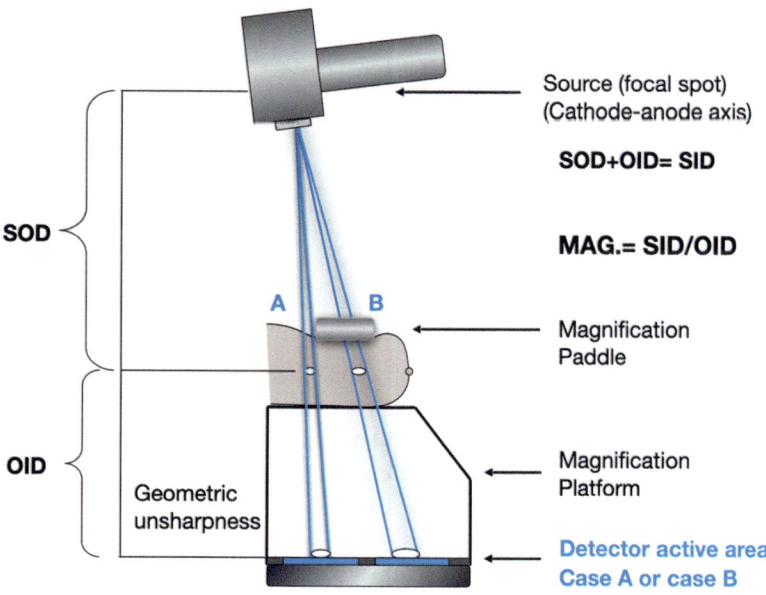

**Fig. B.1** Parameters influencing magnification view in mammography recall

Source (focal spot)
(Cathode-anode axis)

**SOD+OID= SID**

**MAG.= SID/OID**

SOD

OID

A   B

Magnification Paddle

Magnification Platform

Detector active area
Case A or case B

Geometric unsharpness

**Fig. B.2** Spatial
distortion: objects that
are not at the same
distance from the
detector are not
represented as in reality
in terms of their spatial
relationships

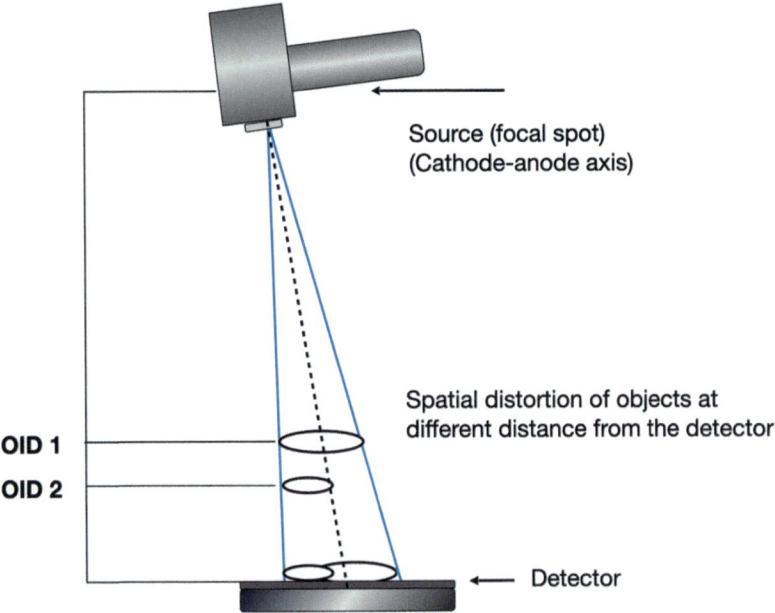

Source (focal spot)
(Cathode-anode axis)

Spatial distortion of objects at
different distance from the detector

OID 1

OID 2

← Detector

**Fig. B.3** Example of
spatial distortion in
mammography:
relationships between
findings at different
distances shown

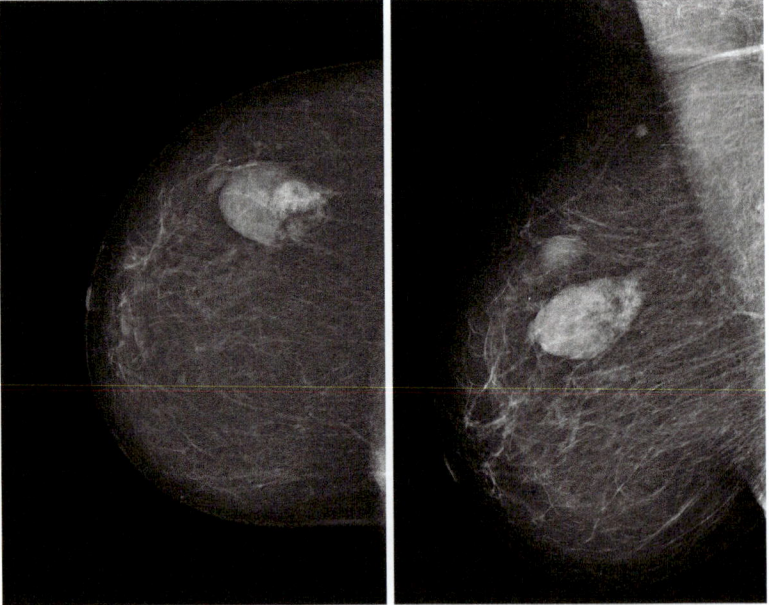

large findings, given the relatively small size of the breast. However, in the case of a suspicious finding of significant size and not parallel to the sensitive plane, it will certainly be distorted. And it will be equally so when the object is far from the central axis of the beam. Another interesting aspect is the *relative position of several objects* at different distances from the detector. This leads to spatial distortion and possible overlapping along the beam direction (Figs. B.2 and B.3).

The obliquity of the beam itself leads to a distortion of the internal structures, as can be observed by comparing the MLO projection (at 45°) with the ML (at 90°). See Chaps. 10 and 25.

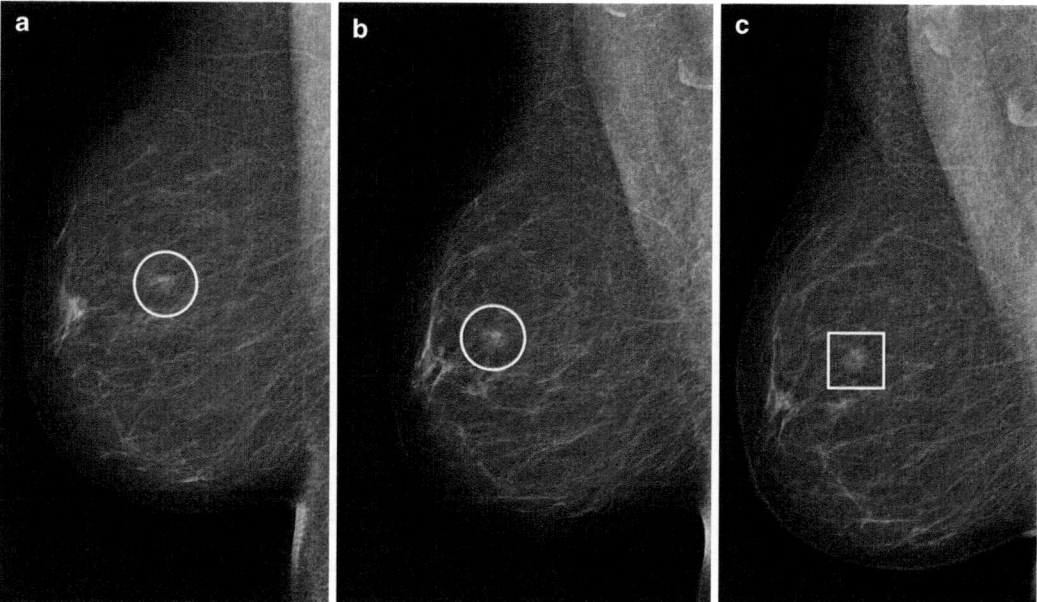

**Fig. B.4** Projections done on the same patient: (**a**) ML correctly performed; (**b**) MLO correctly performed; (**c**) MLO (incorrectly performed), compared, same patient. Note in (**a** and **b**) shape and width of the pectoralis muscle and IMF and different visualisation of the glandular tis- sue, between lateral and oblique projection; (**c**) presence of a finding in the upper quadrants (white square), later found to be a false positive, almost not detectable in the ML, and present but less suspicious in the MLO projection, correct positioning (white circle in **b**)

Note in fact in Figs. B.4(a and b), ML and MLO, respectively, same person, the different localisation of the glandular condensation highlighted (white circles). In ML projection, it appears more posterior and superior than in MLO. In Fig. B.4(c), MLO not perfectly executed, the condensation (white square) totally changes its appearance, despite being the same projection as in Fig. B.4(b) (correctly executed). The finding in Fig. B.4(c) mimicked a lesion, but was a *false positive*, caused also by the incorrect execution of the UP&OUT manoeuvre (Chap. 9).

3. **The Intrinsic Characteristics of the Mammographic Unit: Geometric Unsharpness or Penumbra**

The X-ray source is not point-like (Chap. 7): this means that the margin of the object will be degraded, blurred, to a greater extent the larger the source and the closer the object is to it, and away from the sensitive plane. This phenomenon is called *geometric unsharpness or penumbra.* It is very important in the radi- ology realm, as it contributes to the degradation of image quality, with loss of margins definition. In addition, it should be borne in mind that the focal spot has different dimensions along the cathode-anode axis *(line focus principle,* Chap. 7). That is to say, the *penumbra will be greater on the cathode side* (Figs. B.5 and B.6).

4. **The Characteristics of the X-ray Beam: Radiation Inverse Square Law**

The magnification examination is a second-level examination (Chap. 13), or recall, or callback. It involves obtaining an enlarged image of the studied object, by increasing the OID. This undoubtedly impacts the geometric unsharpness, which increases (Fig. B.5). It also requires an increase in the dose delivered, due to the radiation *inverse square law.* However, the dose is decreased by deactivating the grid. Another aspect to evaluate is the fact that the quality of the image improves, from the point of view of SNR: as can be seen from Fig. B.7, the breast in position 1 will receive more photons than the one in contact with the detector, in position 2. More precisely, a given portion of the breast, the one corresponding to the mag spot view compression paddle, will intercept more photons than the same portion in contact with the detector.

The grid in this examination can be switched off because the air gap between the breast and the detector prevents scattered radiation from reaching it. It is the purpose of the grid in the first place. See also Fig. B.1.

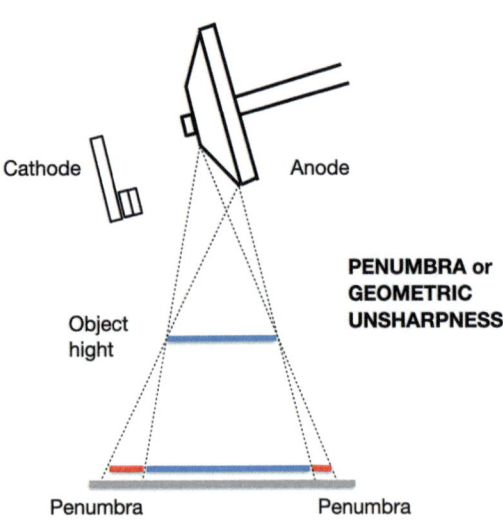

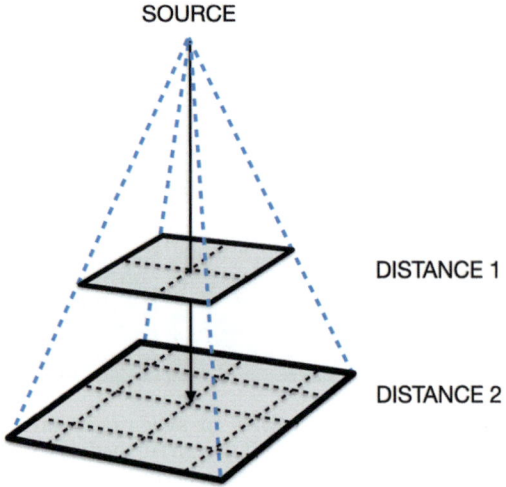

**Fig. B.5** Penumbra or geometric unsharpness and linear focus principle: penumbra is greater on the cathode side

**Fig. B.7** Radiation inverse square law: objects that are at distance 1 from the image plane are magnified, have greater edge blurring, but the image results in a higher SNR

**Fig. B.6** (**a**) Example of microcalcifications in a L CC view; (**b**) Magnified microcalcifications seen in a, with loss of resolution at the deepest part

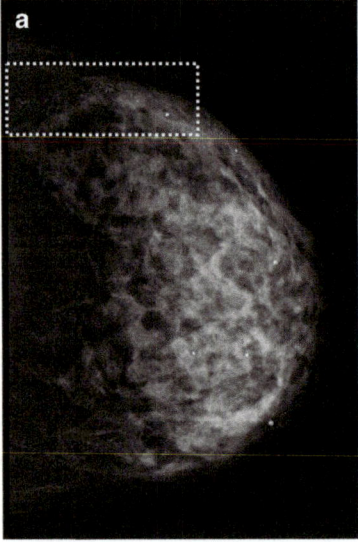

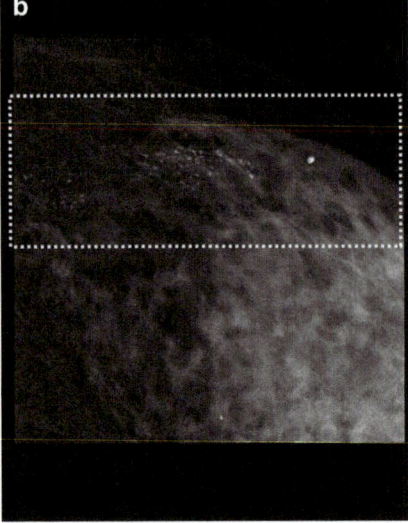

# Annex 3

## Data Collection Sheet for Breast MRI Examination

See Fig. C.1

## DATA COLLECTION SHEET BREAST MRI

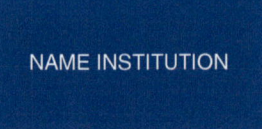

NAME INSTITUTION

| | | |
|---|---|---|
| DATE OF EXAMINATION, HOSPITAL | | |
| PATIENT'S FULL NAME | | |
| PATIENT DATE OF BIRTH | | KG (OZ.) |
| RADIOLOGIST | RADIOGRAPHER | Menstrual (first day of last cycle) 7-14th |
| Menopause (year) | FASTING 4-6 HOURS: YES | NO |
| ALLERGY YES: PROFILAXIS OR PRE-MEDICATION FOLLOWED | PROFILAXIS OR PREMEDICA TION NON FOLLOWED | NO ALLERGY |
| CYTOLOGICAL ASPIRATION YES | RESULT | NO CYT. |
| HISTOLOGICAL SAMPLING YES | RESULT | NO HIST. |
| PROVISIONAL DIAGNOSIS: (mark with X) | Pre-operative assessment | Follow up |
| Familiarity | | Mutated genes |
| Control in chemo neoadjuv. | | More |
| | | |
| | | |

| PREVIOUS SURGERY FOR BC: RIGH SIDE DATE | PREVIOUS SURGERY FOR BC: LEFT SIDE DATE |
|---|---|
| QUADRANTECT | QUADRANTECT |
| MASTECT | MASTECT |
| RT | RT |
| CHEMOTERAPHY | CHEMOTHERAPY |
| ENDOCRINE THERAPY | ENDOCRINE THERAPY |
| ALNB                    SLNB | ALNB                    SLNB |
| ANALOGUES | ANALOGUES |
| BIOLOGICAL THERAPHY | BIOLOGICAL THERAPHY |
| OTHER (other interventions, for benign lesions) | OTHER (other interventions, for benign lesions) |
| | |

**Fig. C.1** BMRI data collection sheet

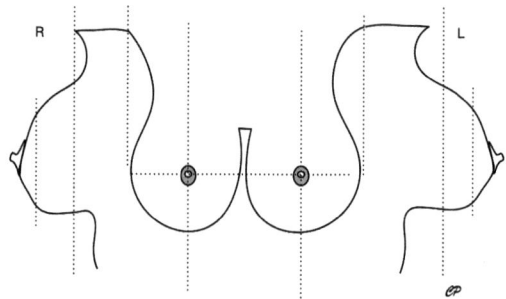

**Scar to mark**

| **IMPLANTS** | R | L |
|---|---|---|
| **NIPPLES** (report if inverted) | R | L |

| **PREVIOUS EXAMINA-TIONS** | ON-SITE | OFF-SITE  (to be uploaded on Pacs) |
|---|---|---|
| MX: DATE | | |
| US: DATE | | |
| MRI: DATE | | |

**SEQUENCES USED**: indicate name, scanner company; if the non-dynamic sequences are or not fat saturated, weighting; mark with X

| DYN | | PHASES N. | T2W | T1W |
|---|---|---|---|---|
| STIR | SILICONE ONLY | SUPPR SILICONE | OTHER | |
| | | | | |
| DWI | b value | | ADC VALUE | |
| CM | | ml | Injection rate ml/sec | |

| **POST-PROCESSING** | | | |
|---|---|---|---|
| LESION A | MAXIMUM DIAMETER (mm) | QUADRANT AND SIDE | CURVE TYPE (1, 2, 3) |
| LESION B | MAXIMUM DIAMETER (mm) | QUADRANT AND SIDE | CURVE TYPE |
| LESION C | MAXIMUM DIAMETER (mm) | QUADRANT AND SIDE | CURVE TYPE |
| | | | |

**Fig. C.1**  (continued)

**NOTES FOR THE READER**

Eco second look

**NOTES FOR THE RADIOGRAPHER (ARTIFACTS, RELATIVE CONTRAINDICATIONS...)**

**Fig. C.1** (continued)

**Supplementary material open access on Cristina Poggi YouTube channel and on FaceBook profile: the links**

https://www.youtube.com/channel/UCbFBVx8D1WHzeEEK4-pnqQA
   @cristinapoggi7579
https://www.facebook.com/cristina.poggi.528

On **artifacts** (2021):

1. https://youtu.be/ojaxqorf_6l
2. https://youtu.be/G_fAmZDt7ms
3. https://youtu.be/RVhPZUqp-rs
4. https://youtu.be/3HCivhdMEfQ

On **compression** (2021):

1. https://youtu.be/LxSuhj8Gbqk
2. https://youtu.be/aHAxFZFCHQ8

On **pectoralis major muscle documentation** (2021–2022):

1. https://youtu.be/TvYITfNNPKU
2. https://youtu.be/9kDcWmalQhY
3. https://youtu.be/lREhJKwooTE
4. https://youtu.be/fN-hRRJcCNE

On **localisation of a finding on mammographic images** (2022–2023):

1. https://youtu.be/fHiX8YhMBe8
2. https://youtu.be/OnNpSSuwmV8
3. https://youtu.be/mKtqr7LXoHk

The same lessons are available also in Italian.

# Index

GPSR Compliance

*The European Union's (EU) General Product Safety Regulation (GPSR)*
*is a set of rules that requires consumer products to be  safe and our*
*obligations to ensure this.*

*If you have any concerns about our products, you can contact us on*
*ProductSafety@springernature.com*

In case Publisher is established outside the EU, the EU authorized
representative is:

Springer Nature Customer Service Center GmbH
Europaplatz 3
69115 Heidelberg, Germany

**Batch number: 10091959**

Printed by Printforce, the Netherlands